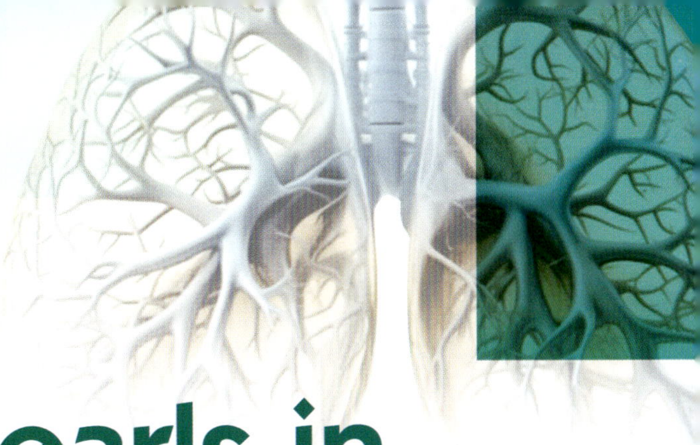

Clinical Pearls in Pulmonary Medicine

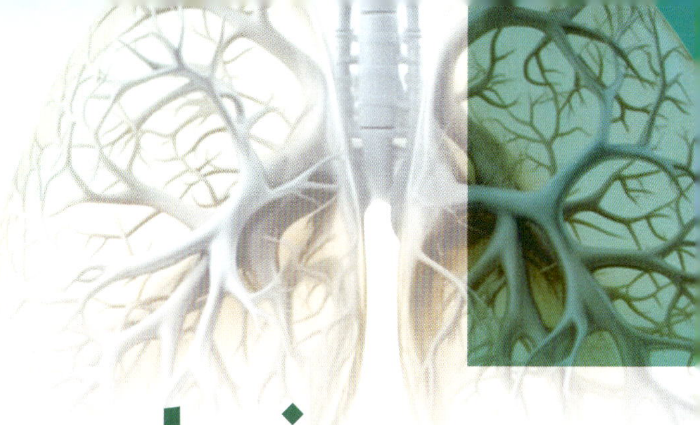

Clinical Pearls in Pulmonary Medicine

Editor

Venkata Nagarjuna Maturu
MBBS, MD, DM, MRCP (SCE), FCCP (USA), FAPSR
Senior Consultant and Head
Department of Pulmonary Medicine
Yashoda Hospitals, Hitec City
Hyderabad

Co-Editors

V Pratibh Prasad
MBBS, DNB, MRCP (SCE), FIP(IAB)
Consultant
Clinical and Interventional Pulmonologist
Department of Pulmonary Medicine
Yashoda Hospitals, Hitec City
Hyderabad

Vipul Kumar Garg
MBBS, DNB, FIP
Associate Consultant
Department of Pulmonary Medicine
Yashoda Hospitals, Hitec City
Hyderabad

CBSPD

CBS Publishers & Distributors Pvt Ltd

New Delhi • Bengaluru • Chennai • Kochi • Kolkata • Lucknow • Mumbai
Gujarat • Hyderabad • Jharkhand • Nagpur • Patna • Pune • Uttarakhand

Disclaimer

Science and technology are constantly changing fields. New research and experience broaden the scope of information and knowledge. The editors have tried their best in giving information available to them while preparing the material for this book. Although all efforts have been made to ensure optimum accuracy of the material, yet it is quite possible some errors might have been left uncorrected. The publisher, the printer and the editors will not be held responsible for any inadvertent errors or inaccuracies.

Clinical Pearls in Pulmonary Medicine

ISBN: 978-93-5466-898-2

First Edition: 2026

Published by Satish Kumar Jain and produced by Varun Jain for

CBS Publishers & Distributors Pvt Ltd

4819/XI Prahlad Street, 24 Ansari Road, Daryaganj, New Delhi 110 002, India
Ph: 011-23266838, 23289259
Website: www.cbspd.com
e-mail: delhi@cbspd.com

Corporate Office: 204 FIE, Industrial Area, Patparganj, Delhi 110 092, India
Ph: 011-49344934 Fax: 011-49344935
e-mail: publishing@cbspd.com
publicity@cbspd.com

Branches

- **Bengaluru:** Seema House 2975, 17th Cross, KR Road, Banasankari 2nd Stage, Bengaluru 560 070, Karnataka, India
  Ph: +91-80-26771678/79 Fax: +91-80-26771680 e-mail: bangalore@cbspd.com
- **Chennai:** 18/8B, Subbarayan Street, Shenoy Nagar, Chennai 600 030, Tamil Nadu, India
  Ph: +91-44-42032115, 45022115 e-mail: chennai@cbspd.com
- **Kochi:** 42/1325, 1326, Power House Road, Opposite KSEB, Kochi 682018, Kerala, India
  Ph: +91-484-4059061–65 Fax: +91-484-4059065 e-mail: kochi@cbspd.com
- **Kolkata:** 147, Hind Ceramics Compound, 1st Floor, Nilgunj Road, Belghoria, Kolkata 700056, West Bengal, India
  Ph: +91-33-25633055/56 e-mail: kolkata@cbspd.com
- **Lucknow:** Basement, Khushnuma Complex, 7 Meerabai Marg (behind Jawahar Bhawan), Lucknow 226001, UP India
  Ph: +91-522-4000032 e-mail: tiwari.lucknow@cbspd.com
- **Mumbai:** PWD Shed, Gala No. 25/26, Ramchandra Bhatt Marg, Next JJ Hospital Gate No. 2, Opp. Union Bank of India, Noorbaug, Mumbai 400009, Maharashtra, India
  Ph: +91-22-66661880/89 e-mail: mumbai@cbspd.com

Representatives

- **Gujarat** • **Hyderabad** • **Jharkhand** • **Nagpur** • **Patna** • **Pune** • **Uttarakhand**

For trade terms please contact customercare@cbspd.com
For general enquiries please contact info@cbspd.com

Printed at: Goyal Offset Works Pvt. Ltd., Kundli, Haryana, India

List of Contributors

Section Editors

Abhishek Goyal MD, DM
Additional Professor
Department of Pulmonary Medicine
All India Institute of Medical Sciences
Bhopal

Deepak Talwar MD, DM, FCCP
Chair and Director
Metro Centre for Respiratory Diseases
Noida, UP

Inderpaul Singh Sehgal MD, DM
Associate Professor
Department of Pulmonary Medicine
PGIMER, Chandigarh

Nishant Gupta MD
Associate Professor
Clinical Director-University of Cincinnati Interstitial Lung Disease Program
The LAM Foundation Endowed Professor for LAM Research, USA

Rakesh K Panchal MB ChB (Hons), MRes, MRCP (UK), FRCP (London)
Consultant Respiratory Physician and Honorary Associate Professor
University Hospitals of Leicester NHS Trust
Glenfield Hospital, Leicester, UK

Sahajal Dhooria MD, DM
Associate Professor
Department of Pulmonary Medicine
PGIMER, Chandigarh

Valliappan Muthu MD, DM
Assistant Professor
Department of Pulmonary Medicine
PGIMER, Chandigarh

Vijay Kumar Chennamchetty MD, IDCC, FSM, FCCP
Senior Consultant Pulmonologist
Apollo Hospitals, Hyderabad

Vishwanath Gella MD, DM
Director and Senior Consultant
Department of Pulmonology and Sleep Disorders
AIG Hospitals, Hyderabad

Authors

Abhishek Goyal MD, DM
Additional Professor
Department of Pulmonary Medicine
All India Institute of Medical Sciences
Bhopal

Alekhya Iakkam DNB
Associate Consultant Pulmonologist
Yashoda Hospitals, Hyderabad

Amrutha P DNB
Resident
KIMS Health, Trivandrum

Anand Vijay DNB, FIP(IAB)
Consultant, Interventional Pulmonologist
Rajagiri Hospital, Kochi

Arjun P MD, DTCD, DNB, FRCP
Senior Consultant and Head
Department of Respiratory Medicine
KIMS Health, Trivandrum

Arun K Rajan DNB
Resident
Yashoda Hospitals, Hyderabad

Arun R Thomas MD, FIP(IAB)
Consultant, Interventional Pulmonologist
Aster MIMS Hospital, Kannur

Arvindran Alaga FRCP (UK), FAPSR, FIP (Japan)
Consultant and Head
Respiratory Department
Hospital Sultanah Bahiyah, Alor Setar Kedah
Head, Respiratory Services, Kedah, Malaysia

Ashwini Chawhan MD, IDCCM
Clinical Assistant
Department of Pulmonary Medicine
PD Hinduja National Hospital and Medical Research Centre, Mumbai

Avishek Kar MD, PDCC, EDARM
Associate Consultant
Institute of Pulmocare and Research, Kolkata

BR Rinoosha MD, FIP(IAB), FSM
Associate Consultant
Interventional Pulmonologist
Yashoda Hospitals, Hyderabad

Chan Tha A Hing MRCP (UK)
Consultant Respiratory Physician
Respiratory Department
Hospital Sultanah Bahiyah, Kedah, Malaysia

Deepak TH MD, IDCCM, Fellow in Thoracic Endoscopy (Japan)
Consultant, Clinical and Interventional Pulmonology
Kovai Medical Center and Hospital, Coimbatore

Hari Prasad Kalpakam MD, DM
Consultant Department of Pulmonary and Critical Care, Apollo Hospitals, Bengaluru

Hasha Thankam Somson MD, DNB
Consultant, Department of Pulmonary Medicine
Rajagiri Hospital, Kochi

Kaumudi Devi MD
Clinical Associate and IP Fellow
Apollo Specialty Hospitals, Bangalore

Kedar Hibare DNB, FCCP
Consultant, Interventional Pulmonologist
Narayana Hrudayalaya, Bangalore

Khushboo Saxena DNB, FCCP, PDCC sleep medicine, FSM, MNAMS
Consultant, Pulmonary and Sleep Medicine
Apollo Sage Hospitals, Bhopal

Kirti Kadian MD, DM
Senior Resident
Department of Pulmonary Medicine
All India Institute of Medical Sciences, Bhopal

Maj Kunal Kumar MD
Consultant Pulmonologist
Military Hospital, Namkum, Ranchi

Lakshmi Narasimhan R MD, DM, MRCP
Consultant, Pulmonology
Manipal Hospitals, Mysore

Lakshimikant Baburao Yenge MD, DM
Consultant Pulmonologist
Deenanath Mangeshkar Hospital and Research Center, Pune

Lekshmipriya Raj DTCD
Resident
Narayana Hrudayalaya, Bangalore

Madhuri Batyala MD
Consultant, Pulmonary Medicine
Apollo Hospitals, Bangalore

Melcy Cleetus DTCD, DNB, EDARM
Consultant
Department of Pulmonary Medicine
Rajagiri Hospital, Kochi

M Punita DTCD
Resident
Apollo Hospital, Bangalore

Murali Mohan BV MD, MRCP(UK), SCE, FRCP (Glas)
Senior Consultant, Pulmonologist
Narayana Hrudayalaya, Bangalore

Narendra Kumar Narahari MD, FCCP
Additional Professor
Department of Pulmonary Medicine
Nizam's Institute of Medical Sciences
Hyderabad

Naresh Chandra DNB, IDCCM
Consultant, Critical Care Medicine
Yashoda Hospitals, Hyderabad

Nitesh Gupta MD, DM
Associate Professor
Department of Pulmonary
Critical Care and Sleep Medicine
VMMC and Safdarjung Hospital
New Delhi

Pooja Bajaj MD
Consultant
Pulmonary Medicine
Apollo Hospitals, Bangalore

Prakhar Agarwal MD, DM
Senior Resident
Department of Pulmonary Medicine
All India Institute of Medical Sciences, Bhopal

Radhika Banka DNB, MRCP
Consultant
Department of Respiratory Medicine
PD Hinduja National Hospital & Medical Research Centre, Mumbai

Rajesh Venkat MD, DNB, IDCCM
Senior Consultant and Head
Department of Pulmonary Medicine
Rajagiri Hospital, Kochi

Rakesh Kodati MD, DM
Assistant Professor
Department of Pulmonary Medicine
Nizam's Institute of Medical Sciences, Hyderabad

Ravi Gupta MD, PhD
Professor
Department of Psychiatry
All India Institute of Medical Sciences, Rishikesh

Ravi Teja Kalavakollu MD, FIP(IAB)
Consultant Pulmonologist
Raviteja Chest Hospitals, Ongole

Ravindra M Mehta MD, FCCP
Chief, Clinical
Interventional Pulmonology and Sleep Medicine
Apollo Specialty Hospitals, Bangalore

Sameer Bansal MD, DNB, EDRM, IDCCM
Consultant, Clinical and Interventional Pulmonology
Apollo Specialty Hospitals, Bangalore

Santhakumar Subramanian MD, DNB, IDCCM, FCCP
Consultant, Clinical and interventional Pulmonology
Kovai Medical Center and Hospital
Coimbatore

Shamil PK MD, DNB, DM
Senior Specialist
Department of Pulmonary Medicine
Aster MIMS, Calicut

Shikha KC DNB
Resident
KIMS Health, Trivandrum

Sravan Kumar DTCD, DNB
Resident
KIMS Health, Trivandrum

Sricharan G MD, IDCCM, ECMO Physician
Consultant, Critical Care and ECMO Physician
Yashoda Hospitals, Hyderabad

Srikant Kashinath Malegaonkar MD, DM
Consultant
Department of Pulmonary and Critical care
Apollo Hospitals, Bengaluru

Srinivas Rajagopala MD, DM
Senior Consultant, Pulmonary Medicine, and Director
Transplant Pulmonology and Lung Failure Unit
Kauvery Group of Hospitals, Chennai

V Nagarjuna Maturu MD, DM, FCCP, FAPSR
Senior Clinical and Interventional Pulmonologist
Yashoda Hospital, Hyderabad

Venkat Raman Kola MD, DNB, IDCCM, EDIC, FICCM, HCM (ISB)
Clinical Director
Department of Critical Care Medicine
Yashoda Hospitals, Hyderabad

Venugopal Jagannathan MD, DNB, EDARM, FCCP
Consultant, Clinical and Interventional Pulmonology
Kovai Medical Center and Hospital
Coimbatore

Vidya B Nair DTCD, DNB
Resident
KIMS Health, Trivandrum

Vikas Marwah MD, MRCP SCE (Resp Med)
Senior Registrar
150 General Hospital, Rajouri

Vipul Kumar Garg DNB, FIP
Associate Consultant, Pulmonologist
Yashoda Super Speciality Hospital, Hyderabad

Foreword

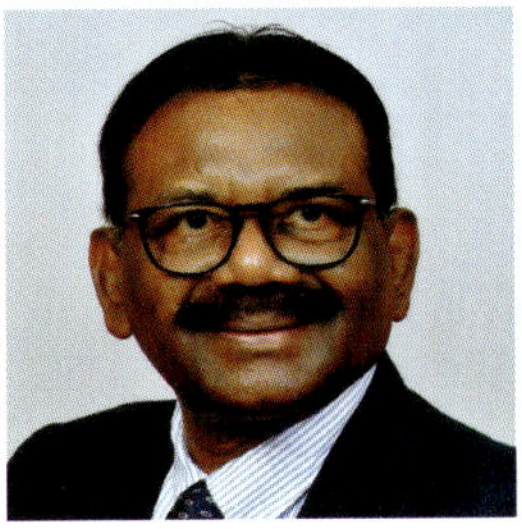

I am elated to pen a few lines as Foreword to the book *Clinical Pearls in Pulmonary Medicine* edited by V Nagarjuna Maturu.

Almost a year ago the idea of making a practical book on various aspects of pulmonary medicine took shape, and I zeroed on Nagarjuna Maturu. I am grateful to him that he agreed to bite the bullet, and produced a spectacularly memorable book. As Iris Murdoch said, between saying and doing many a pair of shoes is worn out. This book took nearly 8 months from concept to counters.

Sir William Osler (1849–1919), British (Canadian-born) physician, and one of the greatest clinicians ever had said "The good physician treats the disease; the great physician treats the patient who has the disease". *Clinical Pearls in Pulmonary Medicine* deals with looking at patient in a holistic fashion, using logic and common sense to manage a variety of lung diseases.

This book caters to the appetite of a young and newly qualified pulmonary clinician, as much as a pulmonologist practicing over several years, and still retains the curiosity to keep learning.

Over the last 44 years, that I have been in practice of pulmonary medicine, treating, training, and teaching in this specialty, I had always felt that after acquiring the specialty qualification, one should be an apprentice under a senior clinician who is academically mature. Again, to quote Sir William Osler "to study medicine without books is to sail an uncharted sea, but to study books alone is not to go to sea at all."

Clinical Pearls in Pulmonary Medicine is a power packed handbook with neatly divided 7 sections, touching almost every aspect of day-to-day pulmonary practice (airway diseases to critical care).

The book has clinical scenarios, real-life case examples, clinical algorithms to evaluate/manage patients, and for the hurried reader key learning points are summarized for each chapter. A rather unique feature of the book is an embedded direct QR code-based links to 110 original articles for those who believe that God is in detail. It was a humongous job for the editor to rope in 50 internationally renowned pulmonary clinicians.

This book is not to be kept in the glass covered cupboards but on the doctor's table for quick reference. To be kept on every clinician's table, as it is a conflation of ideas and a trove of information with cutting edge practices.

Clinical Pearls in Pulmonary Medicine will take you into a trajectory with highly focused thought processes, much like a laser. It is said that a laser is monochromatic and can cut even a diamond, although the sun is a billion trillion times powerful, it cannot match the laser, because it is polychromatic.

I can assure you that, the money will be well spent when you buy one book of *Clinical Pearls in Pulmonary Medicine* for yourself, and a dozen more as a gift for your colleagues and students.

The popularity of the book is sure to spread like a prairie fire and create a new metric in pulmonary medicine.

R Vijai Kumar MD
Director
Hyderabad Chest Center
Vice Chairman
TB Alert (India)

Foreword

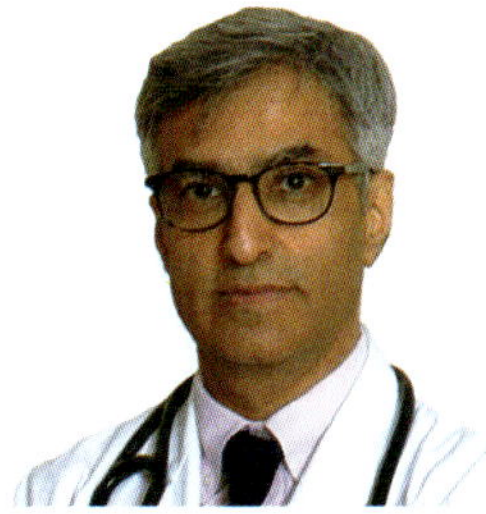

I am deeply impressed that the best teachers in pulmonary medicine who have shaped learnings of thousands of pulmonologists including me, have given their deep learnings in a collection of 31 chapters in this book. This is a unique book as it dwells on the uncharted grounds of difficult but common case scenarios and would help us to navigate with precision when encountered with these puzzling situations in our practice. This book would meet the requirements of our young and senior pulmonologists alike for years. This treasure is a must for all of us to keep it handy to guide us regarding how to approach these 31 challenging clinical situations in pulmonary medicine in our day-to-day practice, where no set guidelines exist.

All authors of the individual chapters are experienced pulmonologists and have shared the unique algorithms which will help readers to use as ready reckoners. I have been involved in teaching postgraduates in pulmonary medicine for last 35 years and always thought that textbook readings give in-depth knowledge to our postgraduate students but does not help them to translate it to bedside applications. This book fills up the 'gap' and I am proud that many of authors and co-authors have been mentored by me.

This book successfully provides small bits of free standing, clinically relevant information based on experience by the experienced and validate its title. This is truly a domain of experience-based medicine, and will be helpful in dealing with clinical problems for which controlled data do not exist.

I hope you all will find its place in your clinics or workplaces and close to heart. Teachings and learning never end and I myself too has found this book to enthuse me as much as it will do to my juniors.

Deepak Talwar MD, DM
Chair and Director
Metro Centre for Respiratory Diseases
Noida

Foreword

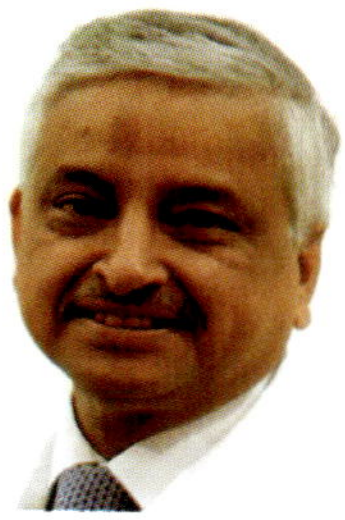

The landscape of medical knowledge is constantly changing with rapid developments in the field of diagnosis and therapeutics. The field of pulmonary medicine has seen major developments in the last decade and it is essential for all practicing physicians to be updated on these developments. As we embark on a journey through the pages of *Clinical Pearls in Pulmonary Medicine*, we find ourselves in the capable hands of experts who have carefully curated a collection of insights, knowledge, and clinical wisdom.

The authors of this book have skilfully woven together a tapestry of pearls—problem-based cases with invaluable pieces of information that shimmer with significance and enhance our understanding of pulmonary medicine. These pearls are not just isolated pieces of information; rather, they form a necklace of enlightenment, guiding healthcare professionals and enthusiasts alike through the labyrinth of respiratory challenges.

Clinical Pearls in Pulmonary Medicine is more than just a compendium of cases and facts; it is a guide for clinicians, educators, and students navigating the vast seas of respiratory medicine. Each symptom or problem-based chapter serves as a lighthouse, casting light on crucial aspects of pulmonary health and also gives references and additional reading material for those interested in more information.

In conclusion, *Clinical Pearls in Pulmonary Medicine* is a beacon of knowledge, offering a comprehensive and insightful exploration of the intricacies of respiratory health. Whether you are a seasoned pulmonologist, a healthcare professional seeking to expand your expertise, or a student eager to grasp the essentials of pulmonary medicine, this book is a valuable companion on your journey. Each case is unique and reflects the vast experience of the authors and provides a real-life experience with challenges faced in day-to-day practice.

Randeep Guleria MD, DM, FAMS, DSc (Honoris Causa)
Chairman, Institute of Internal Medicine, Respiratory and Sleep Medicine
Director, Medanta Medical School
Former Director, All India Institute of Medical Sciences
New Delhi, India

Preface

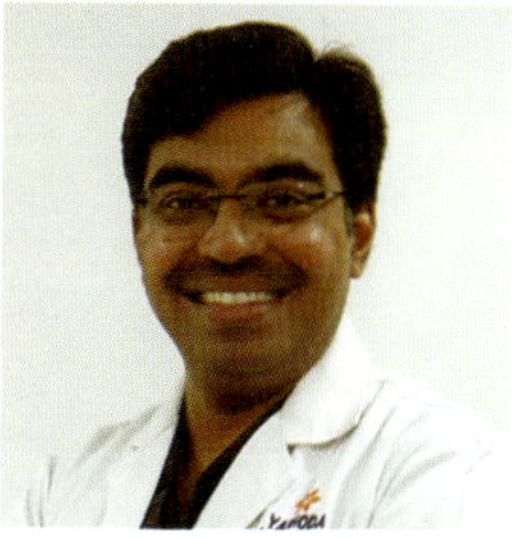

The field of pulmonary medicine has undergone a sea of change over the last two decades. With science evolving, we are now diagnosing new diseases and understanding and characterizing older ones better. The advent of new diagnostic tests and treatment options makes it important for all clinicians to update themselves regularly. A good doctor learns from each of his patients and uses this information to treat his future patients better.

While there are several textbooks in pulmonary medicine, most of these books are disease-centric, which describe the clinical features of a disease. In clinical practice, patients come with a symptom or a clinical syndrome and not with a labelled diagnosis of a disease. It is important for the clinicians to understand how to evaluate this clinical symptom/syndrome and arrive at a correct diagnosis. This book *Clinical Pearls in Pulmonary Medicine* gives a patient centric approach instead of a disease centric approach.

This book was conceived with the idea of providing a wide array of interesting case discussions for the students of pulmonary medicine. It is meant to be a ready reckoner which can be referred to during evaluation of commonly encountered cases. For this, some of the best doctors around the country and the world were approached to share their experience and knowledge. I am grateful to each one of them for taking time out for their busy schedules and writing such detailed and lucid chapters.

Each clinical pearl consists of a case description of a patient including all the laboratory data and clinical images. The author then explains the differential diagnosis and as to how he evaluated that case to come to a final diagnosis. This is followed by a detailed yet lucid discussion of an important clinical entity and its treatment. The discussion focusses on a practical approach to a case scenario, rather than theoretical discussion. Through these 30+ cases we have attempted to cover the diverse spectrum of respiratory diseases to the best of our ability.

I would like to thank Dr R Vijai Kumar, Senior Consultant and Director, Hyderabad Chest Center for giving me the opportunity to compile and edit the book. Pulmonary Medicine, for giving me the opportunity to compile and edit the book. A special thanks to my parents Lt Smt Poornima Maturu and Dr Satish Maturu for molding the best in me and for making me what I am. This book would not have been possible without the support of my wife Mrs Sindhu Maturu, and children. The support of my co-editors who have stayed awake several nights to ensure the book gets ready on time is invaluable.

Happy Reading.

Venkata Nagarjuna Maturu MD, DM, FCCP (USA), FAPSR, FICS
Senior Consultant and Head
Department of Pulmonary Medicine
Yashoda Superspeciality Hospitals
HiTec city, Hyderabad, India

Contents

SECTION 3: PLEURAL DISEASES

Section Editor: Rakesh K Panchal

SECTION 4: CRITICAL CARE MEDICINE

Section Editor: Inderpaul Singh Sehgal

SECTION 5: INTERSTITIAL LUNG DISEASES

Section Editors: Sahajal Dhooria, Nishant Gupta

SECTION 6: SLEEP DISORDERS

Section Editor: Abhishek Goyal

SECTION 7: MISCELLANEOUS

Section Editor: Vishwanath Gella

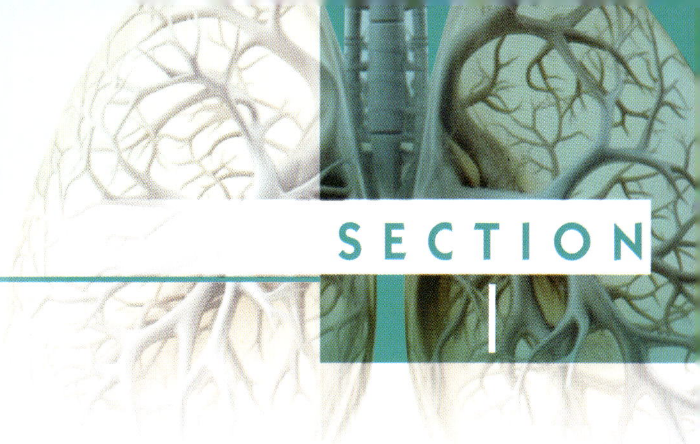

SECTION I

Approach to a Clinical Symptom

1. Approach to a Case of Orthopnea
2. Approach to a Case of Platypnea Orthodeoxia Syndrome
3. Approach to a Case with Massive Hemoptysis
4. Approach to a Case of Bronchorrhea
5. Approach to a Case of Chronic Cough with Normal Chest Radiograph

Chapter 1

Approach to a Case of Orthopnea

• Arun R Thomas • Arun K Rajan • V Nagarjuna Maturu

LEARNING POINTS

1. Orthopnea is a condition where dyspnea worsens in supine position, and improves in the sitting or propped up position.
2. Etiology for orthopnea is varied and it requires a detailed clinical examination and evaluation to ascertain the correct cause.
3. Common causes of orthopnea include volume overload states, neuromuscular diseases, anterior mediastinal masses, morbid obesity and other causes of raised intra-abdominal pressure.

INTRODUCTION

Orthopnea is a clinical condition, defined as increased sensation of breathlessness in a recumbent position which is relieved by sitting or standing. Etiology for orthopnea is diverse, and includes cardiac dysfunction, diaphragmatic disorders, mechanical causes like mediastinal masses, and severe obstructive airway disease. Here we present a case of orthopnea secondary to diaphragmatic weakness due to motor neuron disease (MND).

CASE VIGNETTE

A retired male, mechanic by profession, in his early sixties presented to us with a history of shortness of breath, dry cough, decreased appetite, unexplained weight loss of around 12 kilograms, severe weakness, significant decline in functional status since last four months. Breathlessness was insidious in onset and gradually progressive. It was aggravated on lying flat and was partially relieved on sitting position. Since one month, he was unable to sleep in recumbent position due to severe distress. He did not have any pedal edema or abdominal distension.

Patient is a known diabetic for 20 years, well controlled on regular medication. He is a reformed smoker, with a 10 pack-year history. He underwent cholecystectomy 10 years ago for cholelithiasis.

At presentation, he had severe orthopnea and was breathless even on minimal exertion. On physical examination, he was afebrile and his vital parameters were within normal range. His room air oxygen saturation in sitting position was 95%. Respiratory system examination revealed bilateral, normal vesicular breath sounds. Cardiac examination revealed normal heart sounds and there were no signs of venous congestion. On lying down, he had paradoxical thoracoabdominal movement, suggestive of diaphragmatic weakness, and he could not lie supine for more than a minute.

Central nervous system (CNS) examination showed wasting of proximal muscles in both upper and lower limbs with spontaneous fasciculations. He also had an exaggerated knee reflex, suggesting upper and lower motor neuron involvement. Head and neck examination revealed bulbar weakness, wasting of muscles and tongue fasciculations. No sensory deficits were observed.

Arterial blood gas analysis on room air (at sea level) revealed presence of compensated chronic type 2 respiratory failure (pH: 7.43; pCO_2: 63 mm of Hg; pO_2: 56 mm of Hg; Bicarbonate: 34 mEq/L). Alveolar-arterial oxygen gradient (A-aDO2) was calculated and was found to be normal (15 mm Hg). Normal A-aDO2 ruled out any significant airway/interstitial or parenchymal disease as the cause of his type 2 respiratory failure. Other laboratory workup were within normal range.

Spirometry showed probable severe restriction with a reduced forced expiratory volume 1 (FEV1) of (1.32L, 42%), forced vital capacity (FVC) of (1.39 L, 35%), and a normal FEV1/FVC ratio (95.35%) (Fig. 1.1). Supine pulmonary function testing and magnetic resonance imaging (MRI) brain and spine could not be done because of severe dyspnea in the recumbent position. Ultrasonography (USG) chest showed elevated left hemi diaphragm with absent movements, and reduced movements on the right side.

Nerve conduction study (NCS) was suggestive of moderate symmetrical sensory and motor axonal polyradiculoneuropathy involving the lower limbs more than the upper limbs. Electromyography study (EMG) was suggestive of preganglionic neurogenic lesion with evidence of active denervation and reinnervation in the muscles tested. A diagnosis of motor neurone disease was confirmed. Orthopnea was attributed to bilateral diaphragmatic paresis, and type 2 respiratory failure was attributed due to respiratory muscle weakness.

To rule out secondary causes of motor neuron disease, antinuclear antibody (ANA) profile, autoimmune encephalitis panel, and rheumatoid factor were done and found to be negative. Serum protein electrophoresis and cerebrospinal fluid (CSF) analysis were within normal limits. A final diagnosis of primary motor neuron disease with respiratory muscle involvement was made.

Patient was initiated on non-invasive positive pressure ventilation with an intelligent volume assured pressure support (IVAPS) mode. Minute ventilation was set at 9 L/minute with an expiratory positive airway pressure (EPAP) at 6 cm H_2O. He was advised to use IVAPS continuously during nighttime and intermittently during daytime, with which he was comfortable and able to lie supine. He was also initiated on tablet Riluzole (a benzothiazole derivative) at 50 mg twice a day. In the initial review visit after four weeks, the patient was symptomatically better. Orthopnea had significantly reduced with the use of assisted ventilation. Patient was continued on IVAPS and Riluzole and was advised to be on regular follow up.

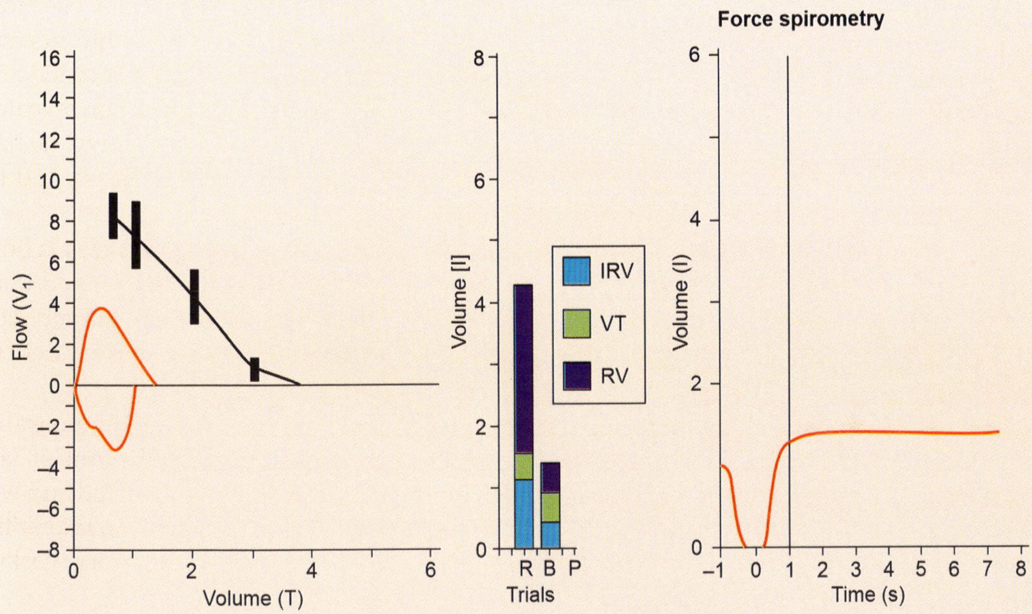

		Pred	LLN	Pre	%Pred	Z-Score
FVC	[L]	4.01	3.08	1.39	35%	-4.7
FEV 1	[L]	3.13	2.32	1.32	42%	-3.5
FEV1% FVC	[%]	78.04	66.59	95.35	122%	2.9
PEF	[L/s]	8.19	6.20	3.69	45%	-3.7
MMEF	[L/s]	2.60	1.23	2.49	96%	1-0.1
FET	[Sec]	-	-	7.34	-	
EV	[L]	-	-	0.08	-	

Fig. 1.1: Spirometry showing preserved FEV1/FVC ratio with severely reduced FEV1 and FVC which may be suggestive of a restrictive ventilatory defect.

DISCUSSION

Orthopnea refers to the sensation of breathlessness in recumbent position, relieved in the sitting or standing position. Spontaneous respiration is controlled by neural and chemical mechanisms. There are varied causes for orthopnea, and each cause has a unique mechanism which contributes to orthopnea (Tables 1.1 and 1.2). The most common causes of orthopnea encountered in routine practice includes heart failure, obesity, diaphragmatic weakness (either due to phrenic nerve damage or due to intrinsic muscle or a motor neuron diseases [MND]), advanced chronic obstructive pulmonary disease (COPD) and anterior mediastinal masses.

A. Orthopnea due to Left Heart Disease/Volume Overload States

The most common cause of orthopnea encountered in clinical practice is due to left heart dysfunction. Whenever a patient complains of orthopnea, it is important to assess for features of volume overload state (pedal edema, elevated JVP, bibasal fine end inspiratory

Table 1.1: Causes of orthopnea

Pathophysiologic condition	*Diseases*
Left heart failure (pulmonary edema)	Left ventricular systolic failure Left ventricular diastolic dysfunction Left heart inflow or outflow tract obstruction
Other causes of pulmonary edema	Kidney failure Chronic liver disease Capillary leak syndromes
Diaphragmatic paralysis	Bilateral diaphragmatic paralysis (neurogenic or a muscular cause) Unilateral diaphragmatic paralysis associated with other pulmonary/cardiac pathology Motor neuron diseases
Elevated abdominal pressure	Massive ascites Large intra-abdominal masses Morbid obesity
Anterior mediastinal masses	Thymoma Lymphoma Any anterior mediastinal mass
End stage respiratory failure	Any cause of end stage respiratory failure (severe COPD, ILD)

Table 1.2: Causes of orthopnea and physiologic mechanisms for orthopnea

Disease condition	*Pathophysiologic mechanism for orthopnea*
Left heart failure	Redistribution of blood from lower extremities and splanchnic beds to the pulmonary vasculature leads to development of pulmonary congestion in the presence of a poorly functioning left heart.
Bilateral diaphragmatic paralysis	Movement of diaphragm more cephalad due to lack of gravity leads to a fall in forced vital capacity and leads to orthopnea. This happens only when the diaphragm is paralyzed/paretic and cannot contract to maintain its position.
Anterior mediastinal masses	Direct compression of the trachea when in supine position
Abdominal masses/raised abdominal pressure	Any cause of raised abdominal pressure will push the diaphragm more cephalad in supine position leading to worsening dyspnea
End stage respiratory failure	Inspiratory respiratory muscles have a mechanical advantage in sitting and tripod position. This is lost in a lying position, and in the presence of a compromised respiratory reserve, can lead to orthopnea.

crepitations). Presence of such features should prompt immediate evaluation for cardiac status by 2D echocardiography, electrocardiography and a serum N-terminal pro B-natriuretic peptide (NT pro BNP) level. If cardiac function is normal, other causes of a volume overload state like renal failure or liver failure have to be considered.

Mechanism of orthopnea in left ventricular failure (LVF) is the development of pulmonary vascular congestion during recumbency. In the horizontal position there is redistribution of blood from the lower extremities and splanchnic beds to the lungs. In normal patients this has little or no effect. In case of patients with LVF, as the additional volume cannot be pumped out by the left ventricle, there is significant reduction in vital capacity and pulmonary compliance resulting in shortness of breath. Pulmonary congestion decreases when the body assumes a more erect position, and this is accompanied by an improvement in the symptoms.

B. Orthopnea due to Neuromuscular Diseases

Mechanism of dyspnea in neuromuscular diseases is attributed to weakness of the inspiratory muscles (diaphragm, external intercostals, scalene, sternocleidomastoids and trapezii). This results in a decline in tidal volume with an increase in respiratory frequency to compensate and maintain alveolar ventilation. Patients with respiratory muscle weakness rely on gravity to assist in diaphragmatic movement. When lying down, gravity assisted caudal movement of the diaphragm is lost, and the position of the diaphragm becomes more intrathoracic. This leads to a further loss in FVC and results in orthopnea. Inadequate ventilation during sleep (nocturnal hypoventilation) is the initial symptom to manifest in diseases affecting respiratory muscles. Inspiratory muscle weakness as it worsens, produces shortness of breath and hypoventilation when awake also.

C. Orthopnea due to Respiratory Diseases

Dyspnea is one of the most common symptoms in a patient with COPD and in patients with other causes of severe airflow obstruction. In such patients breathing discomfort can be further amplified in the supine position. Though the exact mechanism of orthopnea is unknown, the following mechanism has been proposed. This includes impedance of diaphragmatic motion in the supine position, which results in further mechanical disadvantage requiring compensatory increase in ribcage and accessory muscle activity to maintain ventilation. Studies have shown lower maximum inspiratory mouth pressure (MIP) and lower expiratory mouth pressure (MEP) in supine versus sitting position in patients with advanced COPD, reflecting functional weakness of various respiratory muscles in the supine position.

In addition to the above, worsening pulmonary gas exchange abnormalities due to gravitational effect and cephalad shift of abdominal contents, could potentially stimulate chemoreceptors to increase inspiratory neural drive (IND), further compounding respiratory discomfort in some patients. Advanced COPD showed higher rates of IND at rest (estimated by diaphragm electromyography) compared to healthy individuals. Thus, it is postulated that orthopnea in advanced COPD is secondary to acute amplification of IND and neuro-mechanical dissociation (NMD) due to sudden deterioration of load capacity ratio of already compromised inspiratory muscles in supine position.

D. Orthopnea due to Anterior Mediastinal Masses

Any large anterior mediastinal mass (thymoma, lymphoma, germ cell tumors, etc.) can cause direct compression of the large airways which is aggravated in the lying down position (due to assisted gravity). In any individual with unexplained orthopnea or associated stridor, we must examine the mediastinum on chest X-ray. A contrast enhanced CT chest will confirm the presence of anterior mediastinal mass and help characterize the lesion.

E. Orthopnea due to Morbid Obesity/Raised Intra-abdominal Pressure

Morbid obesity is another reason for orthopnea in some individuals. Morbidly obese patients breathe at a low lung volume with a reduced expiratory reserve volume (ERV). Hence during tidal breathing expiratory flow volume is decreased promoting expiratory flow limitation which is further exacerbated in supine position when the functional residual capacity(FRC) decreases because of the gravitational effect of the abdominal contents.

Any cause of raised intra-abdominal pressure (ascites, large masses) can cause a sensation of orthopnea due to a more cephalad position of diaphragm secondary to the raised abdominal pressure.

Approach to a Case of Orthopnea

A detailed history and clinical examination often is helpful in identifying the possible cause of orthopnea. An algorithm for evaluating the cause is proposed in Fig. 1.2. Focussed investigations are helpful in confirming the etiology.

Of the causes of orthopnea, neuromuscular causes of orthopnea are often missed/under diagnosed. Initial diagnostic tests in patients with motor neuron disease (MND)/suspected neuromuscular diseases include pulmonary function testing (PFT) (spirometry–supine and sitting, maximal inspiratory and expiratory pressures (MIP, MEP), and sniff nasal inspiratory pressure (SNIP)), radiology (chest X-ray, fluoroscopic assessment of diaphragmatic motion and ultrasound of diaphragm), and arterial blood gas analysis (ABG) analysis.

A restrictive defect is typical in case of patients with respiratory muscle weakness, identified by reduced forced expiratory volume in one second(FEV1), reduced forced vital capacity (FVC) and with a normal FEV1/FVC ratio (more than 70% predicted) and a reduced total lung capacity(TLC). Spirometry is to be performed in supine and upright position. Though obtaining a supine PFT in these patients can be practically challenging, a fall in VC greater than 30% in the supine as compared to the upright position is suggestive of bilateral diaphragmatic weakness.

A brief summary of investigations which help in confirming the diagnosis are listed in Table 1.3.

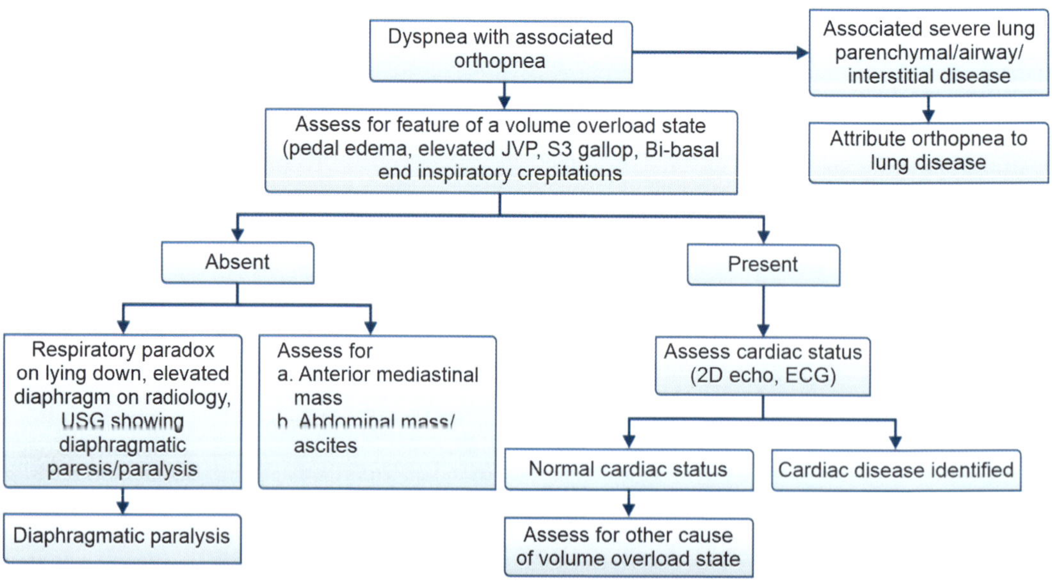

Fig. 1.2: Algorithmic approach to orthopnea

Table 1.3: Investigations and interpretation in a case of orthopnea	
Chest radiograph	Often the first test performed. Careful examination of the mediastinum, diaphragmatic position and costo-phrenic angles (for effusion) is needed. Presence of cardiomegaly and features of pulmonary edema point towards a cardiac cause of orthopnea. Most causes of orthopnea except COPD will have reduced lung volumes on a chest radiograph
Spirometry	Most causes of orthopnea will show a restrictive defect on spirometry (except COPD and airway diseases). A supine spirometry will be helpful when suspecting diaphragmatic weakness as the cause of orthopnea. Fall in FVC by 30% or more points to bilateral diaphragmatic weakness/dysfunction as the possible cause. Flow volume loops may show flattening of one or more limbs when there is a central airway obstruction due to compression by anterior mediastinal masses.
Arterial blood gas analysis	Will help in identifying associated hypercapnia. A normal (A-a) DO2 will help in ruling out significant airway/parenchymal or vascular causes of dyspnea. Hypoxemia/hypercarbia with a normal (A-a) DO2 will point towards a central/neuromuscular cause of respiratory failure
High resolution CT (HRCT) of the chest	Will help in identifying most causes of orthopnea. Features of pulmonary edema (smooth interlobular septal thickening, bilateral pleural effusion) point towards a volume overload state. Lung parenchymal/airway changes (emphysema, small airway disease and interstitial lung diseases) can be identified. A contrast scan is necessary in cases of anterior mediastinal masses for detailed assessment. A normal HRCT chest can indicate a neuromuscular/abdominal cause of orthopnea.
Other tests for assessment of diaphragm	a. Ultrasonography of diaphragm (diaphragmatic thickness and movement with respiration). b. Fluoroscopic assessment of diaphragmatic motion (Sniff test–useful in unilateral diaphragmatic paresis). c. Respiratory muscle strength assessment (MIP, MEP and SNIP test*)

*SNIP test is useful in patients with bulbar weakness who have difficulties in creating a tight seal around the mouth piece to perform routine PFT or MIP or MEP.

FURTHER READING

1. Panchabhai TS, Cabodevila EM, Pioro EP, Wang X, Han X, Aboussouan LS. Pattern of lung function decline in patients with amyotrophic lateral sclerosis: implications for timing of noninvasive ventilation. ERJ Open Research. 2019 Jul 1;5(3).

2. Parshall MB, Schwartzstein RM, Adams L, Banzett RB, Manning HL, Bourbeau J, Calverley PM, Gift AG, Harver A, Lareau SC, Mahler DA. An official American Thoracic Society statement: update on the mechanisms, assessment, and management of dyspnea. American journal of respiratory and critical care medicine. 2012 Feb 15;185(4):435–52.

3. Elbehairy AF, Faisal A, McIsaac H, Domnik NJ, Milne KM, James MD, Neder JA, O'Donnell DE. Mechanisms of orthopnoea in patients with advanced COPD. European Respiratory Journal. 2021 Mar 1;57(3).

4. Perino E, Nesme P, Germain M, Guérin C. Mechanisms of orthopnea in stable obese subjects. Respiratory Care. 2016 Aug 1;61(8):1015–22.

Chapter

2

Approach to a Case of Platypnea-Orthodeoxia Syndrome

• *Vipul Kumar Garg* • *V Nagarjuna Maturu*

LEARNING POINTS

1. Platypnea-orthodeoxia syndrome (POS) is an uncommon clinical condition characterised by breathlessness and hypoxemia that worsen (evidenced by a fall in SpO_2 of more than 5%) in the sitting position and improve in the supine position.
2. It can be caused by an intracardiac or an intrapulmonary shunt, with selective shunting occurring in the sitting position.
3. The evaluation of POS requires a bubble contrast transthoracic echocardiogram (ECHO), which demonstrates a selective shunt occurring in the sitting position.

INTRODUCTION

Platypnea-orthodeoxia syndrome (POS) is a rare clinical entity characterised by dyspnea which worsens in sitting/upright position (platypnea) and arterial desaturation when in the upright position (orthodeoxia). It is an often overlooked cause of dyspnea. The causes can be broadly classified into cardiac POS or pulmonary POS. Here, we present a patient who developed platypnea-orthodeoxia syndrome one month after right pneumonectomy.

CASE VIGNETTE

A female homemaker in her early fifties presented to us with a one-month history of palpitations, breathlessness, and generalised weakness. The breathlessness was insidious in onset and gradually progressive. It worsened when sitting or standing and was partially relieved in a recumbent position.

The patient had hypertension, well controlled on telmisartan. She was diagnosed with pulmonary tuberculosis thirty years ago. Four months ago, she had an episode of massive hemoptysis. A computed tomography (CT) scan of the chest at that time revealed post-tuberculous fibrotic sequelae in the right upper lobe and bronchiectasis in the right lower lobe. The patient then underwent bronchial artery embolization. However, after another episode of massive hemoptysis three weeks later, she underwent a right pneumonectomy to manage the hemoptysis. She remained well for one-month post-pneumonectomy, after which she developed gradually worsening breathing difficulty and platypnea. She was prescribed inhaled bronchodilators and oxygen by local doctors, which did not provide relief.

At presentation, she had respiratory failure. Finger pulse oximetry showed an oxygen saturation of 85% on 10 litres in the supine position. The patient was unable to sit erect due to severe dyspnea. She was started on oxygen via a high-flow nasal cannula. Oxygen saturation remained the same with an FiO_2 between 0.40 and 0.85, suggesting a shunt physiology (Fig. 2.1). There was a significant worsening in dyspnea associated with a 14% fall in SpO_2 upon sitting upright, confirming the diagnosis of POS.

Physical examination revealed volume loss over the right side, with the pneumonectomy scar visible. Auscultation revealed decreased air entry over the right hemithorax and normal vesicular breath sounds on the left. The heart sounds were normal, and no murmurs were heard. Other systemic examinations were normal.

Transthoracic echocardiography confirmed the presence of a 0.8 cm patent foramen ovale (PFO) with a bidirectional shunt worsening in sitting position. Right heart catheterization revealed an elevated mean right atrial resting pressure of 18 mmHg, a normal mean pulmonary artery pressure of 15 mmHg, and a normal pulmonary capillary wedge pressure of 5 mmHg. CT pulmonary angiography did not reveal any intrapulmonary shunt and was negative for pulmonary thromboembolism. The left lung parenchyma was normal.

Thus, a diagnosis of PFO with a positional right-to-left shunt, secondary to right pneumonectomy causing platypnea-orthodeoxia syndrome, was made. A transesophageal echocardiography-guided Amplatzer device closure of the PFO was performed (Fig. 2.2). Post-procedure, the platypnea resolved, and her oxygen saturation improved to 92% on 1 litre of oxygen.

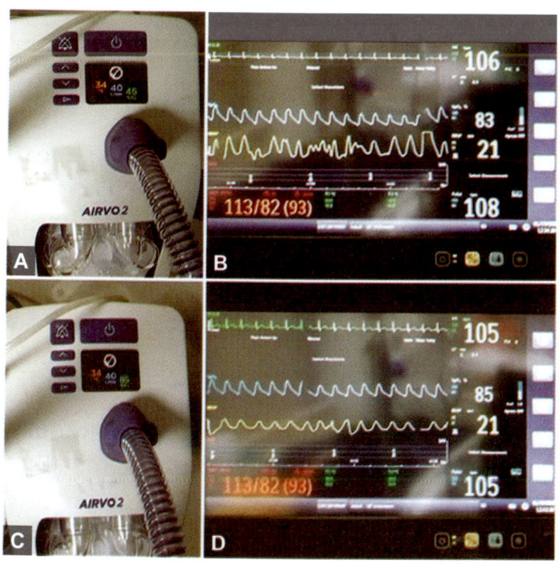

Fig. 2.1: Demonstration of shunt physiology (failure of hypoxemia to be corrected with increasing FiO_2). (A) High flow nasal cannula (HFNC) with FiO_2 set at 0.45; (B) SpO_2 of 83% on FiO_2 of 0.45; (C) HFNC with FiO_2 set at 0.85; (D) SpO_2 of 85% on FiO_2 of 0.85.

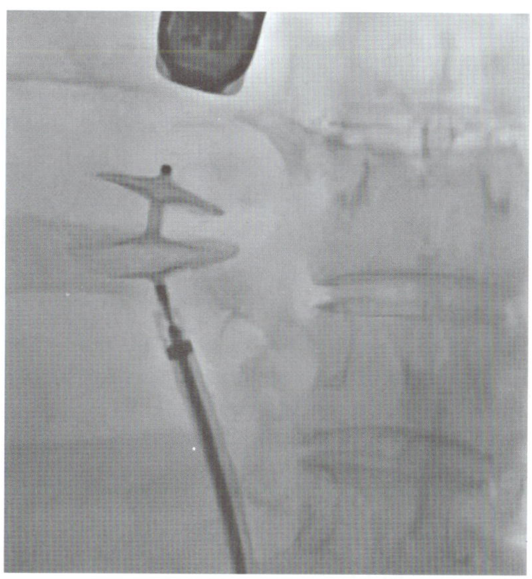

Fig. 2.2: Transesophageal echocardiography guided Amplatzer device closure of persistent foramen ovale (PFO).

At a two-week follow-up, the patient showed substantial improvement and was able to perform her daily activities without any discomfort. She maintained an oxygen saturation of 95% on room air. Transthoracic echocardiography confirmed the position of the Amplatzer device and demonstrated no active shunting across the interatrial septum.

DISCUSSION

Platypnea-orthodeoxia syndrome (POS) is a rare clinical condition characterised by a combination of platypnea and orthodeoxia. Platypnea refers to breathing difficulty that worsens in a sitting position and is relieved by lying down. Orthodeoxia is defined as a decrease in oxygen saturation (SpO_2) of five percent or more, or a fall in the partial pressure of oxygen in arterial blood (PaO_2) of at least four mm of mercury when moving from a lying to a sitting position. The primary mechanisms of POS are broadly classified based on their origin, either intracardiac (cardiac POS) or extracardiac (pulmonary POS or miscellaneous).

Intracardiac POS is the most common cause of POS. For cardiac POS to occur, there must be an anatomical defect that allows right-to-left shunting of blood (such as a patent foramen ovale (PFO), atrial septal defect (ASD), fenestrated atrial septal aneurysm, etc.) and a functional or an associated secondary structural component that contributes to preferential shunting of blood from right to left when the patient moves from lying to sitting/standing. Cardiac POS can occur with either normal or elevated right atrial pressure (Table 2.1).

Pulmonary POS is associated with intrapulmonary shunts, such as pulmonary arteriovenous malformations (PAVM), hepatopulmonary syndrome, or a ventilation-perfusion mismatch (Table 2.1).

The pathophysiology of post-pneumonectomy POS is complex and may involve multiple mechanisms. In our patient, spontaneous mediastinal counterclockwise rotation and diaphragmatic elevation, which usually occur 3 weeks to 7 months post-pneumonectomy, cause stretching and distortion of the interatrial septum. This repositioning of the interatrial septum directs blood flow from the vena cavae towards the interatrial septal defect. The upright position further exacerbates this stretching, orienting the interatrial septum directly in the axis of inferior vena caval flow, resulting in a right-to-left shunt.

The diagnosis of POS requires a high degree of suspicion. The first step in diagnosing POS is the clinical assessment of the patient and identification of platypnea and orthodeoxia. In the presence of a right-to-left shunt, there is no significant improvement in oxygen saturations even after increasing the FiO_2 to 1.0, as observed in this case. Since intracardiac POS is most common, an echocardiogram with or without bubble contrast with intravenous agitated saline should be the first test in the diagnostic algorithm. This study can identify the right to left shunt as well as help differentiate patients with an intracardiac shunt from those with an extracardiac shunt.

Visualisation of a direct shunt or the appearance of bubbles in the left atrium within three cardiac cycles suggests an intracardiac shunt. A delayed microbubble opacification of the left atrium (between three and six cardiac cycles) suggests an extracardiac shunt, most commonly in the pulmonary vasculature. Transesophageal echocardiography may be performed for direct visualization of the cardiac defect or aneurysms if a transthoracic echocardiogram is inconclusive.

If an extracardiac shunt is suspected, computed tomography (CT) angiography of the chest is performed to assess for PAVM. Pulmonary arteriography is the reference standard to confirm intrapulmonary shunts where uncertainty still persists. An approach to diagnosis of POS is illustrated in Fig. 2.3.

Table 2.1: Causes and mechanisms of platypnea orthodeoxia syndrome (POS)

Underlying anatomical or functional alteration	*Pathophysiologic mechanism*	*Accompanying pathologic condition*
Intrapulmonary shunt • PAVM at base of lung	Preferential increase in blood flow through basal PAVMs of the lung on sitting upright. This is due to a gravity induced increase in blood flow in the bases of the lung in sitting position.	• Hepatopulmonary syndrome • Pulmonary arteriovenous malformations (PAVM) or fistulae of any cause • Rendu-Osler-Weber syndrome
Intracardiac shunt • Patent foramen ovale (PFO) • Atrial septal defect (ASD) • Atrial septal aneurysm with fenestration	Positional right-left shunt without elevated right-left pressure gradient	• Compression of RA by aortic dilatation, elongation or aneurysm. • Pericardial effusion • Constrictive pericarditis • Post-pneumonectomy • Eosinophilic endomyocardial disease/RA myxoma
	Positional right-left shunt with elevated right-left pressure gradient	• Pulmonary thromboembolism • Idiopathic pulmonary hypertension • Right hydrothorax • Long duration lung disease causing pulmonary hypertension • Post-pneumonectomy
Ventilation perfusion mismatch • Lower lobe predominant structural lung diseases (an uncommon cause of POS)	• Lower lobe diseased regions get better perfused in erect position and this leads to a functional shunt in the bases. • Healthier upper lobes get less perfused in erect position leading to formation of a functional dead space. • In erect position, combination of functional shunt at bases and functional dead space at apices leads to hypoxemia.	• Lower lobe predominant interstitial disease • Lower lobe predominant parenchymal disease • Lower lobe predominant bronchiectasis

COPD: Chronic obstructive pulmonary disease; *PAVM:* Pulmonary arteriovenous malformation; *RA:* Right atrium; *V/Q Ratio:* Ventilation/perfusion ratio

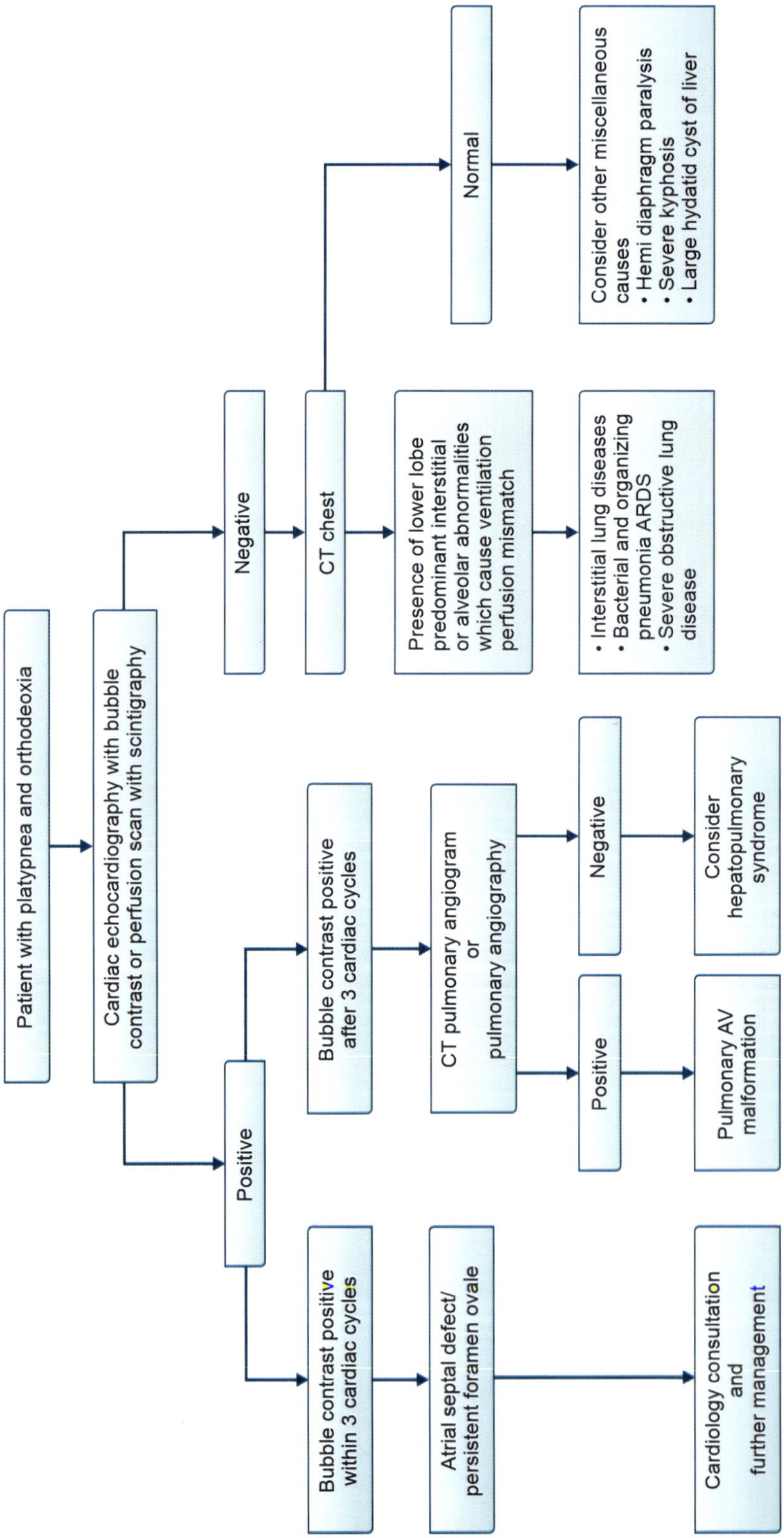

Fig. 2.3: Flowchart for diagnosis of platypnea orthodeoxia syndrome.

Definitive treatment of POS due to an intracardiac shunt involves correction of the primary cardiac anomaly. This may involve closure of the PFO or surgical repair of the ASD. In our case, closure of the PFO was performed with an Amplatzer device, resulting in significant improvement immediately post-procedure.

In patients with PAVM, pulmonary artery embolization, lung resection surgery, or lung transplant may be performed depending on the severity of the disease and the clinical condition of the patient. For patients with underlying parenchymal lung disease, treatment of the pulmonary condition leads to a reduction in V/Q mismatch with subsequent resolution of POS.

FURTHER READING

1. Santos F, Reis AT, Pessoa A, Agudo M, Brigas D, Pessoa AL. Platypnea-Orthodeoxia Syndrome: Two Case Reports. Cureus. 2023 Aug 20;15(8).
2. Agrawal A, Palkar A, Talwar A. The multiple dimensions of Platypnea-Orthodeoxia syndrome: A review. Respiratory medicine. 2017 Aug 1; 129:31–8.
3. Salas-Pacheco JL. Mechanisms of platypnea-orthodeoxia syndrome. Archivos de cardiologfa de Mexico. 2022 Jun;92(2):274–82.
4. Nema R, Rajanna C, Ray A, et al. When sitting suffocates: a rare cause of platypnoea-orthodeoxia syndrome. Breathe 2020; 16: 200205.
5. Lombardi M, Del Buono MG, Princi G, Locorotondo G, Lombardo A, Vergallo R, Montone RA, Burzotta F, Trani C, Crea F, Sanna T. Platypnoea-orthodeoxia syndrome as an uncommon cause of dyspnoea: a literature review. Internal Medicine Journal. 2022 Jun;52(6):921–5.

Chapter 3

Approach to a Case with Massive Hemoptysis

• Sameer Bansal • Kaumudi Devi • Ravindra M Mehta

LEARNING POINTS

1. Massive hemoptysis (MH) is a life-threatening condition, and the initial management priorities include airway protection and stabilising the patient's hemodynamics.
2. Bronchial artery embolization (BAE) is a highly successful first-line option when available for managing massive hemoptysis.
3. Bronchoscopy is valuable but requires the appropriate tools for effective clot and blood clearance, precise lesion identification, and tool deployment.

INTRODUCTION

Life-threatening hemoptysis may be defined as any hemoptysis that causes abnormal gas exchange/airway obstruction, or leads to hemodynamic instability, or exceeds 100 mL in 24 hours. It is a life-threatening emergency, associated with a high mortality rate. Management strategies in a case of massive hemoptysis include bronchial artery embolization, airway protection, endobronchial tamponade, and definitive therapy for the underlying disease. In this case report, we present a case of massive hemoptysis and discuss the approach towards managing hemoptysis.

CASE VIGNETTE

A young man in his early thirties presented with hemoptysis lasting three days, averaging about 100 mL/day of frank bloody expectoration. Upon examination, the patient was hemodynamically stable with a saturation of 95% on room air. Complete blood count, including platelet count and coagulation parameters, were within normal limits.

A computed tomography (CT) angiography of the thorax revealed bronchiectasis in the left lower lobe of the lung with hypertrophic bronchial arteries. There was also a mediastinal soft tissue lesion encircling and compressing pulmonary vessels, suggestive of mediastinitis (Fig. 3.1). The patient underwent bronchial artery embolization (BAE) of the hypertrophied bronchial arteries in the left lower lobe, resulting in a significant reduction of hemoptysis (Fig. 3.2).

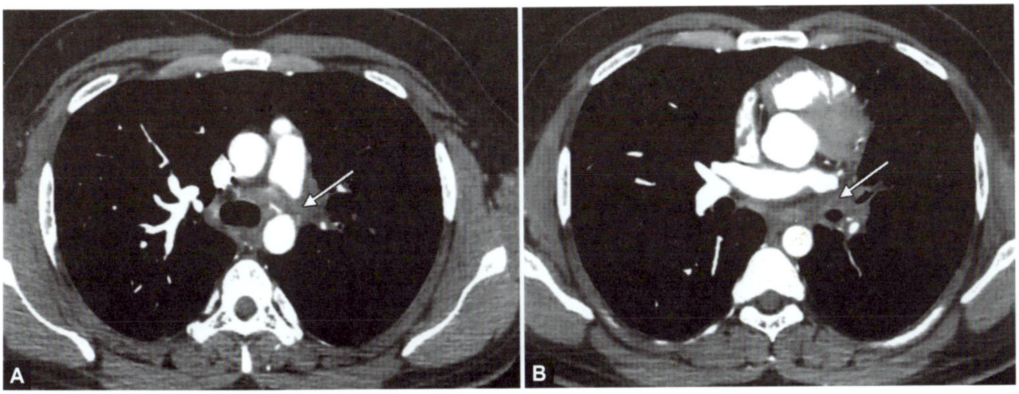

Fig. 3.1: (A) Mediastinal mass like soft tissue encircling the mediastinal structures with a hypertrophied left bronchial artery; (B) Mediastinal soft tissue encircling the left hilum with significant stenosis of the left pulmonary artery and vein.

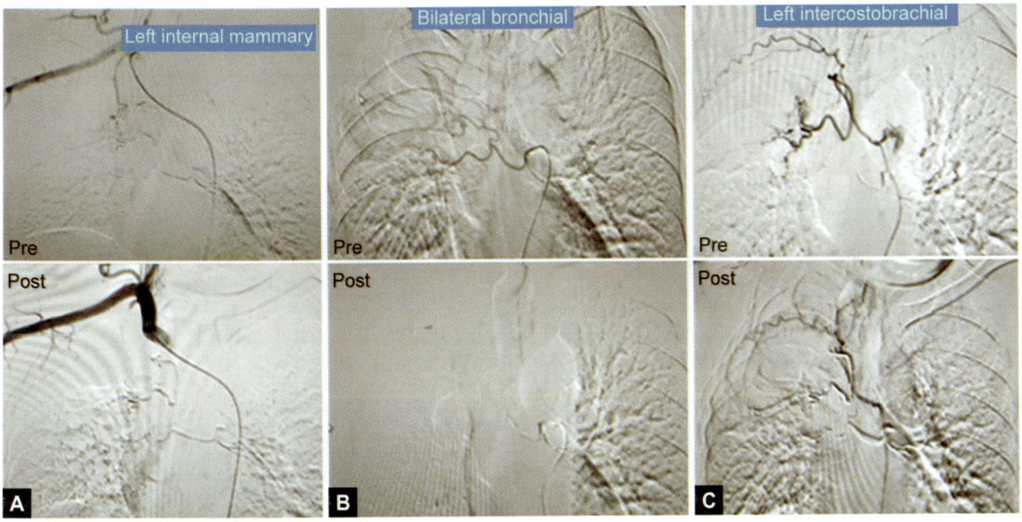

Fig. 3.2: Angiographic runs demonstrating (A) Left internal mammary artery pre- and post-procedure; (B) Bilateral bronchial artery pre- and post-procedure; (C) Left intercostobrachial decreased ooze post-procedure.

Subsequent flexible bronchoscopic evaluation revealed narrowing of the left main bronchus with diffuse nodularity. Mild bleeding was noticed from the inflamed, nodular mucosa. Due to the anticipated high risk of bleeding, the procedure was converted to rigid bronchoscopy under general anesthesia. An endobronchial biopsy from the nodules was performed which led to profuse bleeding. Conservative measures like topical adrenaline and wedging with the scope failed to achieve adequate hemostasis. Balloon tamponade of the left main bronchus using a Fogarty balloon was attempted which improved the ventilatory parameters. Argon plasma coagulation (APC) was performed at the bleeding site after carefully deflating the balloon, but the bleeding continued.

Persistent endobronchial bleeding led to shock and worsening respiratory failure. A customised endobronchial silicone blocker (CESB) was immediately molded and deployed into the left main bronchus and secured with cyanoacrylate glue, achieving hemostasis and improving hemodynamic and ventilatory parameters (Fig. 3.3). Following further discussions

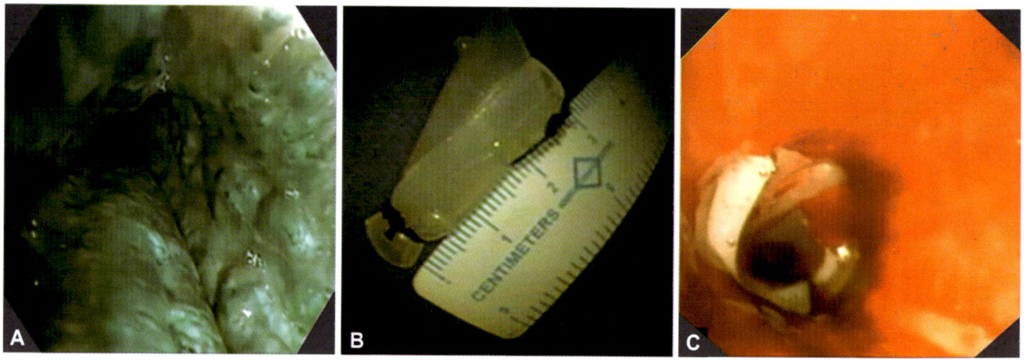

Fig. 3.3: (A) Narrow band imaging showing nodularity and vascularity in the left main bronchus; (B) Customised endobronchial silicon blocker (CESB); (C) CESB *in situ* left main bronchus.

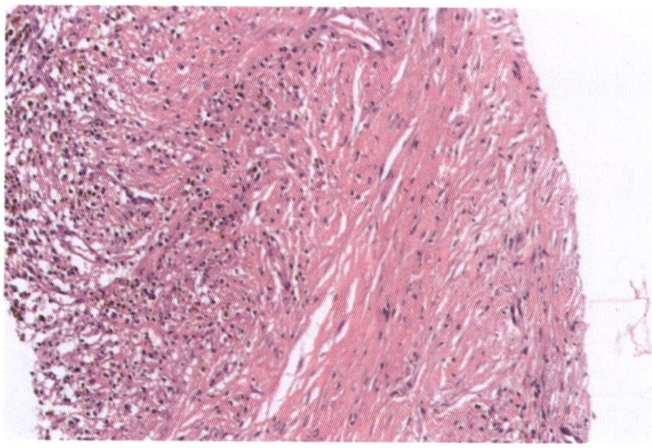

Fig. 3.4: Histopathology photomicrograph (H&E stain; 20X magnification) reveals dense hyaline fibrous tissue with lymphocytic infiltrate.

with the family, a left-sided pneumonectomy was performed as a definitive therapy for hemoptysis control. A final diagnosis of idiopathic fibrosing mediastinitis was made on histopathology (Fig. 3.4).

DISCUSSION

Massive hemoptysis is a potentially life-threatening condition commonly caused by tuberculosis (TB), bronchiectasis, aspergilloma, and malignancy. In addition to the above causes, several diseases can lead to hemoptysis (Table 3.1). Iatrogenic hemoptysis, resulting from diagnostic bronchoscopies, has an incidence rate of approximately 0.26 to 5%.

A prompt assessment of the patient's history and clinical examination is crucial to identify the etiology and source of hemoptysis. In life-threatening cases, airway management is paramount. Establishing vascular access, identifying the bleeding side for patient lateralization, correcting coagulopathies, and administering blood products are essential steps.

For hemodynamically unstable and hypoxic patients, immediate endotracheal intubation with a tube larger than 8 mm in diameter is advised for effective clearance of secretions and blood clots. Selective bronchial intubation may be advantageous if bleeding is localized to any one side.

Chest radiographs (CXR) can localise the bleeding source in about 70% of cases, though they may appear normal in 30% of cases. Computed tomography (CT) of the chest is highly sensitive

Table 3.1: Etiology of hemoptysis	
Category	***Conditions/Diseases***
Airway diseases	• Bronchitis • Bronchiectasis* • Bronchogenic carcinoma* • Bronchial carcinoid tumor • Metastatic cancer to bronchus or trachea • Bronchovascular fistula (e.g. aortic aneurysm with airway erosion) • Dieulafoy disease • Foreign body in airway • Broncholith
Pulmonary parenchymal diseases	• Infection (necrotizing pneumonia, lung abscess) • Bacterial infections (anthrax, leptospirosis, plague, tularemia) • Tuberculous* and nontuberculous mycobacterial disease • Mycetoma and other fungal infections* • Parasitic infections (e.g. paragonimus westermani, strongyloides) • Viral infections (e.g. herpes simplex, dengue fever) • Rheumatic diseases (Goodpasture disease, vasculitides, Behçet disease, antiphospholipid syndrome,systemic lupus erythematosus)
Pulmonary vascular diseases	• Heart failure (acquired or congenital) • Mitral stenosis • Pulmonary arteriovenous malformation • Pulmonary artery pseudoaneurysm • Pulmonary embolism (fat, septic, thrombotic) • Pulmonary veno-occlusive disease • Pulmonary and bronchial artery aneurysms (Hughes Stovin syndrome)
Bleeding disorders	• Anticoagulant and antiplatelet medications • Disseminated intravascular coagulation (DIC) • Platelet dysfunction (e.g. renal failure) • Thrombocytopenia • von Willebrand disease
Trauma	• Blunt trauma chest • Interventional pulmonology procedures
Drugs and toxins	• Cocaine use • Argemone alkaloid-contaminated cooking oil (epidemic dropsy) • Bevacizumab treatment, hydralazine, riociguat • E-cigarette or vaping product use associated lung injury (EVALI)
Idiopathic/miscellaneous	• Idiopathic pulmonary hemosiderosis • Amyloid • Fibrosing mediastinitis

*The most common causes of life-threatening hemoptysis are marked with an asterisk.

for identifying the bleeding site and underlying cause. The diagnostic accuracy of combining CT scanning and bronchoscopy is 83.9%. A dual-phase CT with angiogram can further pinpoint active bleeding, reveal hypertrophied bronchial arteries, and detect aneurysms. Management strategies include bronchoscopic, radiologic, or surgical interventions.

A. Bronchial Artery Embolization

Bronchial artery embolization (BAE), utilizing materials like glue, coils, or gel foam, is established as an effective treatment modality for immediate management of any life threatening hemoptysis. Most causes of massive hemoptysis arise from bronchial or systemic vessels and hence BAE is often successful in controlling the bleed.

A systematic review and meta-analysis by Zheng et al. demonstrated its high efficacy, with technical success and immediate control rates surpassing 99%. However, it also reported a recurrence rate of 23% and a mortality rate around 2%. In situations lacking the necessary infrastructure or expertise for BAE, or when bleed recurs after BAE, exploring alternative therapies becomes essential. These include bronchoscopic or surgical interventions.

B. Bronchoscopic Therapies for Massive Hemoptysis

In managing massive hemoptysis (MH), selecting the appropriate bronchoscope is critical. The flexible bronchoscope, though widely available and easier to train on due to its sub-segmental reach, faces limitations in MH management. The limitations include restricted suctioning capacity, a single small port for interventions, potential ventilation obstruction, and frequent clouding of the lens. Hence a rigid bronchoscope is the preferred scope while managing a case with MH. The rigid bronchoscope, with its dual ports for ventilation and a therapeutic multi-instrument port, offers significant advantages, although it cannot access segmental airways. A hybrid approach of using a flexible bronchoscope through the rigid can help overcome this issue.

Various bronchoscopic techniques are employed in MH management, such as balloon tamponade, APC, laser photocoagulation, and mechanical occlusive devices like glue, Endobronchial Watanabe Spigot (EWS), and CESB. Conservative treatments, including topical vasoconstrictors and secondary fibrinolytics, have limited roles in MH but are more effective in mild hemoptysis cases.

Balloon tamponade is a vital initial strategy for endobronchial bleed control. It helps in tamponading the bleed site, aiding in hemostasis and preventing blood spill-over into healthy lung segments. A Fogarty occlusion balloon, particularly useful for intra-procedural bleeding, is often used in conjunction with other modalities as it is not a stand-alone definitive therapy.

The modality of choice to control bleed while performing bronchoscopy would depend on the source of bleed (proximal airways versus distal parenchymal source) and whether or not the source of bleed is visible on bronchoscopy.

1. **Proximal airway source of bleed:** In cases where the source of bleed is visualized, endobronchial hot therapies such as APC, electrocautery (EC), and laser photocoagulation are commonly employed. These methods have proven effective in managing hemoptysis resulting from various tumors, Dieulafoy's lesions, and hemangiomas. APC and EC probes, readily accessible and compatible with a flexible bronchoscope, enable precise, targeted application. An effective suction is used to clear the visual field, then APC or EC is applied via a flexible bronchoscope passed through a rigid bronchoscope. Laser photocoagulation has demonstrated high efficacy, with success rates up to 94% in controlling hemoptysis across studies. However, its application, similar to APC, is confined to lesions visible through bronchoscopy. A crucial precaution with hot therapies is maintaining the fraction of inspired oxygen (FiO_2) below 40% to mitigate the risk of endobronchial fire.
2. **Distal parenchymal source of bleed:** In cases where the source of bleed is from the lung parenchyma, the aim is to block the segment (s) which are the cause for bleed. Once the

segment is identified, several techniques have been proposed to occlude the segments. Glue therapy, including options like cyanoacrylate glue, Tisseel glue, and fibrin glue, offers a safe and effective treatment for mild to moderate hemoptysis. However, its use is less common in massive hemoptysis due to its temporary presence, typically lasting only a few days, and the risk of overflow into adjacent lung segments. Additionally, it can cause local irritation, potentially leading to cough and expectoration of the glue, with a chance of hemoptysis recurrence.

EWS is utilized as a solid material for bronchial occlusion. The segments which are the source of bleed are blocked by using one or more spigots. EWS is advantageous for occluding multiple segments, thereby controlling parenchymal bleeding. These can be removable via both flexible and rigid bronchoscopy once the definitive therapy of the source of bleed is performed. However, utility is somewhat limited by the availability of only a few sizes (5, 6, and 7 mm), which may not adequately block larger bronchial segments. Mehta et al. introduced a novel approach in managing hemoptysis with CESB. These blockers are tailored to the specific bronchial segment's size, ensuring effective occlusion and a precise

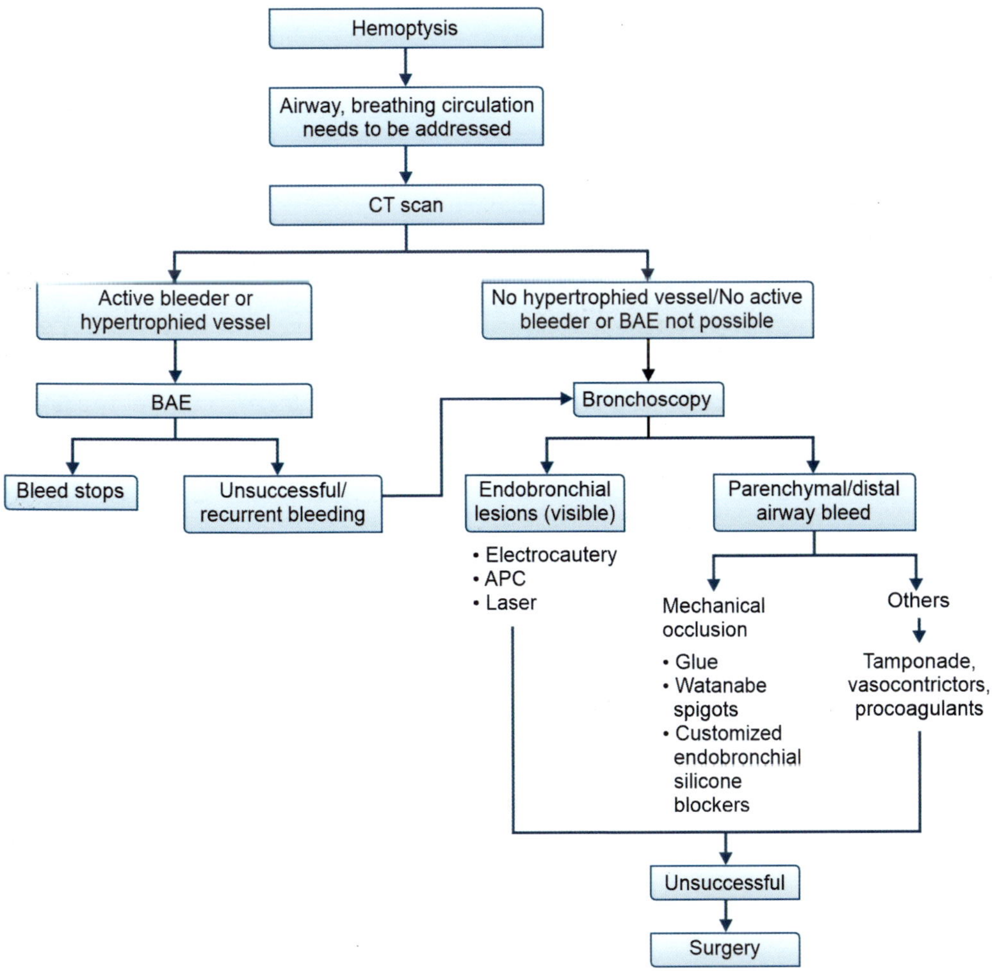

Fig. 3.5: Suggested algorithm for massive hemoptysis management.

fit. Equipped with a bucket handle tag, CESBs are easily removable. A rigid bronchoscope is preferred for their deployment due to its accuracy in placement.

C. Surgical Management

Surgical intervention remains vital for patients with recurrent or intractable hemoptysis unresponsive to bronchoscopic or radiologic treatments. When the disease leading to hemoptysis cannot be reversed by medical therapies, and if the source of bleed can be localized, surgical resection (when feasible) will offer a chance for cure, and must be offered. Surgical options range from lobectomy to pneumonectomy, though postoperative morbidity, which is significant, must be considered.

An algorithm, as in the referenced Fig. 3.5, would effectively encapsulate these diverse treatment modalities and their clinical applications.

FURTHER READING

1. Ibrahim WH. Massive haemoptysis: the definition should be revised. European Respiratory Journal. 2008 Oct 1;32(4):1131–2.
2. Davidson K, Shojaee S. Managing massive hemoptysis. Chest. 2020 Jan 1;157(1):77–88.
3. Zheng Z, Zhuang Z, Yang M, Luo J, Zhang W, Yan Z, Wang X. Bronchial artery embolization for hemoptysis: A systematic review and meta-analysis. Journal of Interventional Medicine. 2021 Nov 1;4(4):172–80.
4. Sakr L, Dutau H. Massive hemoptysis: an update on the role of bronchoscopy in diagnosis and management. Respiration. 2010 Jan 8;80(1):38–58.
5. Koegelenberg CFN, Bruwer JW, Bolliger CT: Endobronchial valves in the management of recurrent haemoptysis. Respiration 2014; 87:84–88.
6. Mehta RM, Godara R, Bhat RS, Loknath C, Singla A. A Novel Technique for the Management of Massive Hemoptysis: The Customized Endobronchial Silicone Blocker. Innovations (Phila). 2020 Mar/Apr;15(2):142–47.

Chapter 4

Approach to a Case of Bronchorrhea

• *Vipul Kumar Garg* • *V Nagarjuna Maturu*

LEARNING POINTS

1. Bronchorrhea, defined as production of copious sputum (>100 ml per day) is an uncommon clinical presentation, and can be classified as purulent or non-purulent bronchorrhea.
2. Presence of a non-purulent bronchorrhea should raise the suspicion of underlying lung malignancy.
3. If left untreated it can lead to dehydration, dys-electrolytemia and rarely hypoxic respiratory failure.
4. There are no specific treatment recommendations and treatment is directed towards managing underlying aetiology, and symptomatic therapy.

INTRODUCTION

Excessive sputum production of more than 100 mL/day is called bronchorrhea. It can result from malignancy, chronic inflammation, or infections. Such large volumes of sputum can result in breathlessness, anxiety, depression and exhaustion. Here we present a case of a middle-aged female who presented with a chronic cough associated with bronchorrhea for over one year before a diagnosis was established.

CASE VIGNETTE

A female homemaker in her fifties, presented with a history of cough and breathlessness for one year. She also complained of generalised weakness and unintentional loss of weight of eight kilograms over the last six months. The cough was insidious in onset, gradually progressive and was associated with copious watery expectoration. There was no diurnal or postural variation. Cough was associated with one episode of streaky haemoptysis one month back. Breathlessness was gradually progressive and she was experiencing breathing difficulty on walking at level ground for a few minutes over the last one month. There was no postural or diurnal variation in breathlessness.

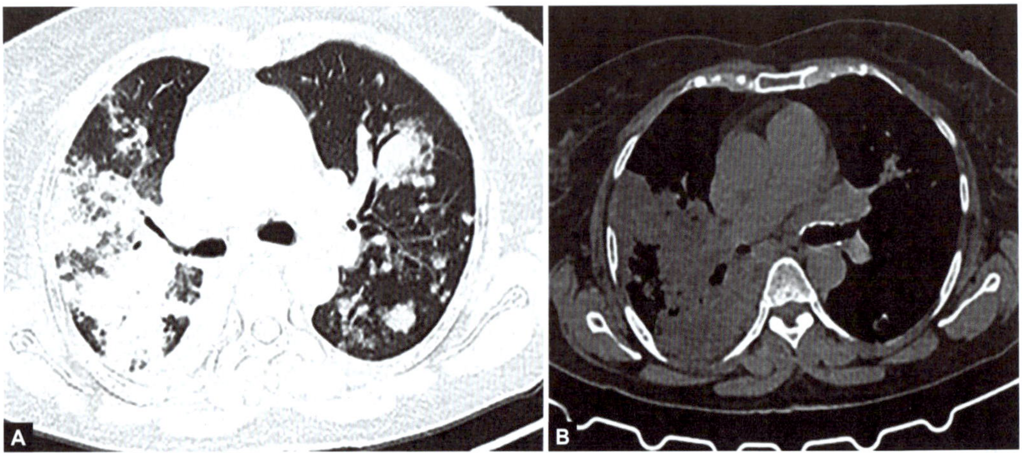

Fig. 4.1: (A) Axial view of HRCT chest, lung window showing right lower lobe consolidation with air bronchogram and bilateral nodular opacities; (B) Axial view of HRCT chest, mediastinal window showing the right mass lesion with soft tissue density.

Patient is known hypertensive and was well controlled on telmisartan. She was diagnosed with severe covid pneumonia two years ago for which she was hospitalised and required oxygen support. In view of her cough and breathlessness, the patient consulted a local physician five months ago and was diagnosed to have right lower lobe pneumonia. Bronchoscopy and bronchoalveolar lavage (BAL) were performed and workup was negative for infective aetiology. Patient was started on anti-tuberculosis therapy on clinicoradiological grounds. Despite treatment, the patient continued to have a severe cough with more than two cups of watery expectoration every day.

At presentation her vitals were as follows: Pulse rate of 78 beats per minute, blood pressure of 110/80 mm of Hg, respiratory rate of 24 per minute, temperature of 98.6°F and finger pulse oximetry saturation of 93% at room air. General examination was normal and respiratory system examination revealed bronchial breath sounds in the right infrascapular and lower interscapular region. Coarse inspiratory crackles were heard diffusely over the left lung. Other clinical systemic examinations were within normal limits.

Complete blood count, renal and liver functions were unremarkable. Echocardiogram showed normal left ventricular function with no valvular abnormalities. Chest radiograph revealed bilateral nodular opacities with largest being in the right lower zone. High resolution computed tomography (HRCT) of thorax revealed large heterogeneous soft tissue density lesions in the right lower lobe with multiple spiculated and coalescing nodules in the right upper lobe, right middle lobe and the entire left lung. No significant mediastinal lymphadenopathy was observed (Fig. 4.1). Sputum Xpert MTB/RIF, smear for acid fast bacilli and fungal smear were negative. Bacterial and fungal cultures were sterile. Antineutrophil cytoplasmic antibodies (ANCA) by ELISA were negative.

On bronchoscopy, the right tracheobronchial tree was found to be flooded with serous secretions extending till the level of carina (Fig. 4.2A and B). After clearance of the secretions, a cryo-biopsy was performed from the right lower lobe and six biopsies were obtained. Histopathological examination of the biopsy revealed presence of moderately differentiated invasive adenocarcinoma with lepidic growth pattern. A diagnosis of bronchorrhea secondary to lepidic adenocarcinoma was confirmed.

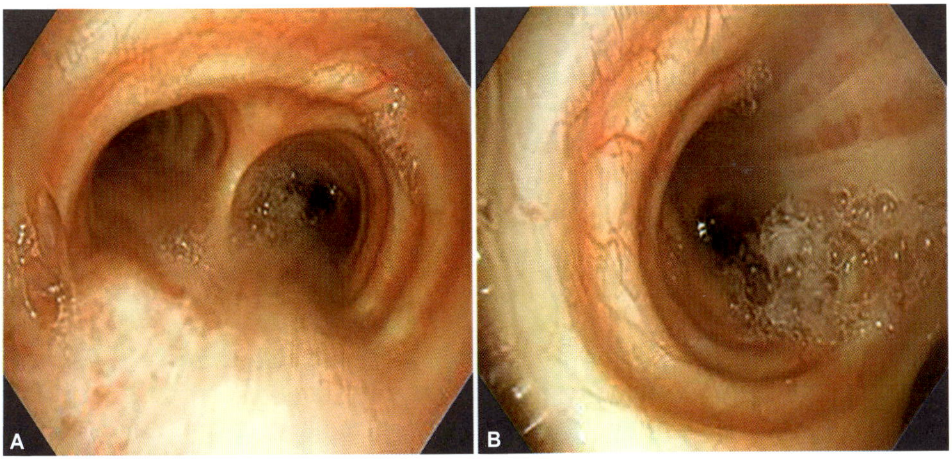

Fig. 4.2: Bronchoscopic image showing copious watery secretions in (A) Right main bronchus at the level of the main carina and (B) The right intermediate bronchus.

DISCUSSION

Bronchorrhea is defined as the production of >100 mL sputum per day. It is an uncommon clinical condition and is described only in a few disease states. It is important to recognize this entity, as it will help in narrowing our differentials. It usually results from chronic inflammation, malignancy or infections and can be due to structural lung abnormalities like lung cavity and bronchiectasis.

Bronchorrhea is a debilitating symptom which is very bothersome to the patient, difficult to manage and occasionally leads to complications. Expectoration of such large quantities is difficult and could be associated with breathlessness, weakness, exhaustion, and anxiousness. If left untreated it leads to dyselectrolytemia, dehydration and in debilitated patients could lead to a functional decline and hypoxic respiratory failure.

Bronchorrhea can be broadly classified into purulent and non-purulent bronchorrhea depending on the presence or absence of purulence in the sputum (Table 4.1).

A. Purulent Bronchorrhea

Purulent bronchorrhea, as the name suggests, is often the result of an untreated/poorly treated bacterial infection of the pre-existing bronchiectasis. The other common causes of purulent bronchorrhea are lung cavity and an empyema with bronchopleural fistula. In the developing world, bronchiectasis remains the commonest cause of purulent bronchorrhea.

Table 4.1: Causes and classification of bronchorrhea

Purulent bronchorrhea	*Non-purulent bronchorrhea*
Bronchiectasis	Lepidic adenocarcinoma of the lung
Lung abscess	Metastasis from adenocarcinoma (colon, pancreas, etc.)
Empyema with bronchopleural fistula	• Asthma (uncommon) • Endobronchial tuberculosis (uncommon) • Organophosphorus poisoning • Ruptured pulmonary hydatid cyst (rare)

Treatment involves identifying the causative organisms and administering appropriate and a longer course of antibiotics (intravenous initially followed by oral maintenance). Addition of nebulized antibiotics to systemic antibiotics may be helpful to eradicate the bacterial pathogen from the bronchiectatic airways.

B. Non-purulent Bronchorrhea

Non-purulent bronchorrhea (also called sterile bronchorrhea) is most often due to lepidic adenocarcinoma of lung or metastasis to lungs from adenocarcinoma elsewhere. It can also be uncommonly seen in asthma, bronchiectasis due to inflammatory bowel disease and organophosphorus poisoning.

Mechanisms of excessive sputum production in bronchorrhea due to malignancy are poorly understood. Major proposed mechanisms are:

1. **Secretory pathway:** Increase in mucin producing goblet cells and metaplasia of non-secretory to secretory cells (driven by EGFR pathway).
2. **Transudative pathway:** Increased inflammatory mediators in response to inflammatory stimuli which leads to excessive transmembrane transudation of secretions.

Management of bronchorrhea is challenging and is primarily aimed at effective management of the underlying disease. There is limited evidence for effective drug treatment of bronchorrhea and there are no established recommendations. Drugs that have been tried to control malignant bronchorrhea are corticosteroids, macrolide antibiotics, octreotide and inhaled indomethacin (Table 4.2).

Table 4.2: Mechanisms of action of medication used for malignant bronchorrhea

Medication	*Mechanism of action*
Corticosteroids	• Inhibit glycoprotein and chloride secretions. • Suppress gene encoding inducible cyclooxygenase. • Directly inhibit glycol-conjugate secretion.
Macrolide antibiotics	• Reduce chloride excretion in airway epithelial cells.
EGFR tyrosine kinase inhibitors	• Inhibit mucin production in lung cancer cells by blocking the epidermal growth factor receptor (EGFR) pathway.
Inhaled indomethacin	• Inhibit cyclooxygenase-2 (COX-2). • Enhance sodium absorption through airway mucosa.
Octreotide	• Reduce secretin-induced chloride efflux from bronchial epithelial cells.

Pharmacotherapy (usually symptomatic management) is chosen considering treatment tolerability, local availability, and treatment cost.

FURTHER READING

1. Bhagat M, Singh A, Bazzi T, Green J. Bronchorrhea, a Rare and Debilitating Symptom of Lung Cancer: Case Report and Review of the Treatment. JTO Clinical and Research Reports. 2022 Oct 1;3(10):100398.

2. Marom ZM, Goswami SK. Respiratory mucus hypersecretion (bronchorrhea): A case discussion—possible mechanism (s) and treatment. Journal of allergy and clinical immunology. 1991 Jun 1;87(6):1050–5.

3. Rémi C, Remi J, Bausewein C. Pharmacological management of bronchorrhea in malignant disease: a systematic literature review. Journal of Pain and Symptom Management. 2016 May 1;51(5):916–25.

4. Zylicz Z. The challenge of bronchorrhea in advanced cancer—a case report with review of literature. Advances in Palliative Medicine. 2010;9(1):9–11.

Chapter 5

Approach to a Case of Chronic Cough with Normal Chest Radiograph

• *Vidya B Nair* • *Sravan Kumar* • *Arjun P*

LEARNING POINTS

1. Chronic cough (cough lasting > 8 weeks) is a common clinical problem, and its management needs a scientific stepwise approach.
2. The three most common causes of chronic cough with a normal chest radiograph are gastro-esophageal reflux disease (GERD), upper airway cough syndrome and cough variant asthma.
3. A failed clinical trial with PPI, does not rule out a significant GERD. An upper GI endoscopy/ 24-hour pH or a pH impedance monitoring will help establish the diagnosis of GERD in such cases.
4. Establishing the right diagnosis, and instituting specific treatment will help patients attain complete symptom resolution and significantly improve their quality of life.

INTRODUCTION

Cough is a protective reflex that clears the respiratory tract and prevents aspiration. Cough is termed as chronic if it lasts for more than eight weeks. Chronic cough has an estimated global prevalence of 2–18% and may be due to a wide array of causes. To identify the potential etiologies, a stepwise approach with detailed history and clinical examination is needed. Here we present a case of an elderly female patient, who presented with chronic dry cough. She was extensively evaluated until the exact cause was identified.

CASE VIGNETTE

A 63-year-old home-maker, with no prior history of respiratory illness or other medical comorbidities, presented with a history of dry cough of seven months' duration. Cough was intermittent and more at night. It starts a while after going to bed and was reported to be more after having spicy food. There was no seasonal variation in cough. She also gave a history of heartburn. There was no history of breathlessness, wheeze, chest pain, palpitation, pedal edema, orthopnea, or rhinitis. There was no history of fever, loss of weight or loss of appetite. There was no history of joint pain/rashes/photosensitivity/exposure to pets/birds.

Family history was non-contributory. On presentation, her vitals were stable and general examination was within normal limits. Examination of the chest was also normal with normal breath sounds heard over all lung fields on auscultation.

The following differential diagnosis were considered:

1. Gastroesophageal reflux disease (GERD)
2. Cough variant asthma
3. Upper airway cough syndrome (UACS)
4. Excessive dynamic airway collapse

Complete blood count, renal and liver functions were within normal limits. Chest radiograph showed normal lung fields (Fig. 5.1). Induced sputum smear for acid fast bacilli (AFB) and Xpert TB/Rif were negative. Spirometry was done to rule out airway disease, which was normal (Fig. 5.2). She was treated initially with a two-week trial of proton pump inhibitors (PPI), considering a possibility of reflux related cough based on her history and normal examination findings. After a short asymptomatic period, she again presented with a persistent cough. In view of persistent symptoms, a methacholine challenge test was done, which was negative (Fig. 5.3). This ruled out cough variant asthma. However, she was initiated on trial of inhaled corticosteroid, considering the possibility of non-asthmatic eosinophilic bronchitis, but symptoms persisted.

To rule out upper airway causes of cough, a flexible laryngoscopy was done which showed restricted adduction of vocal cords with bilateral arytenoid asymmetry. There was postnasal drip with mucopurulent discharge in the right middle meatus tracking to the nasopharynx. She was then treated for upper airway cough syndrome, but the cough was incessant. Dynamic CT chest was normal, ruling out the possibility of excessive dynamic airway collapse (EDAC) or any small airway disease (Fig. 5.4). Meanwhile, the patient was continued on PPIs.

Due to persistent coughing, an esophago-gastro-duodenoscopy (EGD) was performed. This revealed a hiatus hernia and Barrett's esophagus, accompanied by antral erythema and a hyperplastic fundic gland polyp. Notably, there was no evidence of esophagitis.

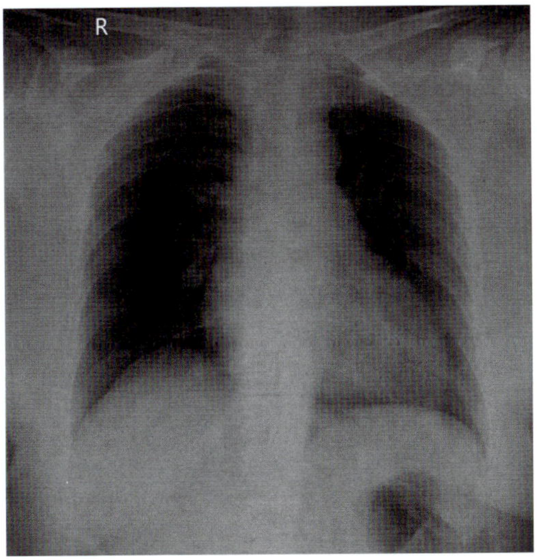

Fig. 5.1: Chest radiograph PA view.

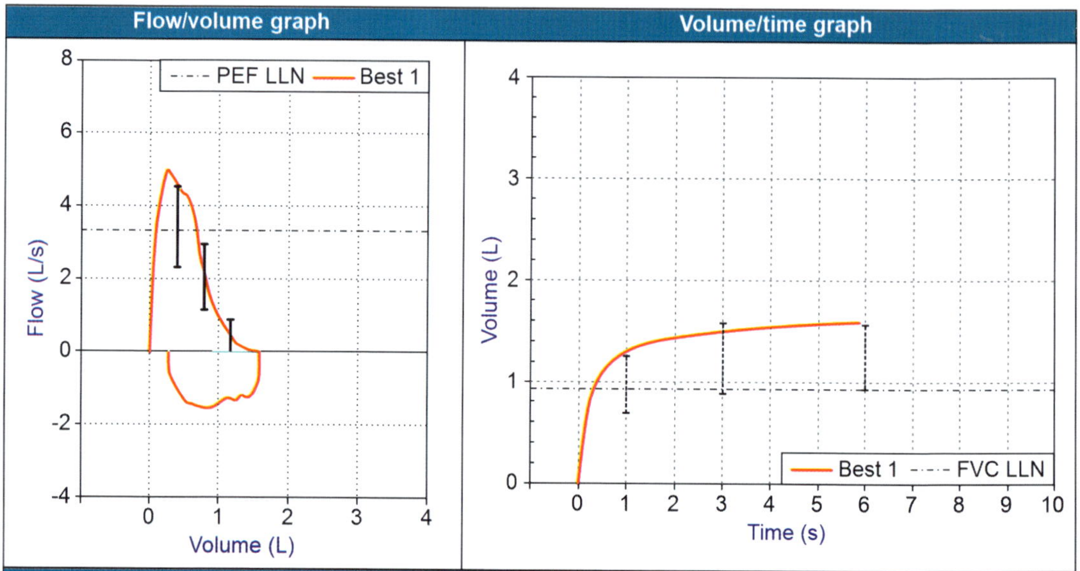

Results

Parameter	Pred	LLN	ATS/ERS best	% Pred.	Z-score
FVC (L)	1.56	0.92	1.59	102	0.08
FEV1 (L)	1.25	0.69	1.30	104	0.15
FEV1 ratio	0.76	0.65	0.82	108	0.89
PEF (L/min)	287	199	3.29	115	0.78
FEF 25-75 (L/s)	2.33	0.94	1.46	63	-1.03

Session quality and repeatability information

Session grade	FVC rep:	FEV1 rep:	FET (s)	Slow start to test	End of test criteria not achieved	Cough detected in 1st second
B	0.07 L (4.4%)	0.05 L (3.8%)	5.86	0 blow (s)	5 blow (s)	0 blow (s)

Fig. 5.2: Pulmonary function test (spirometry).

Indication for test: Cough
Bronchodilator Administered and Dose: Levolin 1.25 mg
Baseline FEV1: 1.18 L
Target 80 of FEV1: 0.94 L

Time	*Concentration*	*FEV1 30 sec*	*FEV1 90 sec*
0–5 min	0.03 mg/mL	1.05	1.14
5–10 min	0.06 mg/mL	1.15	1.14
	0.125 mg/mL	–	–
10–15 min	0.25 mg/mL	1.16	1.12
	0.5 mg/mL	–	–
15–20 min	1 mg/mL	1.1	1.13
20–25 min	2 mg/mL	1.07	1.14
25–30 min	4 mg/mL	1.12	1.08
30–35 min	8 mg/mL	1.13	1.12
35–40 min	16 mg/mL	1.06	1.05

Signs and symptoms after final dose: Nil

Fig. 5.3: Methacholine challenge test.

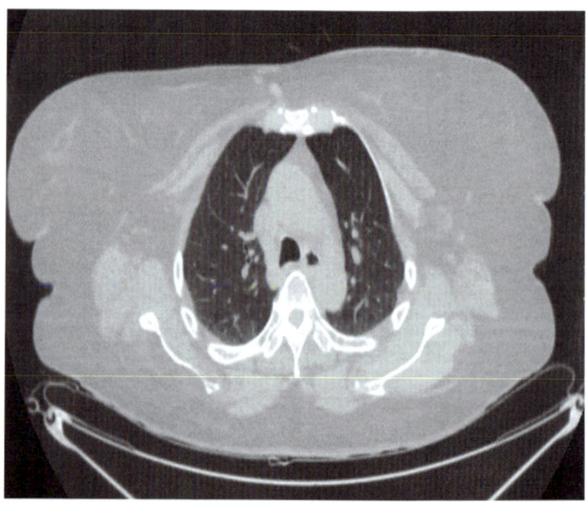

Fig. 5.4: Axial images of high resolution CT chest (expiratory image) ruling out excessive dynamic airway collapse and small airway disease.

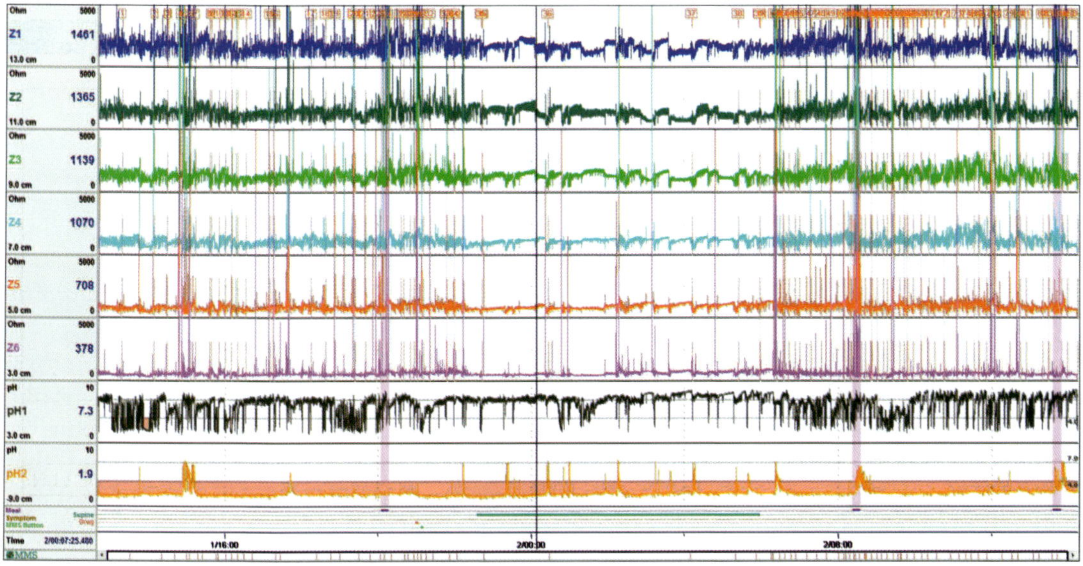

Fig. 5.5: 24 hours esophageal pH and impedance study.

Subsequently, a 24-hour esophageal pH and impedance study was conducted, confirming severe gastroesophageal reflux, as indicated by a DeMeester score of 40 (normal score is < 14.7) (Fig. 5.5). Esophageal manometry demonstrated normal esophageal motility. Based on these findings, a diagnosis of GERD-related chronic cough was confirmed.

Based on the flexible laryngoscopy findings, along with the upper gastrointestinal endoscopy showing gastroesophageal reflux, with a DeMeester score of 40 in 24-hour pH study, surgical management was planned, considering the refractory nature of cough. A definitive treatment with laparoscopic Floppy Nissen's Fundoplication was performed. The patient was advised on lifestyle modifications and diligently continued to adhere to them. On postoperative review, the patient was completely asymptomatic and is currently on regular follow up.

DISCUSSION

The commonly attributed causes of chronic cough are mainly three:

a. Upper airway cough syndrome (previously referred to as postnasal drip syndrome)
b. Cough variant asthma, and
c. Gastroesophageal reflux disease (GERD).

They should always be suspected when individuals present with chronic cough and have a normal chest X-ray. A stepwise empirical trial of medications is a cost-effective approach which can be tried in such patients, when there is no prevailing diagnosis.

In any patient who presents with chronic cough and normal chest radiograph, two questions have to be asked at the outset itself:

1. Is the patient a smoker?
2. Is the patient on any Angiotensin converting enzyme (ACE) inhibitor?

If the answers to these two are "NO", then the most likely diagnosis is either GERD, cough variant asthma or Upper airway cough syndrome (UACS). A few red flags should always be kept in mind whilst evaluating any patient having chronic cough. These include fever, hemoptysis, weight loss, hoarseness of voice, excessive dyspnea or sputum production, smoker (> 45 years of age) or smoker with smoking history of > 20 pack years. These patients need further detailed investigations including sputum examination, high resolution computed tomography (HRCT) thorax and bronchoscopy to rule out malignancy or tuberculosis.

A. Gastroesophageal Reflux Disease

Gastroesophageal reflux disease (GERD) is defined as "a condition which develops when the reflux of stomach contents causes troublesome symptoms and/or complications". Risk factors recognized for GERD include obesity, genetics, tobacco smoking, pregnancy, hiatus hernia, and certain medications and foods.

Heartburn, a burning sensation in the chest, is the classic and most commonly reported symptom of GERD. There may also be a spectrum of nonspecific esophageal symptoms like regurgitation, dysphagia and extra esophageal symptoms like laryngitis, dental problems, chronic cough, adult-onset asthma, and/or aspiration pneumonia. Some studies report that GERD is one of the common causes of persistent cough. GERD related cough is usually nocturnal and worse after meals. Symptoms commonly associated with GERD (e.g.heartburn, or a sour taste in the mouth) are absent in more than 40 percent of patients in whom cough is thought to be attributable to reflux. Potential mechanisms by which GERD might contribute to chronic cough are shown in Fig. 5.6:

1. An esophageal-tracheobronchial cough reflex induced by reflux of acid into the distal esophagus (intraesophageal reflux).
2. Stimulation of receptors on vagal afferent nerves in the upper respiratory tract (laryngo-pharyngeal reflux).
3. Aspiration of gastric contents, leading to stimulation of receptors in the lower respiratory tract and inflammation in the airways.

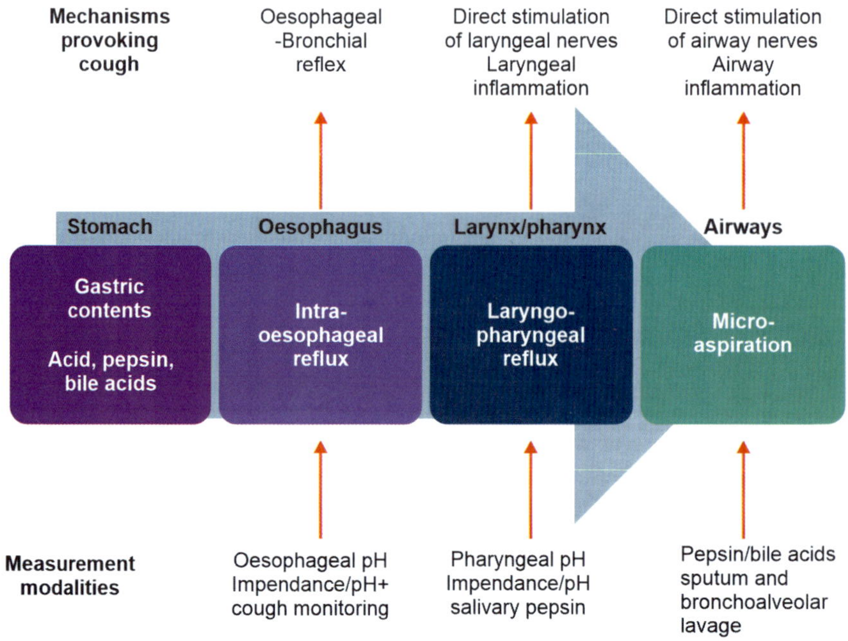

Fig. 5.6: Mechanism of cough in gastroesophageal reflux disease.

Most often, the diagnosis of cough due to GERD is based on clinical features (cough with reflux symptoms) and a response to PPI therapy. Despite adequate lifestyle modifications and maximal anti-reflux therapy, some patients with positive results on esophageal pH monitoring continue to cough. Endoscopy may show erosive esophagitis and Barrett's esophagus which are specific for GERD. Ambulatory esophageal pH monitoring/24-hour pH impedance monitoring can help clinch the diagnosis, especially in those with normal endoscopy findings. It is reserved for patients with persistent symptoms of GERD despite optimal trial of anti-reflux therapy.

Surgical management for reflux disease is generally reserved for patients with hiatus hernia or patient's preference for single time surgical management over long term PPI. Anti-reflux surgery may be performed for atypical (non-gastrointestinal) symptoms (e.g. chronic cough, laryngeal disease, and asthma) when there is objective evidence to attribute such symptoms to reflux. The original fundoplication as described by Rudolph Nissen in 1956 involved passage of the gastric fundus behind the esophagus to encircle the distal 6 cm of the esophagus. Laparoscopic Nissen fundoplication is highly effective in relieving GERD symptoms and is the most durable amongst all the procedures. It is considered as the current gold standard of anti-reflux procedures. However, it is also associated with the greatest potential for adverse effects, such as dysphagia, difficulty in vomiting, and gas bloating.

B. Upper Airway Cough Syndrome

Upper airway cough syndrome (UACS) is another important cause of chronic cough. The mechanisms of cough in UACS are postnasal drip, direct irritation of nasal mucosa, inflammation in the upper and lower airways and sensitization of the cough reflex. The nasal sensory nerves are stimulated by inflammatory factors like histamine after the nasal mucosa receives an external stimulus. Antihistamines and nasal decongestants are the treatment of choice.

C. Cough Variant Asthma and Non-asthmatic Eosinophilic Bronchitis

Cough variant asthma, eosinophilic bronchitis and atopic cough are also commonly attributed causes of chronic cough. Cough variant asthma should be suspected when physical examination and spirometry findings are non-diagnostic. In those with a normal spirometry, bronchial provocation testing (methacholine inhalation challenge) can confirm the diagnosis. In centers where it is unavailable empiric anti-asthma treatment must be initiated with inhaled corticosteroids. A partial response is seen by one week, although complete response may take as long as two months.

Non-asthmatic eosinophilic bronchitis (NAEB) is a close mimicker of cough variant asthma. It is confirmed by the presence of either sputum or bronchial wash eosinophilia and an improvement in the cough following inhaled corticosteroid therapy. Fractional exhaled nitric oxide (FeNO) may be used as a surrogate for eosinophilic inflammation or before a trial of ICS, although no RCTs have evaluated the role of FeNO in identifying responders to therapy. The points which differentiate NAEB from asthma are the absence of mast cells in airway smooth muscles and lack of airway hyper-responsiveness in NAEB. Inhaled corticosteroids are the treatment of choice of this condition. If a causal allergen is identified, it must be avoided.

A stepwise approach for evaluation of chronic cough is illustrated in Fig. 5.7.

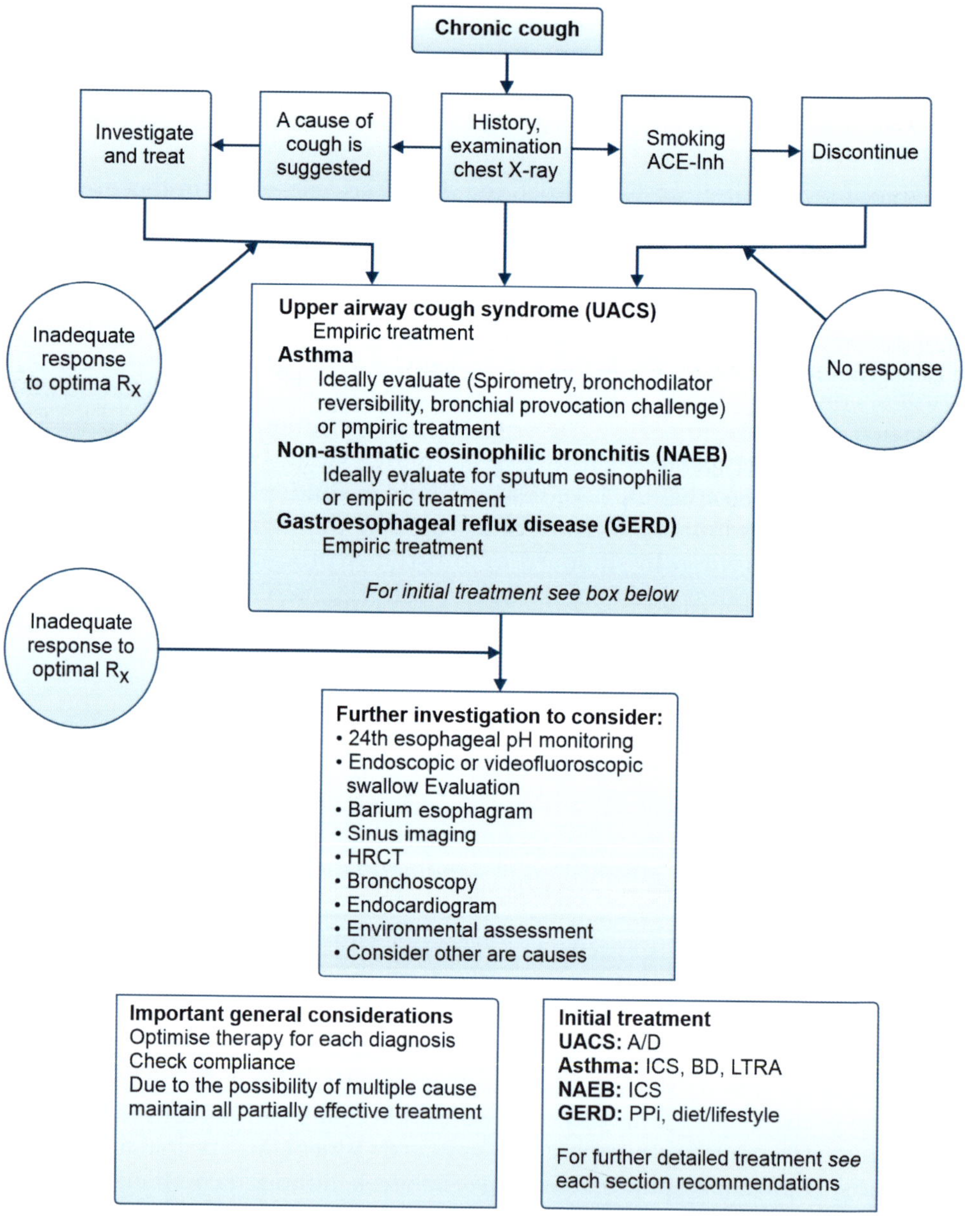

Fig. 5.7: Evaluation of chronic cough: *Adapted from* Irwin et al, ACCP evidence based clinical practice guidelines.

FURTHER READING

1. Morice A, Dicpinigaitis P, McGarvey L, Birring SS. Chronic cough: new insights and future prospects. European Respiratory Review. 2021 Dec 31;30(162).

2. On PC. Overview of chronic cough. The American Journal of Managed Care. 2022 Sep 1;28(9 Suppl):S152–8.

3. Katz PO, Dunbar K, Schnoll-Sussman FH, Greer KB, Yadlapati R, Spechler SJ. ACG Clinical Guideline: Guidelines for the Diagnosis and Management of Gastroesophageal Reflux Disease. Am J Gastroenterol. 2022 Jan 1;117(1):27–56.

4. Lucanska M, Hajtman A, Calkovsky V, Kunc P, Pecova R. Upper Airway Cough Syndrome in Pathogenesis of Chronic Cough. Physiol Res. 2020 Mar 27;69(Suppl 1):S35–42.

5. Irwin RS, Baumann MH, Bolser DC, Boulet LP, Braman SS, Brightling CE, et al. Diagnosis and management of cough executive summary: ACCP evidence-based clinical practice guidelines. Chest. 2006 Jan;129(1 Suppl):1S-23S.

SECTION II

Airway Diseases

Chapter

6

Approach to a Case with Stridor

• *Santha Kumar* • *Venugopal Jagannathan* • *Deepak TH*

LEARNING POINTS

1. Stridor is an alarming and an emergency symptom which requires immediate attention by the physician. It signifies a life-threatening central airway obstruction (airway lumen ≤8 mm in diameter).
2. It is very important to differentiate stridor from wheeze. Misdiagnosis of stridor as wheeze will lead to a delay in initiation of life saving appropriate therapy to the patient.
3. Focussed investigations (CT of the neck and thorax followed by a diagnostic bronchoscopy) will help in establishing the cause in majority of the instances.

INTRODUCTION

Stridor is a high pitched, harsh sound, due to turbulent air flow caused by critical obstruction in the central airways. Presence of stridor indicates a life threatening obstruction of the central airways. Stridor is a symptom, not a diagnosis or a disease, and the underlying cause must be determined, and treatment should be instituted as soon as possible. It is important to prevent morbidity and mortality by diagnosing the cause promptly and managing it appropriately.

CASE VIGNETTE

A man in his mid-thirties presented with progressively worsening shortness of breath, whistling sound during breathing and dry cough for two months duration. Symptoms worsened over the last one week and he also could not lie down flat. There was no diurnal variation in symptoms. He denied fever, chest pain, hemoptysis or any swelling of limbs. He had no comorbid conditions. He was a non-smoker and had no exposure to organic or inorganic dusts at home or at workplace. Since he had wheezing, he had been treated as bronchial asthma before he presented to our facility. On examination, he had a biphasic stridor at rest, more during expiration and rest of the examination was unremarkable. His oxygen saturation on pulse oximetry was 95% on room air.

Index case was suspected to have a central airway obstruction (CAO) based on examination finding of stridor. Spirometry which was performed earlier was reviewed and it revealed a

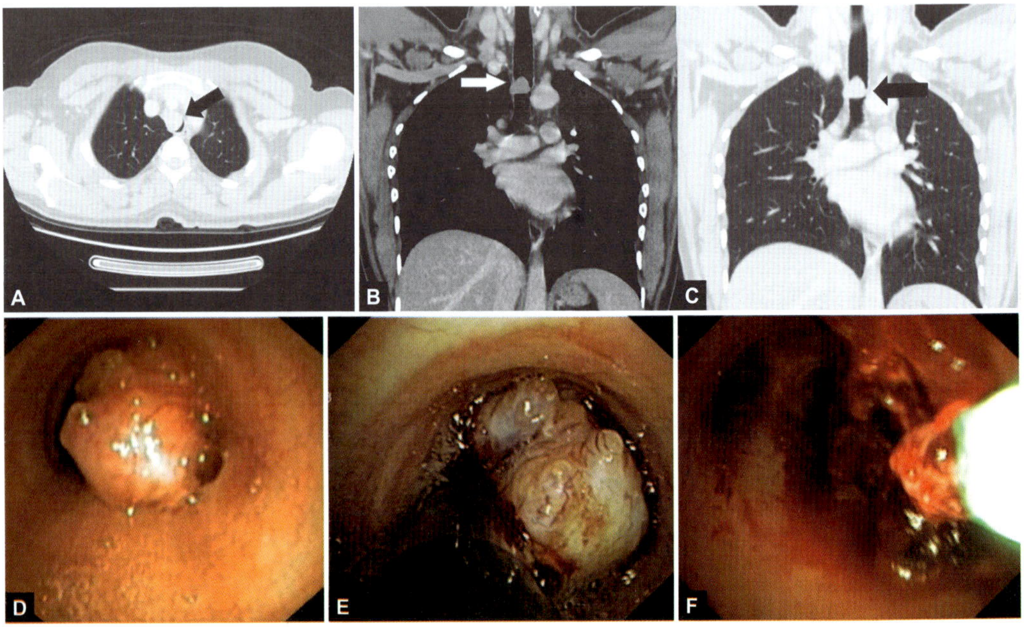

Fig. 6.1: CT scan of the index patient. (A) Axial view shows tumor arising from anterolateral wall occluding more than 80% of lumen (arrow). (B) Tumor visualized in coronal view soft tissue window. (C) Coronal view lung window. (D) Bronchoscopic image of tumor occluding more than 80% of the lumen. (E) Patient was intubated with a micro-laryngeal tube. The tube is passed beyond the tumor and the tip is kept distally. (F) Tumor debulking is done during which the carina is visualised. To achieve hemostasis, argon plasma coagulation is done.

flattening of the expiratory curve of the flow volume loop pointing to the fact that the level of obstruction is in the intrathoracic airways. His chest radiograph showed a soft tissue density inside the lower trachea. A computed tomography (CT) scan of the chest confirmed a soft tissue lesion arising from an anterolateral wall of the lower trachea, with more than 80% luminal obstruction (Fig. 6.1A to C). His blood biochemistry was unremarkable.

He was then subjected for diagnostic bronchoscopy. Bronchoscopy showed a large tumor arising from anterolateral wall of lower trachea with near total occlusion of the lumen (Fig. 6.1D). A 6 mm bronchoscope could not be negotiated beyond the tumor. During diagnostic bronchoscopy he developed severe hypoxia. Immediately he was intubated with a microlaryngeal tube (MLT) under guidance of an ultrathin bronchoscopy. The distal end of the MLT tube was positioned at the carina bypassing the tumor (Fig. 6.1E). Subsequently, the tumor was debulked completely using electrocautery and cryotherapy via a rigid bronchoscope. The tracheal lumen was recanalized (Fig. 6.1F), and he was extubated. The histopathology of the tumor revealed it to be an adenoid cystic carcinoma. Patient was further evaluated for staging and was confirmed as locally advanced adenoid cystic carcinoma. As a definitive therapy, he then underwent tracheal resection and anastomosis. His follow up evaluation up to 3 years did not reveal any recurrence of the carcinoma.

DISCUSSION

A. Definition of Stridor

Stridor is a high pitched, harsh sound, due to turbulent air flow caused by critical obstruction at the level of larynx, trachea or major bronchi. It is a potentially life-threatening problem as

Table 6.1: Stridor versus wheeze–Differences		
	Stridor	***Wheeze***
Location of obstruction	Central airway	Peripheral/small airways
Nature of the sound	• Monophonic • Usually inspiratory. Can be expiratory or biphasic • Harsh noise	• Polyphonic • Usually expiratory • Musical/whistle like in nature
Heard best with	Audible to ear without a stethoscope	Best heard with a stethoscope
Life threatening	Yes	No
Diurnal variability	Absent	May be present
Response to inhaled bronchodilators	Absent	Present

there is a possibility of airway compromise and respiratory arrest. It is very important for the physician to not confuse stridor with wheezing, which is a continuous high pitched expiratory sound, composed of single or multiple notes. Wheezing is a feature of lower/peripheral airway obstruction, whereas stridor is a feature of central airway obstruction (Table 6.1).

Stridor is a symptom, not a diagnosis or a disease, and the underlying cause must be determined as soon as possible. In most cases, a thorough history and physical examination, along with other additional studies (imaging studies and flexible or rigid bronchoscopy) is required to confirm the etiology.

B. Pathophysiology

When air passes through a narrowed flexible airway, the lateral pressure that holds the airway open can drop precipitously (the Bernoulli principle) and cause the tube to close. This process obstructs airflow and produces stridor. Depending on its timing in the respiratory cycle, stridor may be categorized as inspiratory, expiratory, or biphasic.

- Inspiratory stridor suggests a variable extrathoracic (larynx/upper tracheal) obstruction.
- Expiratory stridor suggests a variable intrathoracic (mid/lower tracheal) obstruction.
- Biphasic (inspiratory and expiratory) stridor suggests a fixed central airway obstruction.

C. Etiology

Causes of stridor are numerous and a few are listed in Table 6.2. Based on duration of symptoms, they can be classified as being acute in presentation (days to weeks) or chronic (weeks to months). Laryngeal and vocal cord edema, laryngeal stenosis or tumor (Fig. 6.2A), laryngeal trauma, bilateral vocal cord palsy and goitre (Fig. 6.2B) are the most frequent causes of stridor due to glottic pathologies in adults. At the tracheal level, malignant tumors (Fig. 6.2C), foreign body aspiration (Fig. 6.2D), benign tracheal stenosis (Fig. 6.2E), tracheomalacia, and benign airway tumors are the common causes.

D. Clinical Presentation–History and Clinical Examination

Stridor is an important clinical symptom that every clinician should be aware of, because it is a sign of underlying life-threatening airway obstruction. Indeed, on hearing stridor, the physician should be alert, keeping the tools required for intubation or tracheostomy ready, while simultaneously evaluating the etiology of the stridor.

Table 6.2: Causes of stridor

Duration	*Level of obstruction*	*Causes*
Acute	Nasopharynx or oropharynx	1. Acute tonsillar hypertrophy 2. Peritonsillar abscess 3. Retropharyngeal abscess
	Larynx and vocal cords	1. Anaphylaxis and laryngeal edema 2. Epiglottitis 3. Vocal cord palsy 4. Laryngeal trauma during endotracheal intubation
	Trachea	1. Croup 2. Diphtheria 3. Tracheitis 4. Foreign body aspiration 5. Trauma/Burns
Chronic	Larynx and glottis	1. Post irradiation stenosis 2. Laryngomalacia 3. Laryngospasm 4. Bilateral vocal cord palsy/dysfunction 5. Primary laryngeal carcinoma
	Trachea	1. Tracheal stenosis (post intubation/tracheostomy, irradiation, post tuberculous stenosis, granulomatosis with polyangiitis, relapsing polychondritis). 2. Endotracheal tumors (primary and metastatic tracheal malignancies, tracheal amyloidosis, benign tracheal tumors like papillomatosis, hamartoma). 3. Extrinsic tracheal compression by mediastinal tumors and enlarged lymph nodes, thyroid tumors and goitre 4. Tracheomalacia

To understand the cause of stridor and plan accordingly, we propose using the questions checklist given below.

1. Is the index case an adult or a child? (Children are more likely to have a foreign body aspiration/infective cause of stridor).
2. Is there fever? (If yes, consider infectious causes of stridor: Laryngitis, tracheitis, croup).
3. Is there a witnessed episode of choke? (If yes, a foreign body aspiration should be the first possibility).
4. Are there signs of allergy? (If yes consider angio-edema of the upper airways).
5. Is there any history of trauma? (If yes, a possibility of edema/blood clot or tracheal/laryngeal injury should be considered).
6. Is it acute in onset, or slowly progressive in onset? (If acute in onset, consider infections, allergy/anaphylaxis, foreign body aspiration or airway trauma as the possible causes).
7. Is the stridor present at rest or only on exertion? (When stridor is heard at rest, the airway lumen is usually < 6 mm in diameter and is a medical emergency. If stridor is not present at rest but heard only on exertion, the airway lumen in usually between 6 and 8 mm in diameter).
8. Is the patient using accessory muscles of respiration? (If yes, then it may be a sign of impending respiratory arrest and intervention needs to be done as soon as possible).

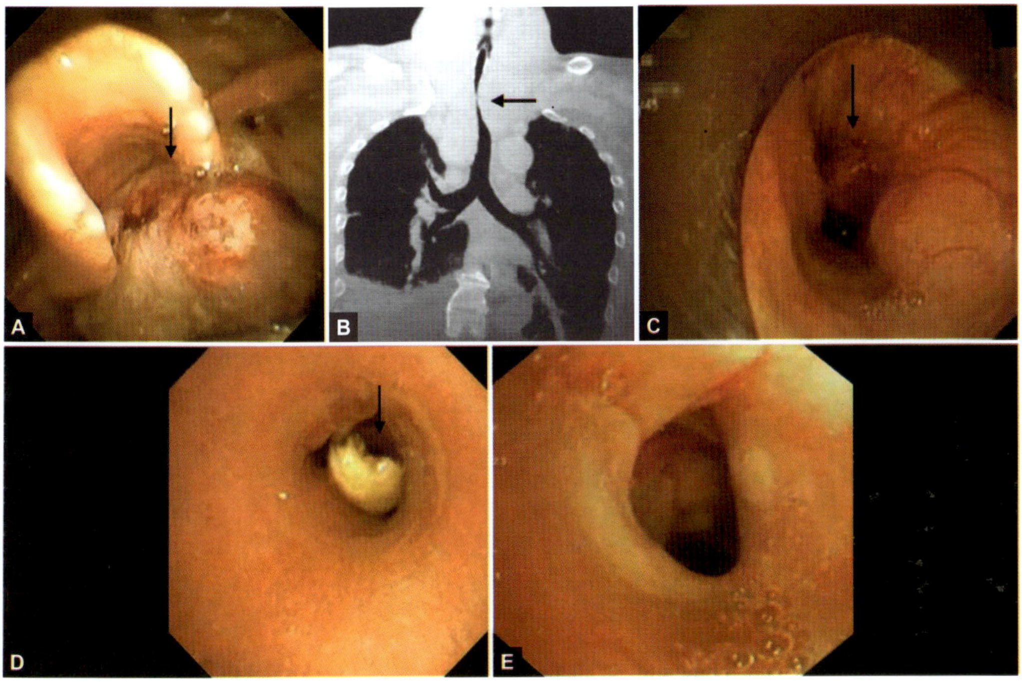

Fig. 6.2: Causes of stridor. (A) A case of laryngeal carcinoma presented with stridor. Tumor (arrow) completely occludes the laryngeal inlet. (B) A 65 years old man presented with stridor and severe hypoxia. HRCT chest coronal view reveals a large goitre with retrosternal extension, compressing the trachea causing near total occlusion of the lumen. (C) Bronchoscopic view of the tracheal tumor causing near total occlusion of the lumen. (D) Bronchoscopic view of the foreign body (peanut). (E) Bronchoscopic view of the tracheal stenosis occluding the tracheal lumen.

Stridor in patients presents a clinical urgency, mandating a prompt and systematic evaluation via an A–E assessment (Airway, Breathing, Circulation, Disability assessment and Exposure) protocol. Initially, the airway assessment should include checking for cyanosis and signs of angioedema. Additionally, the presence of drooling, often linked with epiglottitis, and asymmetrical neck swelling, suggestive of a deep neck space infection, should be meticulously evaluated. The examination should also encompass checking for neck pain or tenderness upon palpation, palpable neck swellings, restricted neck movements, and trismus. Subsequent to the airway evaluation, a comprehensive examination of the patient's breathing is crucial, focusing on the respiratory rate, oxygen saturation levels, respiratory effort, and bilateral air entry. Circulatory assessment involves monitoring the patient's pulse and blood pressure, crucial for evaluating systemic circulation. The disability component entails a thorough mental status examination to discern the extent of hypoxia and hypercapnia. The final aspect, exposure, necessitates a complete physical examination of the patient, with a focus on identifying signs of anaphylaxis, such as an urticarial rash or additional manifestations of angioedema.

Laboratory Investigations

Generally, blood investigations are not essential to diagnose stridor. Arterial blood gas analysis will be useful in patients with respiratory failure. Patients planned for interventions must be investigated with complete blood count, blood urea, serum creatinine, viral markers and for coagulation abnormalities.

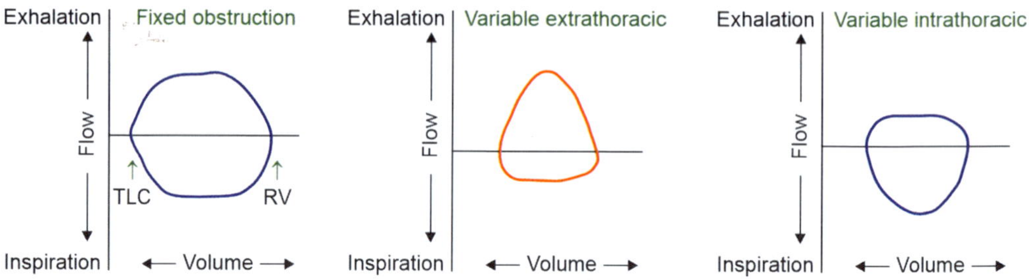

Fig. 6.3: Patterns of flow volume loop (spirometry)in patients with larger airway obstruction. The typical plateau effect on inspiratory and expiratory flow depending on the anatomical level of obstruction is shown.

1. **Imaging studies:** Anteroposterior (AP) and lateral radiographs of the neck and chest are useful for evaluating the airway and lungs. Computed tomography of thorax shows the same lesions as chest radiography, but with better accuracy and better assessment of their nature, origin, shape, vascularisation and relationship with the contiguous structures.
2. **Pulmonary function test (spirometry):** Pulmonary function tests are not possible in acutely ill patients. However, if the patient presents with a chronic or recurrent stridor and dyspnea, the presence of a flattening on either or both of the inspiratory or expiratory flow volume curves is a clue orientating the clinician towards a tracheal obstruction (Fig. 6.3).
3. **Laryngoscopy/bronchoscopy:** Direct visualization of the airway by direct video-laryngoscopy or video-bronchoscopy is the investigation of choice. After radiologic assessment, it should be performed in all cases with stridor. However, the patient's hypoxia must be stabilised and acute epiglottitis must be ruled out before laryngoscopy, as it may worsen the clinical condition in patients with acute epiglottitis/croup.

E. Management of the Cause of Stridor

Initial management of an acutely ill patient: When the patient is in respiratory distress/failure, he/she needs to be stabilised. Supplemental oxygen (in hypoxic patients) in sitting upright position, followed by nebulized short acting beta 2 agonists or nebulised adrenaline and intravenous steroids may be administered. Broad spectrum antibiotics are to be started in suspected infectious etiology. For patients not responding to the initial treatment, an emergency tracheostomy (for laryngeal and subglottic lesions) or rigid bronchoscopic intervention (for tracheal lesions) should be considered. Emergency endotracheal intubation (using a smaller diameter ET tube) by an experienced intensivist with or without bronchoscopy guidance may be an alternative in situations where access to emergency tracheostomy or rigid bronchoscopy is not available to tide over the crisis. Subsequently patient has to be referred to appropriate ENT or interventional pulmonary expert for further management.

Definitive treatment: After stabilising the patient, subsequent definitive treatment (medical management/interventional pulmonology procedure/surgery) depends on the etiology (Table 6.3). When the cause of stridor is infection/anaphylaxis/edema of the airways, medical management will relieve the stridor.

Therapeutic interventional pulmonology procedures will relieve the obstruction and are curative in cases of foreign body aspiration (removal of the foreign body using rigid forceps, cryoprobe, basket or a fogarty balloon), simple tracheal stenosis (one to three sessions of

Table 6.3: Etiology based management of stridor

Cause of stridor	Immediate management	Investigations	Definitive treatment
Foreign body aspiration	Heimlich manoeuvre ± Intubation or tracheotomy/cricothyrotomy (if life threatening)	Chest X-ray, CT scan of thorax and neck	Bronchoscopy and retrieval of the foreign body
Anaphylaxis, laryngeal edema	Intramuscular adrenaline injection, intubation/ tracheostomy/cricothyrotomy	None	Intravenous fluids, systemic corticosteroids, nebulized steroids and bronchodilators. Find out the offending agent and avoid exposure
Acute epiglottitis	Keep in head up position only, No tongue-blade examination ± Intubation or tracheotomy/ cricothyrotomy, empiric antibiotics	Neck soft tissue x-ray/CT neck: thumb sign	Appropriate intravenous antibiotics
Other infections: croup, tracheitis	Oxygen support, nebulised adrenaline, intravenous steroids	Imaging, microbiological diagnosis	Appropriate intravenous antibiotics
Benign tracheal stenosis	Bronchoscopic dilatation, debulking of the granulation/ tracheostomy	CT scan of the chest/neck	Simple stenosis requires tracheal dilation and follow up. In complex stenosis, recurrence is common and needs surgical resection or tracheal silicon stenting (where surgery is not feasible)
Glottic and laryngeal neoplasms	Tracheostomy	CT scan of the Neck	Biopsy and tissue diagnosis followed by definitive surgical resection or palliative chemoradiation in advanced disease
Tracheal tumors	• Purely endoluminal: bronchoscopic intervention/ resection • Purely extrinsic compression: Endoluminal stenting • Mixed: Bronchoscopic intervention ± stenting	CT scan of the chest/ neck	• Definitive treatment based on histopathology • Treatment of the compressing tumor by surgical resection or radiation • Surgical resection/ chemoradiation

tracheal dilation), and benign purely endoluminal tracheal tumors (resection and removal of the tumours). In other scenarios, interventional pulmonology procedures are performed with a palliative intent. Advanced malignancies of the airways/mediastinum can be managed with palliative dilatation and tracheal/tracheobronchial stenting. The initial diagnostic bronchoscopy itself may be escalated to a therapeutic one in the same sitting (as in the index case), or a therapeutic procedure can be planned and performed at a later date (depending on the clinical condition of the patient).

Surgical procedures are curative in certain instances. Localised abscesses (peritonsillar, retropharyngeal or parapharyngeal) in the neck region require surgical incision and drainage along with appropriate antibiotics. Complex tracheal stenosis and localised neoplastic lesions of trachea should be managed by complete resection with appropriate margins and re-anastomosis of trachea. An algorithm to manage the stridor shown here (Fig. 6.4).

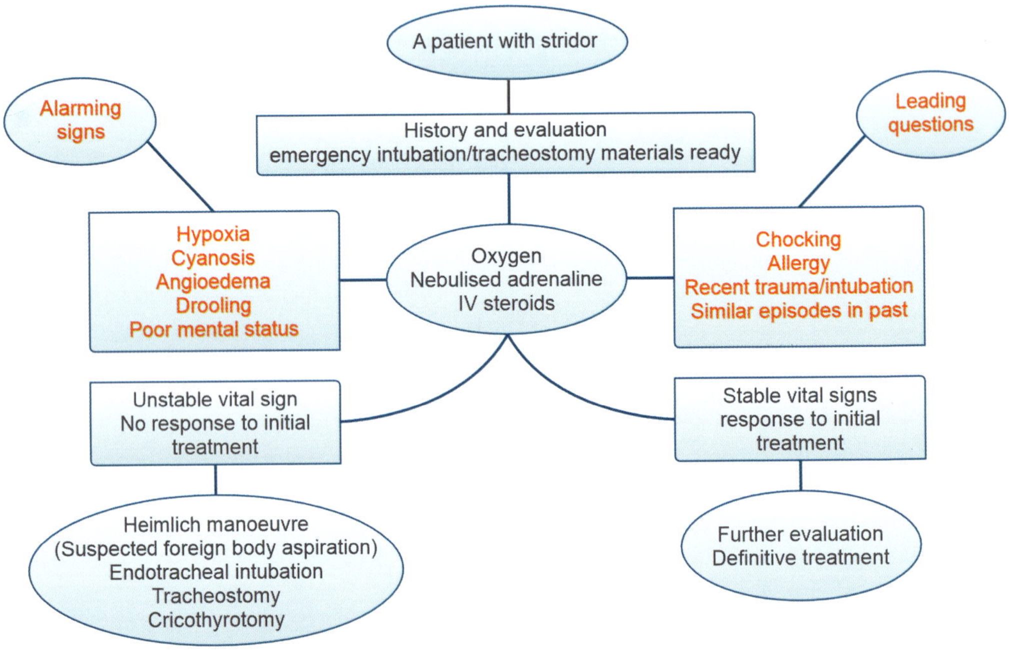

Fig. 6.4: Algorithm for management of stridor.

FURTHER READING

1. Eskander A, De Almeida JR, Irish JC. Acute upper airway obstruction. N Engl J Med 2019; 381: 1940–1949.
2. Ernst A, Feller-Kopman D, Becker HD, et al. Central airway obstruction. Am J Respir Crit Care Med 2004; 169: 1278–1297.
3. Marchese A, Langhan ML. Management of airway obstruction and stridor in pediatric patients. Pediatr Emerg Med Pract. 2017 Nov;14(11):1–24.
4. J. Lynch and S.M. Crawley. Management of airway obstruction. BJA Education, 18(2): 46e51 (2018).
5. Natali D, Le H, Nguyen Ngoc C, et al. A 62-year-old man with stridor and dyspnoea. Breathe 2021; 17: 200201.

Chapter

7

Approach to a Case of Difficult to Treat Asthma

• Vikas Marwah • Kunal Kumar

LEARNING POINTS

1. Difficult to treat asthma is not the same as severe asthma.
2. Always confirm the diagnosis of bronchial asthma objectively in a patient with uncontrolled asthma.
3. A step wise approach focussing on confirming the diagnosis, checking inhaler technique and adherence, identifying and treating comorbidities, identifying and removing potential triggers will help in achieving good symptom control in most cases of difficult to treat asthma.

INTRODUCTION

Chevalier Jackson first recognized that "All that wheezes is not asthma". Other processes that narrow the diameter of an airway like chronic obstructive pulmonary disease, endobronchial or tracheal stenosis, endobronchial tumors, and upper airway obstruction may also present with wheezing. Such patients may be misdiagnosed and treated as having difficult or severe asthma. Herein, we present a case of Hodgkin's lymphoma in a young male who had an initial erroneous diagnosis of bronchial asthma.

CASE VIGNETTE

A 17-year-old young male presented with complaints of gradually progressive exertional shortness of breath, cough, and wheezing of one-month duration. The patient had reduced exercise tolerance (100 meters of slow-paced running) and breathlessness with wheezing triggered by exertional activities like running. His symptoms used to be relieved with rest. He also gave a history of allergic triggers to dust and strong smells. He denied any history of diurnal variation, fever, weight loss, or chest pain. He was initially evaluated by a primary physician who started him on inhaled corticosteroids with long-acting bronchodilators. After two weeks, he was reassessed again, and since he had a sub-optimal response, his treatment was escalated to GINA step 5 which consisted of high-dose inhaled corticosteroids, long-acting β_2 agonists, muscarinic antagonists, and montelukast. He also had received a short course of oral corticosteroids twice in the last month. Since the patient did not achieve the desired level of symptomatic relief, he reported to us for further management.

Table 7.1: Relevant laboratory investigations in the index case

Sl.No.	Parameters (unit)	Index	Reference limits
1.	Haemoglobin (gm/dL)	14.9	12–15.5
2.	White blood cells (× $10^3/\mu L$)	11.1	4–11
3.	Absolute eosinophil count(/cc)	650	<500
4.	Platelets (× $10^3/\mu L$)	404	150–450
5.	Protein (gm/dL)	6.8	5.2–8.5
6.	Albumin (gm/dL)	3.3	3.5–5.5
7.	Albumin: Globulin ratio	0.94	0.8–2.2
8.	Bilirubin (mg/dL)	0.3	0.2–1.0
9.	Creatinine (mg/dL)	1.0	0.6–1.2
10.	Random blood glucose (mg/dL)	109	<200
11.	Erythrocyte sedimentation rate (mm/hr)	08	0–20
12.	Serum lactate dehydrogenase (U/L)	170	225–450
13.	Bronchial wash for MTB GeneXpert	MTB not detected,	
14.	Mantoux test	03 mm × 03 mm induration	<10 mm

On examination, he had a body mass index of 19.5 kg/m^2 and had normal oxygen saturation levels on room air. Chest auscultation revealed bilateral monophonic wheeze equally heard in both phases of respiration. The wheezing was more prominent on the right side of the chest and decreased in intensity towards the infra-axillary region.

He had leukocytosis with raised absolute eosinophil count (Table 7.1). Spirometry showed features of severe obstruction without significant reversibility (FEV1:0.81L, 24.6%). Spirometry also showed flattening of the expiratory limb which raised a suspicion of alternate obstructive pathology. Chest radiograph had widened right paratracheal stripe (Fig. 7.1) and contrast-enhanced computed tomography (CT) of the chest showed a conglomerate of enlarged lymph nodes in prevascular, pretracheal, paratracheal, aortopulmonary window, and subcarinal region with post-contrast enhancement (HU-40 HU). Lymph nodes in the paratracheal region were causing compression and luminal compromise of the trachea (Fig. 7.2A). A positron emission tomography (PET)-CT whole body was suggestive of extensive mediastinal lymphadenopathy and luminal compromise of the trachea (Fig. 7.2B).

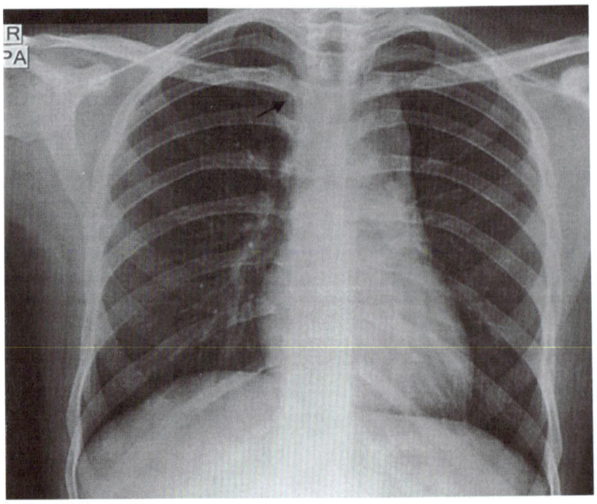

Fig. 7.1: Widened right paratracheal stripe (arrow) seen on the chest X-ray.

This patient most likely had an incorrect diagnosis of severe asthma. The differential diagnosis of mediastinal lymphadenopathy are:

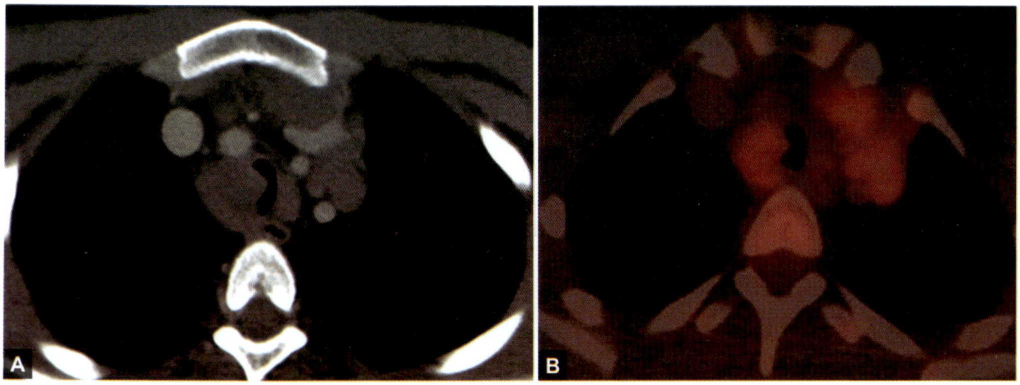

Fig. 7.2: (A) CECT Chest showing mediastinal lymphadenopathy with extrinsic compression and luminal invasion of trachea by the paratracheal lymph nodes. (B) PET CT showing mediastinal lymphadenopathy and luminal compromise of trachea.

1. Lymphoma
2. Tuberculosis
3. Sarcoidosis

The patient underwent flexible fiberoptic bronchoscopy, which revealed a sessile broad whitish mass in the posterior aspect of the middle third of the trachea (Fig. 7.3). Histopathological examination and immunohistochemistry analysis of biopsy specimens of both anterior mediastinal and tracheal mass were consistent with classical Hodgkin's lymphoma. He was started on chemotherapy with ABVD (adriamycin, bleomycin, vinblastine and dacarbazine) regimen. Follow-up PET CT showed metabolic resolution of mediastinal lymphadenopathy with relief of tracheal compression. Repeat spirometry showed significant improvement in lung function (FEV1-3.36 L, 101.3%). He could now comfortably walk without respiratory distress.

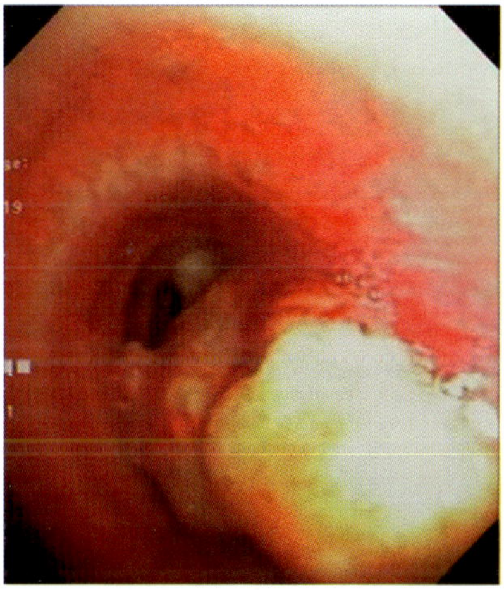

Fig. 7.3: Endotracheal broad based sessile mass visualized on flexible video bronchoscopy.

DISCUSSION

Doctors often use the term "severe asthma" and 'difficult-to-treat asthma" interchangeably. This is a misconception and proper differentiation of these two subsets of patients is essential for patient management. As per GINA 2023, 17% of asthma patients may have difficult-to-treat asthma. Difficult-to-treat asthma is asthma that is uncontrolled despite using medium/high-dose inhaled corticosteroids and a second controller, or maintenance oral corticosteroids, or that requires such high-dose treatment to remain controlled. This difficult to treat asthma may be either due to modifiable factors or because the diagnosis itself is diagnosed incorrectly.

Severe asthma is a subset of difficult-to-treat asthma which remains uncontrolled despite correction of modifiable factors. It is of paramount importance that there is no diagnostic uncertainty when the term severe asthma is used, whereas the same is not true for difficult-to-treat asthma. When a patient presents to the clinic with a label of severe asthma, we propose the five step algorithm to approach.

STEP 1: Confirm the Diagnosis of Asthma

About 12–50% of patients labelled as severe asthma are not actually asthma cases. Whenever a patient is referred with severe asthma, we should first ascertain that the diagnosis is correct. Very often asthma mimics may be erroneously misdiagnosed as asthma due to overlapping clinical features. Respiratory diseases which mimic asthma may be classified based on the location of pathology as extrathoracic upper airway, intrathoracic central airway, intrathoracic lower airway and systemic causes (Fig. 7.4). Patients with chronic obstructive pulmonary disease, cardiac asthma, foreign body in the airway, eosinophilic lung diseases, tracheobronchomalacia, vocal cord dysfunction, and diseases causing airway compression can present with wheezing and are often misdiagnosed and managed as difficult asthma (as in index case).

Objective evidence of asthma (presence of reversible airway obstruction or a positive broncho provocation test) should always be sought. If the initial bronchodilator response on spirometry is inconclusive, we must repeat the test after withholding bronchodilators or try to assess when the patient is acutely symptomatic. This increases the possibility of catching reversible airway obstruction on spirometry. Peak flow charting and broncho-provocation tests are some of the other means to ascertain the diagnosis of asthma. A negative broncho-provocation test in a symptomatic patient almost certainly rules out bronchial asthma though results may be false negative in cases of exercise-induced bronchoconstriction.

Clinical and investigational clues which point to an alternate diagnosis of asthma are mentioned in Table 7.2. Excessive cough and sputum may point toward the presence of bronchiectasis. Presence of stridor may point towards endobronchial/tracheal involvement. Fever, cough, night sweats, and weight loss with wheezing may be seen in endobronchial tuberculosis or lymphoma.

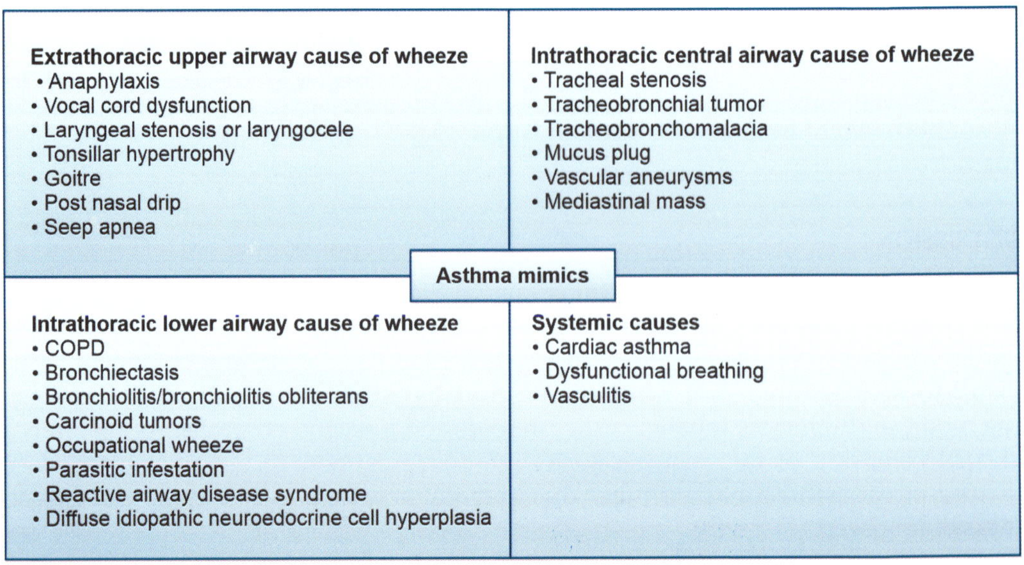

Fig. 7.4: Classification of some of the common asthma mimics.

Table 7.2: Clinical and investigational clues to identifying an asthma mimic		
Sl.No.	***Clinical pointers***	***Comment***
1.	Presence of stridor.	Stridor indicates a critical central airway obstruction.
2.	Presence of monophonic wheeze.	Asthma usually has bilateral polyphonic and an expiratory predominant wheeze. If not, a proximal airway obstruction needs to be considered.
3.	Presence of unilateral wheeze.	
4.	Inspiratory predominant wheeze.	
5.	Lack of response to inhaled bronchodilators or a short course oral corticosteroids.	Most asthmatics responds to inhalers and oral corticosteroids and hence lack of response should raise a suspicion against the diagnosis of asthma.
6.	Lack of variability of symptoms.	Could point towards COPD as the cause of symptoms.
7.	Presence of associated fever, hemoptysis, weight loss or appetite loss.	Endobronchial tuberculosis or an airway malignancy needs to be considered.
8.	Presence of orthopnea or pedal edema.	Should raise the suspicion of a cardiac wheeze.
9.	Presence of copious sputum production.	Raises the possibility of associated bronchiectasis.
10.	Presence of a multi-system involvement.	A possibility of an alternate cause like vasculitis needs to be considered.
	Investigational pointers	
1.	Flattening of one or more limbs of the flow volume loop.	Indicates a central airway obstruction (CAO), not asthma.
2.	Chest radiograph showing a widened mediastinum or narrowed central airway.	A possibility of CAO needs to be considered.
3.	Lack of a positive broncho-provocation test.	A strong pointer against the diagnosis of asthma.
4.	Very high absolute eosinophil count (>1000 cells/mm^3).	Associated diseases like ABPA, EGPA needs to be considered.

ABPA: Allergic bronchopulmonary aspergillosis; *EGPA:* Eosinophilic granulomatosis and polyangiitis.

While interpreting a spirometry, it is important to look at the flow volume loop in addition to the spirometry values. Flow-volume loop on spirometry shows inspiratory flow limitation in cases of extrathoracic central airway obstruction (paradoxical vocal cord dysfunction) whereas in the case of intrathoracic central airway obstruction (tumors, etc.) expiratory flow limitation can be seen. Severe eosinophilia and raised immunoglobulin E(Ig E) levels may point toward eosinophilic lung diseases. Computed tomography of the chest can help in the identification of bronchiectasis, emphysema, tumors, mediastinal lymphadenopathy, and postobstructive pneumonia. Two-dimensional echocardiography and serum N terminal pro B natriuretic peptide (NT pro BNP) levels can be done in an elderly patient with wheezing and features of cardiac dysfunction. Bronchoscopic visualization helps in identifying endobronchial abnormalities and lesions which can mimic asthma (endobronchial tuberculosis, bronchial stenosis or airway tumors).

STEP 2: Check for Inhaler Technique and Adherence

Once we have ruled out asthma mimics and ascertained the diagnosis of asthma we must investigate for modifiable factors. Incorrect inhaler technique is the most common modifiable cause of uncontrolled asthma seen in as high as 80% of the population. Symptomatic relief after regular use of inhalers may prompt patients to skip inhalers and this suboptimal adherence may eventually lead to uncontrolled asthma. Objective measurement of adherence like checking the dose counter on an inhaler device or a mobile application-based survey of dose intake may assist in ensuring adherence. High levels of the fraction of exhaled nitric oxide (FeNO) test despite the patient being on a high dose of inhaled corticosteroids also is a marker of poor adherence. Unintentional barriers to adherence like forgetfulness can be overcome more easily by the patient in comparison to deliberate decisions on the part of the patient to skip drug intake. Intentional non-adherence can be because of socioeconomic factors, secondary gain, or denial of the disease.

STEP 3: Screen for Asthma Comorbidities and Asthma Associated Diseases

Comorbid conditions like gastroesophageal reflux disease, allergic rhino-sinusitis, obesity, obstructive sleep apnea, anxiety and depression can co-exist with asthma and when undiagnosed and untreated lead to poor control of asthma. It is important to screen for the above associations by appropriate history, clinical questionnaires, and when in doubt perform relevant investigations (upper airway examination, CT of nose and paranasal sinuses, upper gastrointestinal endoscopy, 24-hour pH impedance monitoring, overnight polysomnography) to confirm.

Anxiety, depression, and social stress not only cause poor control but are a negative influence on quality of life. The relationship between asthma and gastroesophageal reflux disease (GERD) is bidirectional. Uncontrolled GERD negatively impacts asthma control while medications for asthma can themselves worsen GERD. When we are assessing a patient with uncontrolled asthma, we must look for these modifiable factors before considering dose escalation. Polysomnography should always be done in an uncontrolled asthma patient with clinical features suggestive of sleep apnea.

All patients with uncontrolled asthma need to be screened for the presence of allergic bronchopulmonary aspergillosis by *Aspergillus fumigatus* specific IgE levels. When elevated (>0/35 kUA/L) other investigations (serum total IgE levels, absolute eosinophil count, *A. fumigatus* specific Ig G levels, HRCT chest) need to be performed to confirm the diagnosis of ABPA. When identified, treatment of ABPA will often leads to improvement in asthma control. Other disease which can coexist and worsen asthma control is eosinophilic granulomatosis with polyangitis. When in doubt (clinical history, multiorgan involvement, very high eosinophil counts) serum anti-neutrophil cytoplasmic antibody (ANCA) should be performed.

STEP 4: Identify Asthma Triggers in Home and Work Environments

A thorough history of possible asthma triggers in the home as well as the workplace environment is essential. Attempts should be made to avoid exposure to all potential triggers as ongoing exposure leads to poor asthma control. Concomitant smoking, exposure to certain drugs (non-steroidal anti-inflammatory drugs, non-selective beta blockers) and exposure to aeroallergens often contribute to poor asthma control. A significant proportion of patients have sensitization to indoor allergens such as house dust mites, moulds, and animal dander. Very often a lifestyle modification to avoid undue exposure to these aeroallergens may improve asthma control.

STEP 5: Phenotype the Case of Severe Asthma

If asthma remains uncontrolled despite a certain diagnosis of asthma, optimal and regular use of correct dose inhalers, management of asthma comorbidities, and avoidance of asthma triggers we may label the patient as having severe asthma. Such patients contribute to about 3% of the total asthmatic population. Once labelled as severe asthma, the next step is to phenotype asthma. Asthma can be classified into four phenotypes–T2 high allergic, T2 high eosinophilic, T2 high overlap and T2 low asthma. The ways to phenotype asthma are beyond the scope of this chapter. Once phenotyped, the optimal additional therapeutic strategy (biologics, macrolides, bronchial thermoplasty) needs to be determined.

Severe asthma is essentially a subset of difficult-to-treat asthma. Severe asthma not only affects daily quality of life but also enhances the burden on the overall healthcare system. Proposed management algorithm for uncontrolled asthma is given in Fig. 7.5.

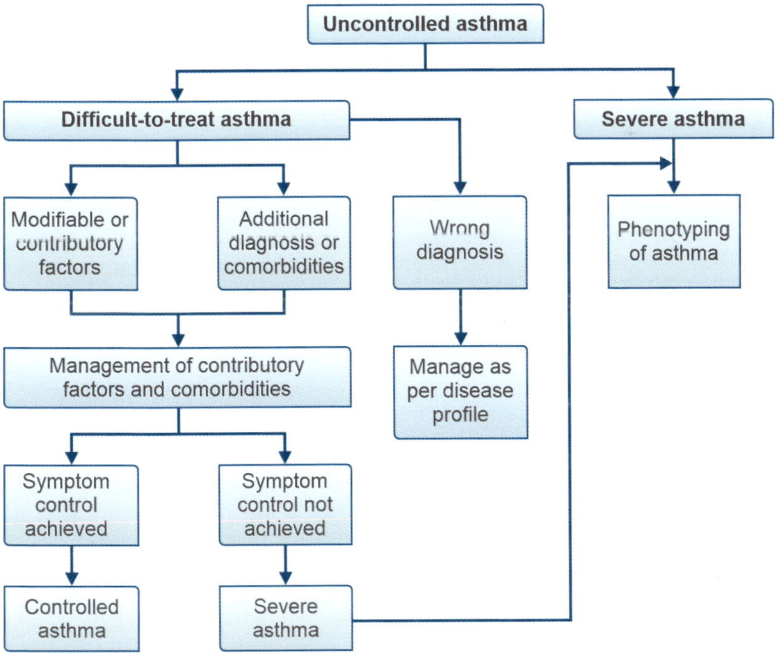

Fig. 7.5: Proposed management algorithm for uncontrolled asthma.

FURTHER READING

1. Global Initiative for Asthma. Global Strategy for Asthma Management and Prevention, 2023. https://ginasthma.org/2023-gina-main-report/.

2. BTS/SIGN guidelines for management of asthma, 2019. www.brit-thoracic.org.uk/quality improvement/guidelines/asthma/.

3. Khurana S, Jarjour NN. Systematic Approach to Asthma of Varying Severity. Clin Chest Med. 2019 Mar;40(1):59–70.

4. Mansur AH, Prasad N. Management of difficult-to-treat asthma in adolescence and young adults. Breathe. 2023 Mar;19(1):220025.

5. Chou EY, Pelz BJ, Chiu AM, Soung PJ. All that Wheezes is not Asthma or Bronchiolitis. Crit Care Clin. 2022 Apr 1;38(2):213–29.

Chapter

8

Approach to a Case with Localized Bronchiectasis

• *Rakesh Kodati* • *Narendra Kumar Narahari*

LEARNING POINTS

1. For patients presenting with focal/ localised bronchiectasis, an early bronchoscopic examination is recommended to rule out any obstructing lesions, particularly when other causes are not apparent.
2. Aspiration events can often be overlooked, leading to a delay in the clinical presentation and development of bronchiectasis.
3. Surgical resection of the affected bronchiectatic segment or lobe should be considered in cases where the disease is refractory, characterized by frequent exacerbations or recurrent hemoptysis, and does not respond to optimal medical therapy.

INTRODUCTION

Localised/focal bronchiectasis (BXSIS) secondary to a proximal airway obstruction is an uncommon cause of bronchiectasis. In this report, we present a case of focal BXSIS characterized by recurrent respiratory tract infections, attributable to a foreign body aspirated in childhood. Additionally, we delineate a comprehensive list of causes and describe our systematic approach to diagnosing and managing a case of focal BXSIS.

CASE VIGNETTE

An 18-year-old male patient was evaluated for a preoperative assessment prior to undergoing lung resection surgery. He had been asymptomatic until the age of 5, after which he started experiencing annual episodes of cough, each marked by purulent expectoration and fever. These episodes, typically lasting one to two weeks, were managed with oral antibiotics.

He denied any history of hemoptysis, ear or sinus infections, or foreign body aspiration. No similar familial medical history was reported. Initially diagnosed with bronchiectasis by a local physician, he frequently required oral antibiotics due to recurrent infections.

Physical examination revealed a thin physique and grade two pan digital clubbing. Vital signs included a pulse rate of 82 beats per minute, a respiratory rate of 20 breaths

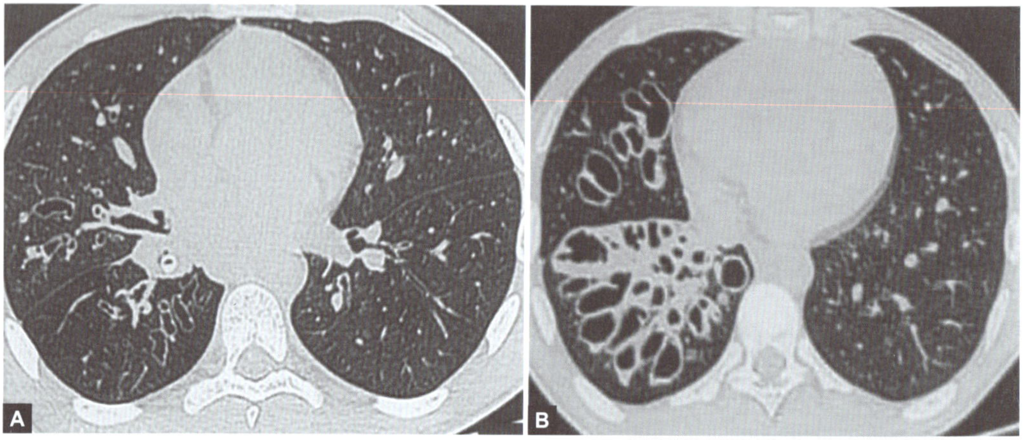

Fig. 8.1: High resolution computed tomographic scan (HRCT) of thorax showing (A) Bronchiectasis in the segments of right middle and the lower lobe along with radiopaque foreign body within the lumen of the right lower lobe bronchus; (B) Bronchiectasis localised to the right lower and middle lobes.

per minute, and an oxygen saturation of 96% on room air. Auscultation identified coarse inspiratory crackles in the right infra-scapular and infra-axillary regions. The cardiovascular examination was unremarkable. A high-resolution computed tomographic (HRCT) scan of the chest demonstrated cystic bronchiectasis predominantly affecting the right middle and lower lobes. Notably, a radiolucent opacity was detected intraluminally in the right lower lobe bronchus (as shown in Fig. 8.1A and B).

Laboratory investigations, including complete blood count and serum creatinine, were within normal limits. His serum IgE and *Aspergillus fumigatus*-specific IgE levels were also normal, along with standard immunoglobulin levels. Flexible bronchoscopy was performed, revealing a stricture with partial luminal occlusion in the right bronchus intermedius (RBI). Additionally, a foreign body was identified in the posterior basal segment of the right lower lobe (RLL). Using rat-tooth alligator forceps, this foreign body was successfully extracted and identified as a rubber cap from a child's whistle toy (as depicted in Fig. 8.2). Bronchoalveolar lavage samples were analysed for tuberculosis, fungal infections, and non-tuberculous mycobacteria (NTM), with all results returning negative.

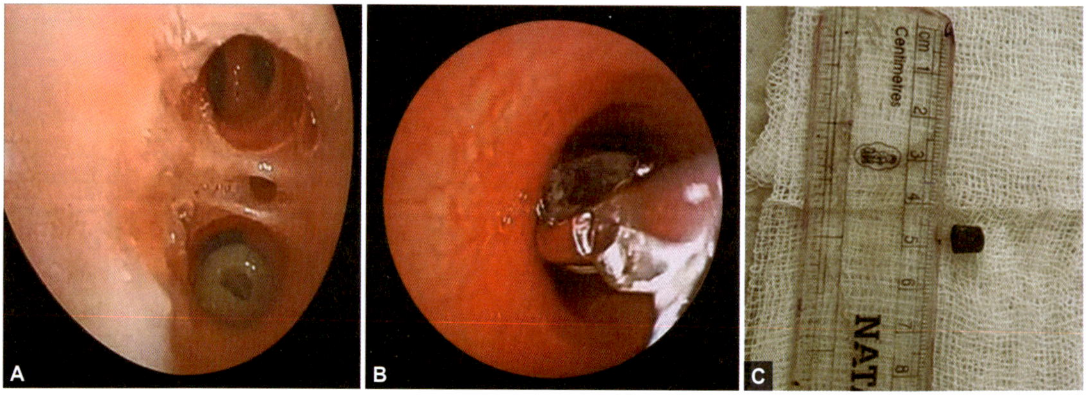

Fig. 8.2: (A) Flexible bronchoscopy showing foreign body in posterior segment of RLL; (B) Removal of foreign body using rat tooth forceps; (C) Foreign body (0.6 × 0.5 cm rubber part of the whistle toy).

Consequently, a diagnosis of post-obstructive bronchiectasis affecting the right middle and lower lobes was established. It is hypothesized that the foreign body initially obstructed the RBI, contributing to the development of bronchiectasis in the two lobes, before eventually becoming dislodged into the segments of the RLL. Given that the patient's exacerbations were not severe, surgical resection was deferred. Airway clearance techniques and postural drainage were advised. At a three-month follow-up, the patient demonstrated symptomatic improvement.

DISCUSSION

Bronchiectasis is typified by a syndrome of productive cough and recurrent respiratory infections, stemming from the permanent dilation of the bronchi. This condition signifies the end stage of various disorders, some of which necessitate specific treatments. Therefore, promptly identifying the underlying etiology is crucial.

The initial step in the diagnostic evaluation of bronchiectasis involves categorizing the disease as either being localized or diffuse. Bronchiectasis is considered to be localized if it is limited to segments of one/two ipsilateral lobes of the lung. Localized BXSIS typically results from an isolated incident, such as intraluminal airway obstruction due to a foreign body or tumor, necrotizing pneumonia, or tuberculosis. An exhaustive list of causes and a systematic approach to managing localized bronchiectasis are detailed in Table 8.1 and illustrated in Fig. 8.3. A brief description of the causes of focal bronchiectasis is provided below.

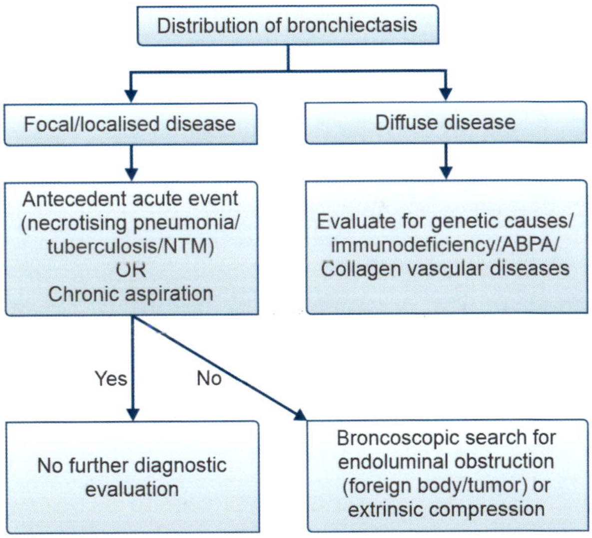

Fig. 8.3: Approach to a case of bronchiectasis.

A. Foreign Body Aspiration

Foreign body (FB) obstruction is a relatively rare cause of BXSIS and is frequently overlooked in cases of localised disease. FB aspiration is more prevalent in children, particularly those under the age of 3 years. Such incidents can occur during choking episodes while eating, in the event of

Table 8.1: Causes of localized bronchiectasis

Category	*Causes*
A. Proximal bronchial obstruction	1. Endoluminal obstruction (neoplasms, foreign body, broncholith) 2. Stenosis of the bronchus 3. Extrinsic compression (lymph nodes, tumors)
B. Sequel of a localized Infection	1. Tuberculosis 2. Necrotizing bacterial pneumonia 3. Non-tuberculous mycobacterial infection
C. Chronic aspiration	
E. Intra-lobar sequestration	

trauma, or due to loss of consciousness. Often, the history of such aspiration incidents is not recognized, and in some cases, the obstructive material, such as peanuts or vegetables, may not be detectable through radiographic studies. Therefore, a thorough patient history and a high degree of clinical suspicion are vital for the timely identification of foreign body-induced bronchiectasis.

In pediatric cases, foreign body (FB) obstruction typically involves a mainstem bronchus, whereas in adults, foreign bodies are more likely to be lodged distally. This difference is attributed to anatomical variations. The right main bronchus is wider and more vertically oriented compared to the left, thereby presenting as the path of least resistance for aspirated materials in adults. However, in children, the main bronchi on both sides are of equal size and have similar angulation. As a result, foreign bodies in children are found with equal frequency in both the left and right main bronchi.

B. Proximal Airway Obstruction (Tumors)

Slow growing tumors, both benign and malignant, can lead to airway obstruction, impaired secretion drainage, recurrent or chronic infections, and consequently, BXSIS. The more frequently encountered tumor types include benign slow growing tumors such as carcinoid tumors and papillomas. Additionally, extrinsic airway compression is often caused by hypertrophic lymphadenitis, typically associated with granulomatous diseases such as sarcoidosis or tuberculosis.

C. Post Infectious Bronchiectasis

In developing countries, post-infective causes, particularly previous tuberculosis, are the most prevalent etiological factors for BXSIS. The pathogenesis is largely attributed to the destruction of the bronchial walls' elastic and muscular components, coupled with traction from parenchymal fibrosis. Non-tuberculous mycobacterial (NTM) infections can either be opportunistic in patients with existing BXSIS or a primary cause of the condition. NTM-associated BXSIS typically localizes to the right middle lobe and the lingular segment of the left upper lobe. Additionally, recurrent aspiration, often due to dysphagia or gastro-oesophageal reflux, is recognized as a cause of BXSIS, usually localizing to the lower lobes.

D. Intra-lobar Sequestration

Intra-lobar sequestration often leads to recurrent respiratory infections in the affected lobe and this can lead to development of a localized bronchiectasis in the affected lobe. It more often affects the lower lobes, and is often diagnosed in young adults or adolescents. It is diagnosed by identifying an aberrant systemic arterial supply from the descending thoracic/abdominal aorta. It is always recommended to perform a thoracic angiogram in cases of lower lobe localized bronchiectasis to identify sequestration. The treatment of choice for sequestration is surgical resection.

Current evidence does not conclusively demonstrate the superiority of surgical intervention over conservative management in bronchiectasis (BXSIS). Indications for considering surgical resection in localized bronchiectasis include:

1. Uncontrolled symptoms despite optimal medical treatment.
2. Severe or frequent exacerbations that significantly disrupt social or professional activities, and
3. Recurrent refractory or massive hemoptysis.
4. Sequestration

FURTHER READING

1. Hill AT, Sullivan AL, Chalmers JD, De Soyza A, Elborn SJ, Floto AR, et al. British Thoracic Society Guideline for bronchiectasis in adults. Thorax. 2019;74(Suppl 1):1–69.

2. Chan ED, Wooten WI, Hsieh EWY, Johnston KL, Shaffer M, Sandhaus RA, et al. Diagnostic evaluation of bronchiectasis. Respiratory Medicine: X. 2019;1:100006.

3. Polverino E, Goeminne PC, McDonnell MJ, Aliberti S, Marshall SE, Loebinger MR, et al. European Respiratory Society guidelines for the management of adult bronchiectasis. Eur Respir J. 2017;50(3).

Chapter 9

Approach to a Case with Bilateral Bronchiectasis

• Rajesh Venkat • Melcy Cleetus • Hasha Thankam Somson

LEARNING POINTS

1. Bronchiectasis (BE) has varied causes, with bilateral multilobar bronchiectasis often indicating systemic diseases rather than endobronchial lesions like tumors or foreign body.
2. Major causes of bilateral bronchiectasis include ABPA, connective tissue diseases, immunodeficiency states, cystic fibrosis, and primary ciliary dyskinesias.
3. Targeted history-taking, physical examination, and specific investigations are necessary to identify the etiology of BE.
4. Follow-up and monitoring are essential, as some cases of initially idiopathic bronchiectasis may reveal their etiology over time as the disease evolves.

INTRODUCTION

Bronchiectasis (BE) is a heterogeneous group of disorders characterized by abnormal, permanent dilation and destruction of the airways. This condition manifests with varying degrees of productive cough, hemoptysis, and dyspnea. Determining the etiology of bronchiectasis is crucial for implementing specific treatment strategies, in addition to general supportive measures commonly used for all BE etiologies. The etiologies differ significantly between localized BE, which affects a single lobe or segment, and bilateral generalized BE, which involves multiple areas. Distinguishing between localized and generalized bronchiectasis is therefore vital for guiding the etiological workup and selecting appropriate diagnostic tests. This review outlines the common causes of BE, details the diagnostic approach, and discusses the prevalent causes of bilateral generalized BE, illustrated with a real-life case example.

CASE VIGNETTE

A 26-year-old male with no known allergies or atopic conditions presented with a chronic history of recurrent respiratory infections dating back to childhood. The frequency and severity of these infections have progressively increased. In the past year alone, he experienced five pneumonia episodes, requiring hospitalization and intravenous antibiotics on two occasions. He also reported recurrent upper respiratory tract infections, characterized by rhinitis and sinusitis. Notably, there were no instances of skin or subcutaneous infections, mucocutaneous infections, middle ear infections, or a history of pulmonary tuberculosis. His gastrointestinal and urinary functions were normal. The patient experienced significant weight loss (16 kg over the last two years). He was born to non-consanguineous parents and has no family history of similar medical conditions. Additionally, there is no reported history of addiction, substance abuse, high-risk sexual behavior, or significant childhood infections such as measles, pertussis, or tuberculosis.

Physical examination revealed a malnourished male with a BMI of 15.9 kg/m^2, indicating severe undernutrition. He appeared pale and had grade 3 digital clubbing in all fingers. Aside from these findings, the general examination was unremarkable. Respiratory assessment indicated distress, as evidenced by an elevated respiratory rate of 24 breaths per minute and the use of accessory muscles for breathing. His oxygen saturation was 92% on ambient air. Chest auscultation revealed bilateral coarse, leathery crackles in the lower lung fields. Additionally, he also had features of situs inversus totalis, including dextrocardia and left-sided liver placement. Cardiac examination revealed a right parasternal heave and an accentuated pulmonary component of the second heart sound, suggesting pulmonary hypertension.

Given the patient's clinical presentation and physical findings, a suspicion of bilateral bronchiectasis with secondary infection and situs inversus totalis was considered, with primary ciliary dyskinesia as a likely underlying etiology. A chest radiograph confirmed the presence of dextrocardia and bilateral bronchiectasis (Fig. 9.1A). Further detailed imaging using high-resolution computed tomography (HRCT) of the thorax confirmed bilateral cystic bronchiectasis affecting both the upper and lower lobes, alongside the dextrocardia (Fig. 9.1B and C). Additional tests were conducted to rule out other causes of bilateral bronchiectasis. These included serum total IgE, Aspergillus-specific IgG and IgE, and peripheral blood eosinophil count, all of which were unremarkable and thus excluded allergic bronchopulmonary aspergillosis. The serum immunoglobulin profile was within normal limits, and the sweat chloride level was also normal, ruling out common variable immune deficiency (CVID) and cystic fibrosis (CF).

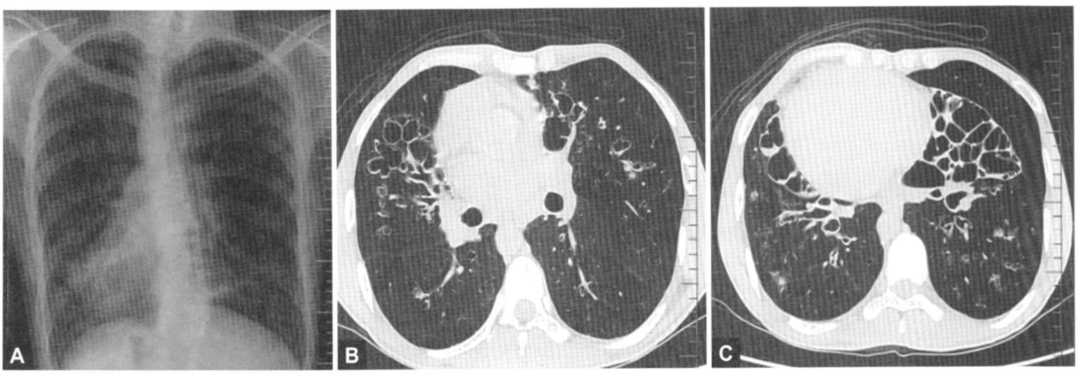

Fig. 9.1: (A) Chest X-ray reveals presence of dextrocardia with bilateral bronchiectasis; (B) HRCT chest reveals cystic bronchiectasis in bilateral upper lobe with dextrocardia; (C) HRCT chest reveals cystic bronchiectasis in bilateral lower lobes with fluid level observed.

Further investigations revealed bilateral sinusitis with mucosal thickening in the maxillary sinuses and narrowed sinus ostia on CT imaging of the paranasal sinuses. A semen analysis indicated oligozoospermia. A two-dimensional echocardiography showed normal left ventricular function and normally functioning valves, and a moderate eccentric tricuspid regurgitation, and moderate pulmonary artery hypertension (PA pressure-36 plus right atrial pressure).

The comprehensive diagnostic process led to a diagnosis of Kartagener's syndrome, characterized by presence of situs inversus totalis, bilateral sinusitis, bilateral cystic bronchiectasis, with secondary respiratory infection, hypoxemia, pulmonary artery hypertension, and protein-energy malnutrition.

For the acute infective episode, the patient was administered systemic antibiotics. Long-term management strategies including airway clearance techniques, pneumococcal and influenza vaccinations, nutritional support, and health education were initiated. The patient continues to receive clinical follow-up for ongoing management of his condition.

DISCUSSION

When to Suspect Bronchiectasis?

Bronchiectasis should be suspected based on clinical presentation. Key symptoms that prompt suspicion include a chronic productive cough, persistent mucopurulent expectoration, and recurrent respiratory infections. Additionally, undiagnosed hemoptysis warrants consideration of bronchiectasis as a differential diagnosis.

It is crucial to acknowledge that many cases of bronchiectasis may not present with these classic symptoms and could be clinically asymptomatic. Other, less prominent manifestations of bronchiectasis may include a cough with scanty phlegm and wheezing. Therefore, a high index of suspicion is necessary, especially in atypical presentations.

Certain patient populations are at an increased risk for developing bronchiectasis. These include individuals with:

- Current or past mycobacterial infections.
- Severe, persistent asthma, particularly with Aspergillus sensitization.
- Chronic obstructive pulmonary disease (COPD) characterized by recurrent exacerbations or chronic expectoration.
- Connective tissue diseases, such as rheumatoid arthritis.
- HIV infection.
- Inflammatory bowel disease.

In patients with these conditions, proactive investigation for bronchiectasis might be warranted, even in the absence of specific bronchiectasis-indicative symptoms. Early identification and management of bronchiectasis in these high-risk groups can be crucial for optimizing outcomes and mitigating disease progression.

Confirming the Diagnosis of Bronchiectasis

In all patients with suspected bronchiectasis, a baseline chest X-ray in an erect patient position, using a posteroanterior projection, is recommended as a minimum initial investigation. However, it is important to note that the sensitivity of chest X-rays in diagnosing bronchiectasis is relatively low. Limitations of chest X-rays include poor localization of lesions, inability to accurately assess the extent and severity of the disease, and limited capacity to suggest an etiology.

Given these limitations, a high-resolution CT scan (HRCT) of the thorax is the diagnostic test of choice for bronchiectasis and should be performed in all suspected cases. HRCT is significantly more sensitive and can provide detailed information about the location, extent, and severity of bronchiectasis, as well as offer insights into possible underlying causes. The optimal scanning protocol is summarized in Table 9.1.

HRCT can reveal both direct and indirect signs of bronchiectasis (Table 9.2). These signs, both direct and indirect, are key indicators for the HRCT based diagnosis of bronchiectasis. Ideally, baseline imaging should be conducted during a period of clinical stability. This approach allows for more effective serial comparisons in future assessments.

Evaluating the Etiology of Bilateral Bronchiectasis

The initial evaluation of bronchiectasis (BE) necessitates a thorough history and a focused physical examination. These steps are instrumental in guiding subsequent targeted testing and in gaining insights into potential etiologies. A detailed exploration of the patient's comorbidities and past medical history is essential, with a focus on identifying diseases that could be causative, such as rheumatoid arthritis, Sjögren's syndrome, asthma, chronic obstructive pulmonary disease (COPD), gastroesophageal reflux disease, and inflammatory bowel disease.

Specific etiologies of bronchiectasis often manifest with associated symptoms, including sinusitis, frequent extrapulmonary infections, and infertility. These associations, particularly

Table 9.1: Scanning CT protocol for bronchiectasis

Parameter	***Value***
Volumetric acquisition	
Tube potential	120–80 kVp: 100 or 80 kVp" to be preferred for small size patients
Tube current	≤240 milliampere (mA):≤100 mAs" or effective mAs"
Slice thickness	≤1.5 millimetres (mm)
Gantry rotation time	As short as possible (e.g. 200–500 ms), always <1 sec
Pitch	1–1.5
Reconstruction algorithm	High spatial frequency
Lung parenchyma windows mean/width	–400 to –700 HU/>1000 HU
Soft tissue windows mean/width	50/350 HU

Table 9.2: Radiologic features of bronchiectasis on a HRCT chest

Category	***Features/Signs***
Direct features of bronchial dilatation	1. Broncho Arterial ratio >1 (internal airway lumen versus adjacent pulmonary artery). 2. Lack of tapering of bronchi. 3. Airway visibility within 1 cm of the costal pleural surface or touching the mediastinal pleura.
Commonly associated indirect signs	1. Bronchial wall thickening. 2. Mucus impaction. 3. Mosaic perfusion/air trapping on expiratory CT. 4. Centrilobular nodules with tree in bud appearance

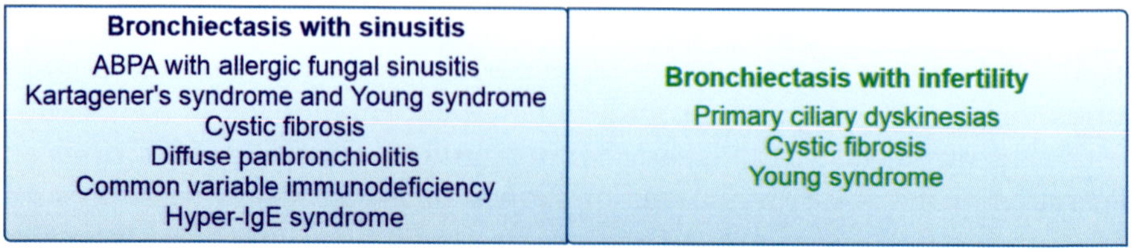

Fig. 9.2: Bronchiectasis with sinusitis and infertility.

the association between bronchiectasis, sinusitis, and infertility (Fig. 9.2), is crucial for narrowing the differential diagnosis.

In all patients diagnosed with bronchiectasis, it is essential to conduct a complete blood count, measure serum total IgE, and assess sensitization to *Aspergillus fumigatus* (either through specific IgE testing or skin prick testing). Routine sputum cultures for bacterial, mycobacterial, and fungal pathogens are recommended for all bronchiectasis patients. Additionally, for those patients whose bronchiectasis etiology remains undiagnosed, a serum immunoglobulin profile is recommended. To detect inborn errors of immunity that are not identifiable via immunoglobulin assays, measuring baseline specific antibody levels against *Streptococcus pneumoniae* capsular polysaccharides can be beneficial. In cases of low pneumococcal antibodies, administering the 23-valent polysaccharide pneumococcal vaccine, followed by re-assessment of specific antibody levels after 4–8 weeks, is advisable.

For patients exhibiting clinical features suggestive of cystic fibrosis (CF) such as a family history of CF, malnutrition, or symptoms originating in childhood–cystic fibrosis testing should be considered. Similarly, testing for primary ciliary dyskinesia (PCD) is advised in patients presenting with clinical features supportive of the diagnosis, including neonatal respiratory distress, childhood onset of symptoms, recurrent otitis media, rhinosinusitis, or infertility.

In patients presenting with concurrent clinical features of arthritis, connective tissue diseases, or systemic vasculitis, tests for rheumatoid factor (RF), anti-cyclic citrullinated peptide (anti-CCP), antinuclear antibodies (ANA), and anti-neutrophil cytoplasmic antibodies (ANCA) are advisable. These tests may also be considered when other diagnostic evaluations yield non-contributory results.

For patients with concurrent basal panacinar emphysema, testing for alpha-1 antitrypsin (A1AT) deficiency is indicated. Assessments for reflux and aspiration should be conducted based on individual clinical judgement. Serum protein electrophoresis is recommended for all bronchiectasis patients with elevated immunoglobulins. Additionally, serological testing for HIV in bronchiectasis patients can be valuable, though this should be tailored based on local HIV prevalence, social factors, and individual risk profiles. Table 9.3 provides a summary of the standard investigations required to determine the etiology of bronchiectasis (BE).

Specific Conditions Associated with Bilateral Bronchiectasis

Some specific conditions associated with BE require special mention as they are more common, require specific diagnostic modalities and have treatment implications. These are discussed in detail below.

Allergic Bronchopulmonary Aspergillosis (ABPA)

Allergic Bronchopulmonary Aspergillosis (ABPA) is an important cause of bronchiectasis in India, primarily resulting from hypersensitivity to *Aspergillus fumigatus*. This condition

Table 9.3: Investigations performed to determine etiology in cases with bilateral bronchiectasis

Investigation	*Indication*	*Expected Result*	*Comment(s)*
HRCT thorax	Investigation of choice for diagnosis of BE	Diagnosis of BE. Also determines the extent, type, and gives specific clues to etiology	Diagnoses Situs inversus, WCS, Mounier-Kuhn syndrome, ABPA, etc.
Tests for ABPA (serum IgE level, Aspergillus specific Ig E and IgG levels, blood eosinophil counts)	All undiagnosed bronchiectasis. All cases of severe asthma	Elevated in ABPA	Prior treatment may alter values
Tests for primary ciliary dyskinesia (nNO, HSVMA, TEM)	BE with situs inversus, onset in childhood, history of neonatal distress syndrome, BE associated with sinusitis or infertility	Depressed level of nNO. Abnormal ciliary structure and beating.	nNO is a good screening test.
Tests for immunodeficiency (CBC, Ig profile, flow cytometry, lymphocyte subset, genetic tests)	Childhood onset, recurrent infections, sinusitis, skin infections, rare infections	Shows specific deficiencies and abnormalities	Interpretation needs thorough knowledge
Tests for cystic fibrosis (sweat chloride estimation, CFTR mutation analysis)	Childhood onset, malnutrition, abdominal symptoms	Elevated sweat chloride, detection of specific mutations	All potential mutations may not be detectable by routine analysis
Other investigations			
Tests for rheumatic/auto-immune diseases (RA, anti-CCP, ANA, ANCAs)	Suspected CTDs based on joint and muscle symptoms, skin lesions	Positivity in significant titres	Needs correlation with clinical criteria for final diagnosis
Alpha 1 antitrypsin levels	Young patient with COPD and BE, lower lobe panacinar emphysema	Low levels clinch the diagnosis	Can guide augmentation therapy
Swallowing evaluation, esophageal pH monitoring	Suspected aspiration syndromes	Direct assessment of aspiration risk	Aspiration as etiology of BE is often a diagnosis of exclusion
Protein electrophoresis	If elevated immunoglobulins	Monoclonal band	Diagnosis of multiple myeloma/MGUS
Colonoscopy	Suspected inflammatory bowel disease	Characteristic lesions on visualization and histopathology	–

ABPA: Allergic bronchopulmonary aspergillosis; *ANA:* Anti-nuclear antibody; *ANCA:* Anti neutrophil cytoplasmic antibody; *BE:* Bronchiectasis; *CBC:* Complete blood count; *CCP:* Cyclic citrullinated peptide; *COPD:* Chronic obstructive pulmonary disease; *CTD:* Connective tissue diseases; *HSVMA:* High speed video electron microscopy; *MGUS:* Monoclonal gammopathy of unknown significance; *nNO:* nasal Nitric Oxide; *RA:* Rheumatoid arthritis; *TEM:* Transmission electron microscopy; *WCS:* William Campbell syndrome.

often complicates the clinical course of patients with asthma and cystic fibrosis. ABPA is characterized by a range of clinical and radiological manifestations, typically including poorly controlled asthma and recurrent/migratory pulmonary infiltrates, which may or may not be accompanied by bronchiectasis. The diagnostic criteria for ABPA have been well-established in the context of asthma and have subsequently been adapted for cystic

Table 9.4: Modified ISHAM-AWG diagnostic criteria for allergic bronchopulmonary aspergillosis (ABPA) diagnosis

Predisposing conditions (One must be present)	• Asthma • Cystic fibrosis • Chronic obstructive lung disease • Bronchiectasis OR • Presence of a compatible clinico-radiological presentation (expectoration of mucus plugs, finger-in-glove and fleeting opacities on chest radiograph, lung collapse, and others)
Essential criteria (both should be present)	• *Aspergillus fumigatus*-IgE ≥0.35 kUA/L • Serum total Ig E ≥500 IU/mL
Other criteria (At least two must be present)	1. Positive IgG against *A. fumigatus* 2. Total eosinophil count >500 cells/microL in glucocorticoid-naïve patients (may be historical). 3. Thin-section chest CT consistent with ABPA (bronchiectasis, mucus plugging, and high-attenuation mucus) or fleeting opacities on chest radiograph consistent with ABPA

IgE: Immunoglobulin E; *ABPA:* Allergic bronchopulmonary aspergillosis

fibrosis. Diagnostic indicators such as transient pulmonary shadows, central bronchiectasis, and high attenuation mucus on CT scans are instrumental in diagnosing and assessing the severity of ABPA.

Furthermore, ABPA is recognized as both a cause and a complicating factor in bronchiectasis. The International Society for Human and Animal Mycology (ISHAM) criteria, illustrated in Table 9.4, provide recommendations for diagnosing ABPA. To diagnose ABPA, the person should have a predisposing condition or compatible clinical presentation. In addition he should demonstrate sensitization to *A. fumigatus* (elevated specific Ig E levels or positive skin test) and should have an elevated serum Ig E level. In addition, they should have any two of the three minor criteria (elevated eosinophil counts (current or in past), the presence of Aspergillus precipitins or IgG, and characteristic radiologic features).

Inborn Errors of Immunity (IEI)

Inborn errors of immunity (IEI) represent a critical aspect of immunodeficiency, with a prevalence of 5% in a comprehensive systematic review of etiological studies. In adults, immune deficiencies are predominantly associated with defects in antibody production. Identifying and treating significant antibody syndromes, such as common variable immune deficiency (CVID), is crucial, as immunoglobulin replacement therapy can markedly reduce exacerbation frequency and enhance clinical outcomes.

Most congenital immunodeficiencies are identified in infancy or childhood, not adulthood, and are often marked by recurrent hospitalizations for serious infections and potential growth retardation due to chronic illness. However, CVID is an exception, occurring in both children and adults, and is characterized by reduced levels of IgG, IgM, or IgA.

The standard diagnostic tests for IEI include a complete blood count (CBC) focusing on lymphopenia (<1500), peripheral smear, immunoglobulin profile, flow cytometry for lymphocyte subset analysis, complement levels, antibody titers to vaccine antigens, and genetic testing. For adults, differentiating primary from secondary immunodeficiencies through appropriate testing is also crucial.

Primary Ciliary Dyskinesias (PCD)

Primary ciliary dyskinesias (PCD) account for 0.9 to 10.3% of bronchiectasis cases in adults, varying with the clinical context. A key screening tool for suspected PCD is the nasal nitric oxide (nNO) measurement test, where PCD patients typically exhibit abnormally low levels. A cutoff value of 30 nL/minute provides a nearly 99% negative predictive value and 76% positive predictive value, making it an effective, office-based screening tool.

Further diagnostic evaluations are recommended at specialized centers focusing on PCD. Nasal brushing, a minimally invasive technique, is used to collect ciliated epithelial samples. These samples are assessed under high-speed video microscopy analysis (HSVMA) to assess ciliary beat frequency and pattern. The normal range for ciliary beat frequency is 11–20 Hz, and qualitative assessment of the beat pattern is also performed. HSVMA has a 100% sensitivity and 93% specificity in diagnosing PCD.

Additionally, transmission electron microscopy (TEM) is utilized to examine ciliary ultrastructure, offering a sensitivity of 79% and a specificity of 100% for PCD diagnosis. Both HSVMA and TEM are highly effective diagnostic tools but necessitate specialised equipment and expertise. Figure 9.3 illustrates a comprehensive algorithm for PCD testing in clinical practice.

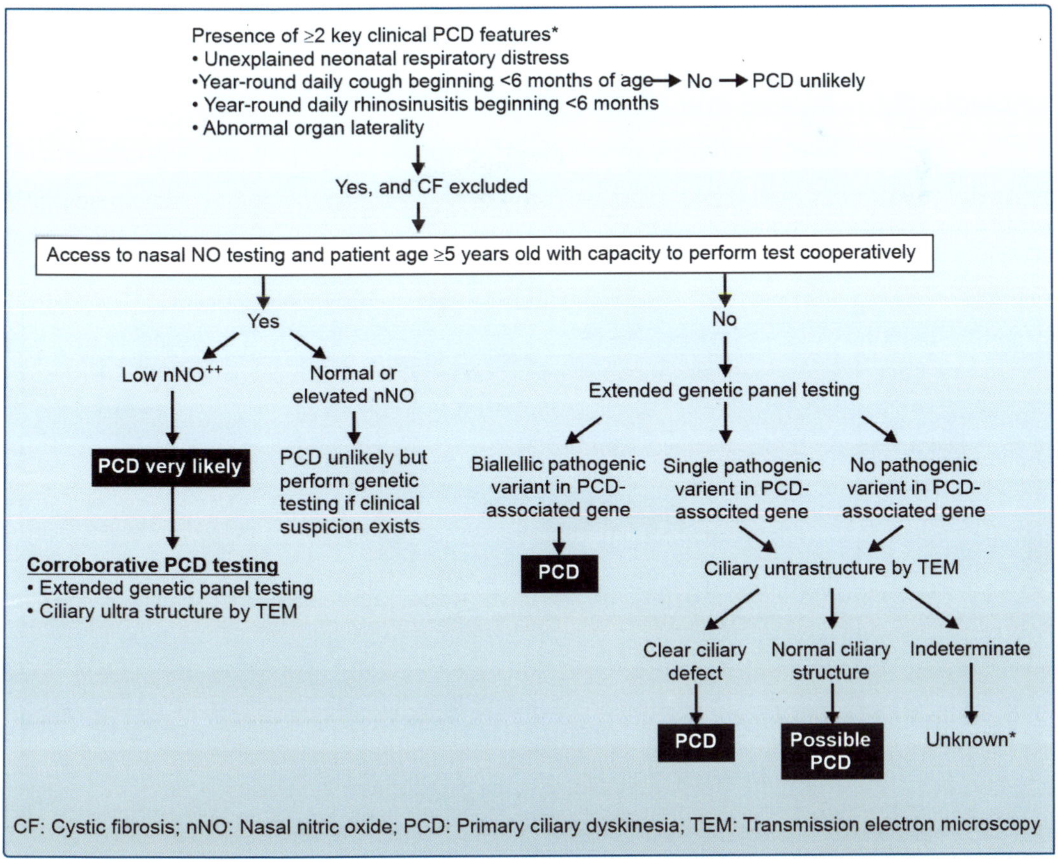

Fig. 9.3: Algorithm for primary ciliary dyskinesia testing (*Adapted from:* Chan ED, et al. Diagnostic evaluation of bronchiectasis. Respiratory Medicine: X. 2019; 1:100006)

Cystic Fibrosis

Cystic fibrosis (CF) accounts for 0.6 to 2.7% of adult bronchiectasis cases, varying by geography. In regions with a high CF prevalence, particularly Western countries, routine newborn screening for CF is a standard practice. CF predominantly affects Caucasian populations and is relatively rare in Asian populations.

Clinicians often suspect CF in cases with early childhood onset, a history of malabsorption leading to failure to thrive, and childhood steatorrhea. It is important to note that the specific CFTR mutation significantly influences clinical manifestations, with some less severe symptoms linked to rarer mutations. Radiological findings typically show upper lobe bronchiectasis, and patients often have a history of *Staphylococcus aureus* in sputum cultures.

Standard diagnostic tests include the sodium chloride sweat test and CFTR mutation analysis. The sweat test, typically conducted using pilocarpine iontophoresis, should be performed twice. The test results are interpreted as follows: less than 30 mmol/L chloride indicates a negative result, 30–60 mmol/L a borderline result, and over 60 mmol/L confirms a positive test. The CFTR gene, located on chromosome seven, has over 2000 identified mutations. Extensive mutation screening has proven effective in identifying more CF cases.

The diagnosis and management of CF necessitate a multidisciplinary approach, including genetic expertise. Figure 9.4 presents a detailed diagnostic algorithm for CFTR gene testing.

Connective Tissue Disease-Rheumatoid Arthritis

BE is an infrequent yet frequently overlooked complication in patients with rheumatoid arthritis (RA), occurring in only a minority of these individuals. Despite this, the significant

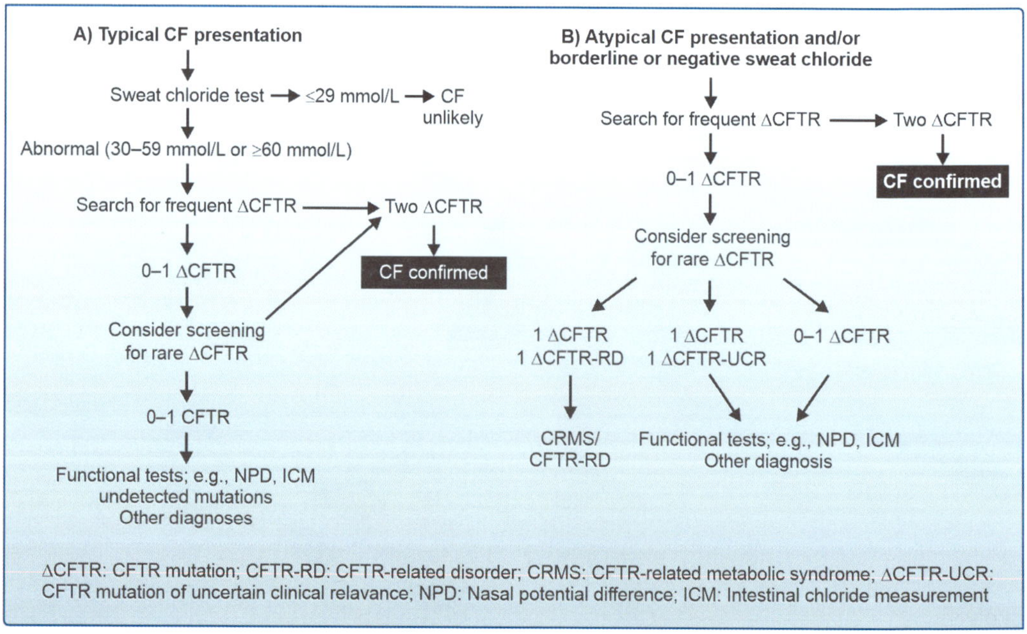

Fig. 9.4: Algorithm for CFTR genetic testing (*Adapted from:* Chan ED, et al. Diagnostic evaluation of bronchiectasis. Respiratory Medicine: X. 2019;1:100006)

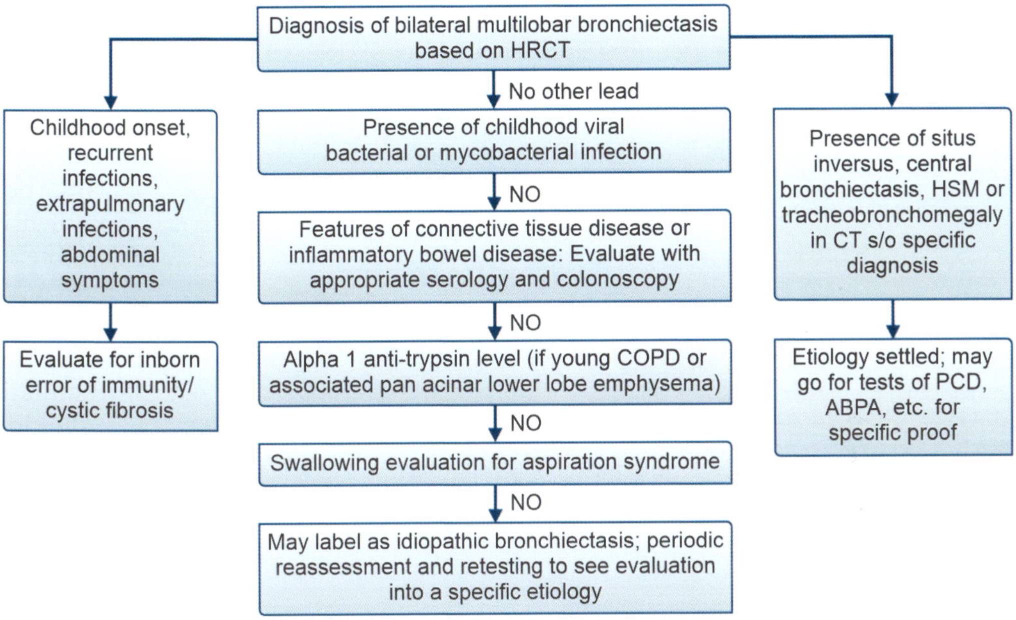

Fig. 9.5: Algorithm for etiological evaluation of bilateral bronchiectasis.

association between RA and BE necessitates the evaluation of auto-antibodies, such as rheumatoid factor (RF) and anti-cyclic citrullinated peptide (anti-CCP) antibodies, in undiagnosed cases of BE. It is crucial to interpret marginal elevations of RF and anti-CCP with discernment, as these increases can also be observed in the general population. Consequently, an isolated elevation in these markers should not deter the investigation of other potential causes for BE.

Inflammatory Bowel Disease (IBD)

There is a well-established link between bronchiectasis and IBD. In IBD, airway involvement is the most common pulmonary complication following infections and drug toxicity. Notably, two-thirds of those with airway inflammation in IBD are found to have BE, but most of these do not have associated symptoms.

A comprehensive, practical algorithm for the etiologic evaluation of bilateral BE is illustrated in Fig. 9.5.

FURTHER READING

1. Hill AT, Sullivan AL, Chalmers JD, De Soyza A, Elborn SJ, Floto AR, et al. British Thoracic Society Guideline for bronchiectasis in adults. Thorax. 2019;74(Suppl 1):1–69.

2. Polverino E, Goeminne PC, McDonnell MJ, Aliberti S, Marshall SE, Loebinger MR, et al. European Respiratory Society guidelines for the management of adult bronchiectasis. Eur Respir J. 2017;50(3).

3. Contarini M, Finch S, Chalmers JD. Bronchiectasis: a case-based approach to investigation and management. Eur Respir Rev. 2018 Jul 11;27(149):180016.

4. Chan ED, Wooten WI, Hsieh EWY, Johnston KL, Shaffer M, Sandhaus RA, et al. Diagnostic evaluation of bronchiectasis. Respiratory Medicine: X. 2019;1:100006.

5. Agarwal R, Sehgal IS, Muthu V, Denning DW, Chakrabarti A, Soundappan K, et al. Revised ISHAM-ABPA working group clinical practice guidelines for diagnosing, classifying and treating allergic bronchopulmonary aspergillosis/mycoses. Eur Respir J. 2024 Apr 4;63(4):2400061.

Chapter 10

Approach to a Case with Airway Foreign Body

• *Srikant Kashinath Malegaonkar* • *Kaumudi Devi* • *Ravindra M Mehta*

LEARNING POINTS

1. Airway foreign bodies even though uncommon, are an important clinical problem for a clinician.
2. History, clinical suspicion, and radiology form the backbone of inital assessment of a case with airway foreign body.
3. In pediatric and asphyxiating cases, rigid bronchoscopy is the conduit of choice; in others flexible bronchoscopy is the preferred modality.
4. Choice of tools to be used to dislodge and remove the foreign body depends on the nature of foreign body and status of airway lodging it.

INTRODUCTION

Foreign body (FB) aspiration, though uncommon, poses a potentially life-threatening situation necessitating immediate intervention. FB aspiration may manifest acutely with respiratory failure, or it can mimic sub-acute and chronic respiratory diseases, which can delay diagnosis, particularly in the absence of a clear history of aspiration. Radiology plays a crucial role in the assessment of FB, aiding in its confirmation, localization, and planning for retrieval. Interventional pulmonologists have access to a broad array of tools, chosen based on the type of FB, the condition of the airway where the FB is lodged, and the patient's clinical profile. The success of FB extraction is significantly influenced by the availability of these tools, the proceduralists' familiarity with them, and their overall expertise. In this report, we present two cases and outline a management approach for airway FBs, drawing conclusions from these case vignettes.

CASE VIGNETTE 1

A 43-year-old woman presented to the outpatient department with a history of aspirating a nose pin two days prior. An initial attempt to retrieve the foreign body was made at a peripheral centre using flexible bronchoscopy, but it was unsuccessful. Upon presentation,

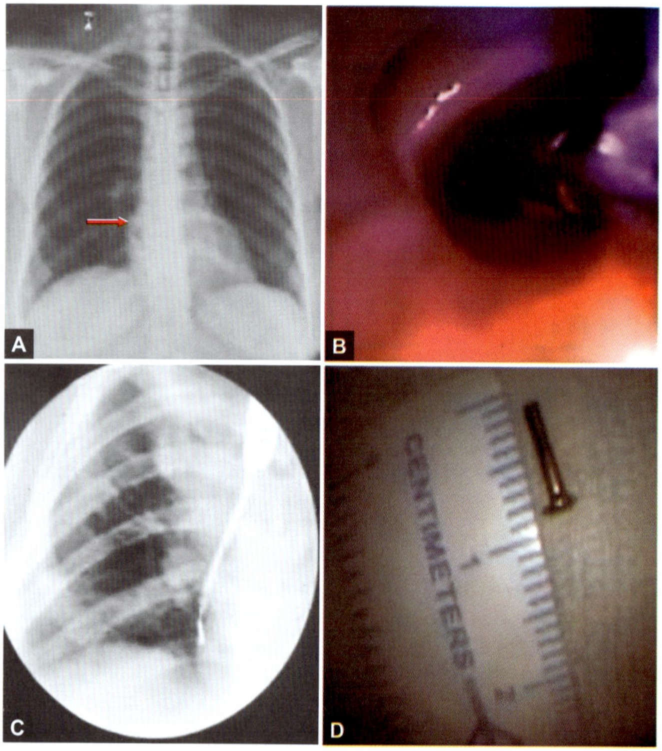

Fig. 10.1: (A) Chest radiograph showing foreign body–nose pin in right lower zone (red arrow); (B) Foreign body being held with flexible forceps; (C) Fluoroscopy image showing flexible forceps grasping pointed end of FB; (D) Nose pin after extraction.

she was hemodynamically stable with an oxygen saturation of 98% on room air. A chest X-ray revealed a linear, radiopaque foreign body in the right lower zone (Fig. 10.1A). Computed tomography (CT) of the thorax confirmed the presence of a linear, radiopaque object, consistent with the nose pin, lodged in the medial basal segment of the right lower lobe. Examination with a thinner bronchoscope showed the foreign body deeply embedded in the medial basal segment of the right lower lobe.

Due to the sharp edges of the foreign body and the risk of injury to the vocal cords, rigid bronchoscopy was employed to ventilate the patient. A flexible bronchoscope was inserted through the barrel of the rigid scope. Flexible alligator forceps were used to securely grasp the foreign body at its pointed tip (Fig. 10.1B), and fluoroscopy assisted in visualizing the disimpaction and retrieval process (Fig. 10.1C). The foreign body was carefully maneuvered into the barrel of the rigid scope and removed en bloc with the scope (Fig. 10.1D). A subsequent examination of the tracheobronchial tree was conducted to ensure there were no remnants and to assess the site of impaction. The patient experienced an uneventful recovery.

CASE VIGNETTE 2

A 50-year-old male presented to our outpatient department with a recurrent history of pneumonia in the right middle lobe (RML). Upon detailed inquiry, the patient recalled a choking episode occurring five years prior to the current presentation. Subsequent to this episode, he underwent rigid bronchoscopy where a foreign body was identified and removed

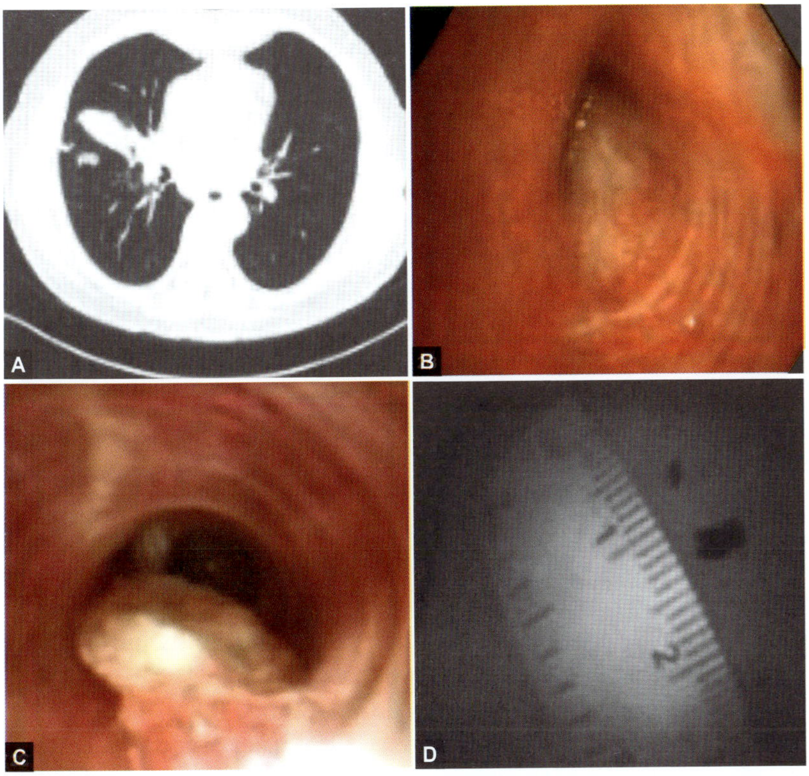

Fig. 10.2: (A) CT thorax axial section showing bronchiectasis of RML; (B) bronchoscopy showing pinhole stenosis of RML bronchus; (C) Thin bronchoscope showing foreign body in distal RML past the stenosis; (D) Picture of foreign body after retrieval.

piecemeal from the right middle lobe bronchus. The foreign body was identified as an areca nut. The patient's condition improved post-procedure.

However, a few months later, the patient experienced a recurrence of symptoms. A CT scan of the chest revealed narrowing of the RML bronchus with bronchiectatic changes in the RML (Fig. 10.2A). The patient then underwent flexible bronchoscopy, during which the narrowing of the RML bronchus was confirmed (Fig. 10.2B). Surprisingly, during the diagnostic bronchoscopy, which navigated the stenotic segment, another foreign body was visualized, deeply impacted beyond the stenotic segment (Fig. 10.2C).

Balloon dilation was performed to widen the stenotic segment, enabling the extraction of the foreign body using rigid forceps (Fig. 10.2D). Following the extraction, a significant amount of purulent secretion was observed emanating from the obstructed segment. These secretions were cleared. The patient has been under follow-up since this procedure and has not experienced any further episodes of pneumonia.

DISCUSSION

Foreign body (FB) aspiration, though relatively rare, is a potentially life-threatening medical emergency, especially when the FB lodges in the trachea and central airways. Epidemiologically, it is most commonly encountered in children and the elderly, with the bimodal distribution largely attributed to immature or uncoordinated swallowing reflexes.

Airway foreign bodies are typically classified into two categories: organic and inorganic. This classification plays a crucial role in determining the management approach.

FB aspiration can present in various ways, ranging from a witnessed episode leading to respiratory failure to more subtle presentations. In some instances, when a clear history of aspiration is absent, cases may be misdiagnosed and treated as asthma, bronchiectasis, or pneumonia. In fact, a clear history of aspiration is not evident in approximately 30–50% of cases. Our second case illustrates this point, where the patient had a chronic history and was initially treated for pneumonia. Chest imaging, particularly computed tomography (CT) of the chest, is instrumental in locating the FB and planning its retrieval. Direct visualisation of the FB or indirect evidence such as collapse, post-obstructive pneumonia, or hyperinflation are common radiological features associated with FB aspiration.

Stepwise Approach to Management of Foreign Body Aspiration

1. **Initial Airway Assessment and Ventilation:** The primary focus is on assessing the patient's airways and ensuring adequate ventilation. In cases of asphyxiation, rigid bronchoscopy is the first-line management tool, if available. If not, noninvasive ventilation, supraglottic devices, or endotracheal intubation may be utilized.
2. **Radiological Assessment:** This is a crucial step as it provides information about the location and type of FB, as well as the status of the airway leading to the FB. Such information is essential for formulating an appropriate management strategy.
3. **Type of Foreign Body:** Understanding the nature of the FB is critical, as it influences the choice of retrieval tools. Inorganic FBs are typically easier to retrieve with grasping tools like forceps. Organic FBs, due to their potential to fragment or their hygroscopic nature, present more challenges. Cryoadhesion using a cryoprobe is often ideal for organic FBs. The shape of the FB also plays a role in the selection of instruments, with baskets and snares being suitable for rounded or oval FBs.
4. **Choice of Conduit:** Rigid *vs* flexible bronchoscope: The decision between using a rigid or flexible bronchoscope for FB extraction depends on various factors. While flexible bronchoscopes have become the preferred choice in most situations, rigid bronchoscopes are favoured in pediatric cases, cases with respiratory failure, or when flexible bronchoscopy fails, as illustrated in Case 1.
5. **Foreign Body Retrieval Steps:** The three cardinal steps for FB retrieval are dislodging, securing, and removing the FB. However, not all three steps are necessary in every case.
6. **Tools for Retrieval:** The choice of tools depends on the nature of the FB and the condition and location of the airway where it is impacted.
    a. For inorganic FBs like pins, screws, pen caps, and whistles, forceps (alligator, rat tooth, shark tooth, and rigid) are commonly used. Caution is advised to grasp pointed ends of FBs to avoid mucosal damage, as demonstrated in Case 1.
    b. Organic FBs are often fragile and hygroscopic, making cryoprobes more effective for establishing firm adhesion and facilitating en bloc retrieval.
    c. Rounded or oval FBs are easier to retrieve with snares and baskets.
    d. Impacted or long-standing FBs, which may cause granulation tissue and airway stenosis, require additional tools. Fogarty balloons, argon plasma coagulation, lasers, and controlled radial expansion balloons can be utilised to dilate the proximal area, as shown in Case 2.

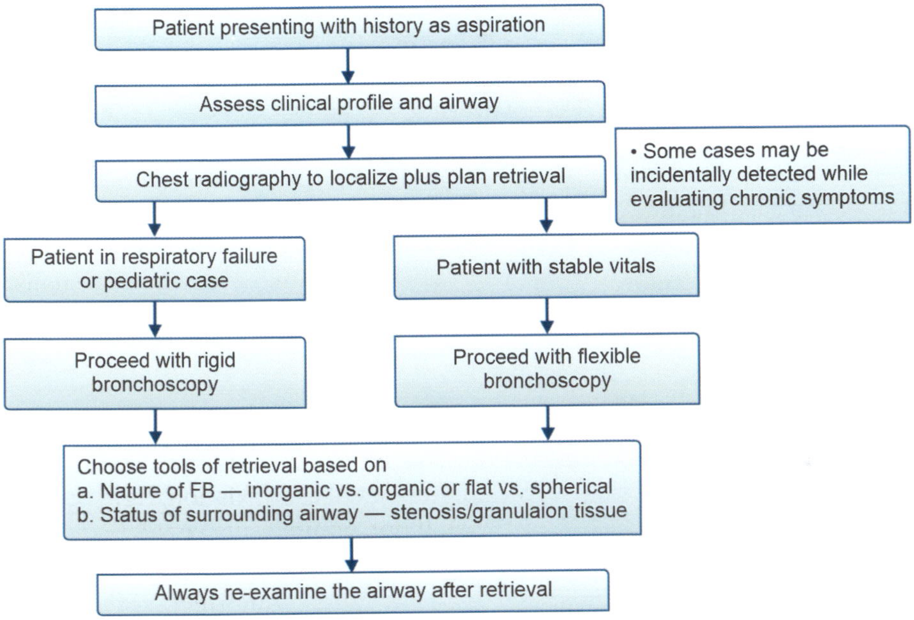

Fig. 10.3: Approach to management of airway foreign body.

7. **Post-retrieval Airway Examination:** Always re-examine the airway after retrieval to check for remnants, aspirate secretions, and examine the site of impaction.

Pediatric FB cases require particular attention due to the higher incidence of acute presentations, smaller airway sizes, and the need for rigid bronchoscopy as conduit. Pulmonologists trained in pediatric bronchoscopies and FB removal, should only attempt as small airway size is unforgiving. The integration of newer technologies like navigation bronchoscopy, thinner bronchoscopes, and advanced tools is anticipated to further improve FB retrieval outcomes.

An algorithm to summarize the approach to a foreign body is depicted in Fig. 10.3.

FURTHER READING

1. Sehgal IS, Dhooria S, Ram B, Singh N, Aggarwal AN, Gupta D, et al. Foreign body inhalation in the adult population: experience of 25,998 bronchoscopies and systematic review of the literature. Respir Care. 2015;60(10):1438–48.
2. Sajawal Ali M, Musani AI, Gaurav K. Pulmonary Foreign Body: An Unusual Cause of Recurrent Pneumonia. Arch Bronconeumol Ed Impr. 2018;39–39.
3. Mehta AC, Rafanan AL. Extraction of airway foreign body in adults. J Bronchol Interv Pulmonol. 2001;8(2):123–31.
4. Mu L, Sun D, He P. Radiological diagnosis of aspirated foreign bodies in children: review of 343 cases. J Laryngol Otol. 1990;104(10):778–82.
5. Sehgal IS, Dhooria S, Goyal R, Agarwal R. Airway foreign bodies: rigid vs flexible approach. Thorac Surg Interv Pulmonol Clin Guide. 2021;91–104.
6. Sehgal IS, Dhooria S, Behera D, Agarwal R. Use of cryoprobe for removal of a large tracheobronchial foreign body during flexible bronchoscopy. Lung India Off Organ Indian Chest Soc. 2016;33(5):543.

SECTION III

Pleural Diseases

Chapter 11

Approach to a Case with Exudative Pleural Effusion and Elevated ADA Level

• *Ravi Teja Kalavakollu* • *V Nagarjuna Maturu*

LEARNING POINTS

1. The three common causes of unilateral exudative pleural effusion in developing countries are tubercular pleural effusion, malignant pleural effusion and syn-pneumonic effusion.
2. Elevated pleural fluid ADA (>70 IU/L) is an useful biomarker for diagnosing pleural tuberculosis. However, it should always be interpreted in the correct clinical context.
3. Other diseases which can have elevated pleural fluid ADA levels are lymphomas, syn-pneumonic effusions and rheumatoid effusions.
4. When in doubt, a thoracoscopic pleural biopsy helps to confirm the diagnosis.

INTRODUCTION

Exudative pleural effusions frequently pose a diagnostic challenge in our routine clinical practice and must be carefully evaluated to determine the underlying cause. Exudative effusions have a varied etiology, with tuberculosis, malignancy, and parapneumonic effusion being the most common. Other less common causes like inflammatory and connective tissue disorders can also cause exudative pleural effusions. Pleural fluid analysis and pleural biopsy may be required to confirm the definitive cause. Exudative pleural effusions with elevated pleural fluid adenosine deaminase (ADA) levels are a common diagnostic dilemma and require a systematic approach to identify the underlying cause.

CASE VIGNETTE 1

A male office worker in his early thirties presented with dry cough, low grade fever and right sided chest pain of three weeks duration. Chest pain was pleuritic in nature and increased on coughing.

There was a past medical history of hypothyroidism and palmoplantar psoriasis. He was hemodynamically stable with reduced breath sounds noted in the right infrascapular region on auscultation. Chest radiograph (CXR) showed blunting of the right costophrenic angle and thoracic ultrasound (TUS) confirmed it to be an effusion. TUS guided right pleural

Table 11.1: Pleural fluid characteristics of the index cases

Pleural fluid analysis	*Case 1*	*Case 2*
Color	Pale straw colour	Pale straw colour
Total cell count (cells/mm^3)	7,000/mm^3	24,521/mm^3
Differential count	95% lymphocytes	90% lymphocytes
Protein (g/dL)	5.88	6.77
Albumin (g/dL)	2.91	3.54
Glucose (mg/dL)	81	67
ADA (IU/L)	104	59
Xpert MTB/RIF	MTB not detected	MTB not detected
RA Factor (U/mL)	176	72.4

ADA: Adenosine deaminase; *MTB:* Mycobacterium tuberculosis; *RA:* Rheumatoid arthritis; *IU:* International units

fluid aspiration demonstrated an exudative lymphocytic effusion with elevated ADA level (Table 11.1). In the absence of any risk factors for malignancy, the possibility of a tubercular pleural effusion was considered and the patient was started on anti-tubercular treatment (ATT). The patient had no symptomatic improvement after one month of ATT with increasing dyspnea, cough and fever spikes. CXR showed an increase in the pleural effusion (Fig. 11.1A).

Medical thoracoscopy was then performed to confirm the diagnosis. On medical thoracoscopy the pleura was found to be thickened (Fig. 11.1B) with few thin adhesions. Pleural biopsy revealed features of fibrinous pleuritis (Fig. 11.1C). On retaking the history, the patient also complained of early morning joint pains and stiffness for the last three months. Serum and pleural fluid for rheumatoid factor were elevated. Further investigations disclosed a markedly elevated serum anti-cyclic citrullinated peptide (Anti-CCP) level at 200 U/ml (normal range: <5 U/ml). Notably, there was also a significant increase in anti-thyroid peroxidase (Anti-TPO) antibodies, measuring 322 IU/ml (normal range: <8 IU/ml).

Based on these findings, the patient was diagnosed with rheumatoid arthritis related pleural effusion and autoimmune hypothyroidism. Patient was started on low dose oral prednisone, methotrexate and hydroxychloroquine. ATT was withheld, and his symptoms gradually improved along with radiological resolution of pleural effusion (Fig. 11.1D).

CASE VIGNETTE 2

A male civil engineer in his early forties, presented with a 20 days history of fever, right sided pleuritic chest pain of two days and three kilogram weight loss over a fortnight.

The patient had a history of seropositive rheumatoid arthritis (RA) and was on maintenance oral methotrexate. He reported similar complaints of cough one year ago, which resolved with over the counter cough suppressants. On examination, breath sounds were reduced on the right infra-scapular area. Chest radiograph (CXR) showed right costophrenic angle blunting (Fig. 11.2A). A computed tomography (CT) of the chest showed right mild pleural effusion with subsegmental atelectasis. Ultrasound guided right pleural fluid aspiration revealed an exudative lymphocytic effusion with elevated ADA levels (Table 11.1).

A differential diagnosis of tubercular pleural effusion, rheumatoid effusion and malignancy were considered. Medical thoracoscopy was performed which revealed the presence of

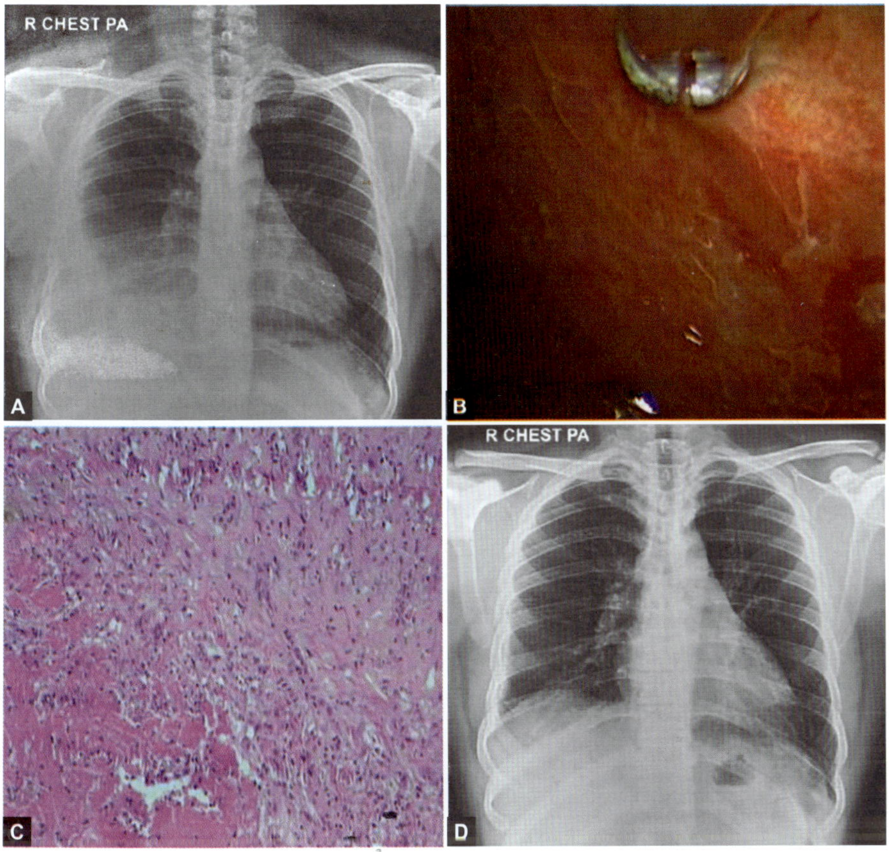

Fig. 11.1: (A) Chest radiograph showing a moderate right pleural effusion; (B) Thoracoscopic image showing dull and thickened parietal pleura; (C) Histopathology image (H&E 40X) of pleural biopsy showing features of fibrinous pleuritis (acute and chronic inflammation with fibrin and proliferating fibroblasts); (D) Chest radiograph showing resolution of pleural effusion.

opaque and thickened pleura (Fig. 11.2B). Pleural biopsy histopathology showed features of chronic pleuritis with lymphoplasmacytic infiltrate favouring an autoimmune etiology (Fig. 11.2C). Pleural fluid for rheumatoid factor assay was positive. A diagnosis of RA associated effusion was made. The patient's immunosuppressive therapy was escalated to a combination of oral corticosteroids, hydroxychloroquine and methotrexate. The patient improved symptomatically and CXR showed radiological resolution (Fig 11.2D).

DISCUSSION

The approach to a case of an exudative pleural effusion should be guided by a detailed clinical history and examination of the patient. The three common causes of unilateral exudative pleural effusion in developing countries are syn/parapneumonic effusions (PPE), tubercular pleural effusion (TPE) and malignant pleural effusion (MPE). In addition to the three common causes, there are various causes of exudative pleural effusions and these are listed in Box 11.1.

The first step in the evaluation of any clinically significant pleural effusion is an ultrasound guided diagnostic thoracentesis. Elevated pleural fluid (PF) protein (>3 g/dL), elevated

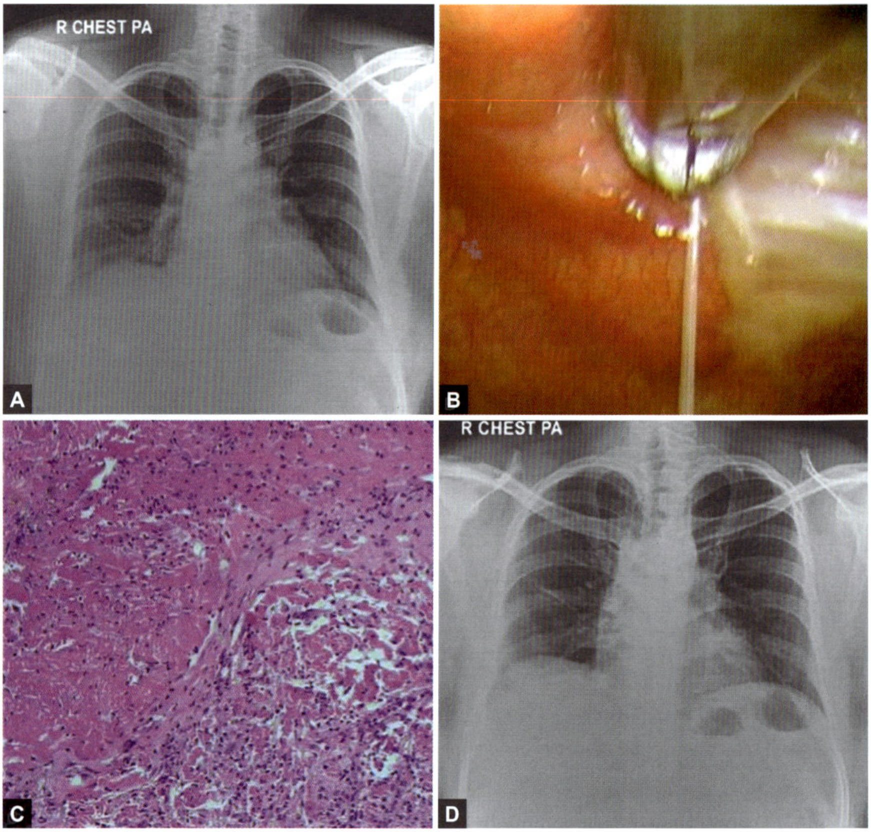

Fig. 11.2: (A) Chest radiograph showing a mild right pleural effusion (blunting of right costophrenic angle); (B) Thoracoscopic image showing a dull thickened parietal pleural surface; (C) Histopathology image (H&E 40X) of pleural biopsy showing features of chronic inflammation with proliferating fibroblasts; (D) Chest radiograph showing resolution of pleural effusion.

Box 11.1: Causes of an exudative pleural effusion

- **Infections:** Tuberculosis, bacterial, fungal, viral pneumonia, septic emboli
- **Malignancies:** Primary pleural neoplasms, metastasis
- **Iatrogenic:** Misplaced catheters, esophageal perforation
- **Connective tissue diseases:** SLE, rheumatoid arthritis, MCTD, granulomatosis with polyangiitis
- Cholesterol effusions and chylous effusions
- **Miscellaneous:** Pancreatitis, pulmonary embolism, uremic pleurisy, sarcoidosis, post-cardiac surgery, ARDS, SVC syndrome, catamenial hemothorax, Meigs syndrome, bilo pleural fistula, radiation therapy

SLE: Systemic lupus erythematosus; *MCTD:* Mixed connective tissue disorder; *ARDS:* Acute respiratory distress syndrome; *SVC:* Superior vena cava.

pleural fluid LDH, a low serum pleural fluid protein gradient (<3.1 g/dL) or low serum pleural fluid albumin gradient (<1.2 g/dL) confirm the effusion to be an exudative effusion. Further evaluation of exudative pleural effusions requires a combination of biochemical, cytological and microbiological pleural fluid analysis. When the etiology remains unclear after initial pleural fluid analysis reports, a pleural biopsy (thoracoscopic or image guided) needs to be performed to establish a definitive diagnosis.

Demonstration of malignant cells on pleural fluid cytology or cell block preparations confirms the effusion to be a MPE. In cases where pleural fluid does not show malignant cells, histological examination of pleural tissue remains the gold standard for diagnosing MPE.

The presence of acute febrile illness, purulent sputum and pulmonary infiltrates in a patient in a patient with radiological evidence of pleural effusion is suggestive of a parapneumonic effusion or empyema. Pleural analysis showing aspiration of frank pus, low pH, low glucose, combined with a positive microbiological analysis can confirm a diagnosis of syn-pneumonic effusion or empyema.

A definitive diagnosis of a TPE can be established when it is confirmed microbiologically (positive AFB smear, MTB culture or a nucleic acid amplification test). Microbiologic confirmation is often not possible due to the paucibacillary nature of disease. Pathologic evidence of granulomas in pleura and absence of other causes of a granulomatous inflammation is the next best confirmatory evidence for TPE. In the absence of a microbiologic or a pathologic diagnosis, PF biomarkers like ADA are often used in the developing world to establish a diagnosis of TPE.

Pleural Fluid Adenosine Deaminase (ADA)

Adenosine Deaminase (ADA) is an enzyme produced by lymphocytes and has been utilized as a biological marker for diagnosing tuberculous pleural effusion (TPE). There is no ideal cut off value for ADA in pleural fluid (PF) for diagnosing TPE. Several cut offs (40 IU/L, 60 IU/L and 70 IU/L) have been tested. The higher the ADA level, the higher is the clinical probability of the diagnosis being a TPE.

Indian guidelines for diagnosing TPE recommend the use of a cut off of 70 IU/L for diagnosing TPE. If the ADA is in between 40 and 70 IU/L, a trial of anti-tubercular therapy may be considered if the clinicoradiologic picture is suggestive of tuberculosis. Otherwise a pleural biopsy is recommended. If ADA is <40 IU/L, a diagnosis of TPE is less likely and hence a pleural biopsy needs to be performed. An algorithm for approach to an exudative pleural effusion based on ADA levels is given in Fig. 11.3.

Although TPE is the commonest cause of an elevated PF ADA level, many diseases other than tuberculosis, such as empyema/parapneumonic effusion (PPE), lymphomas and autoimmune diseases (rheumatoid arthritis) may also have high ADA levels (Table 11.2). Up to two-thirds of empyemas and one-third of syn-pneumonic effusions have elevated ADA levels (>40 IU/L). Differentiation of TPE from a PPE is not difficult as TPE is usually lymphocyte predominant whereas a PPE is neutrophil predominant. Differentiation of TPE from other diseases which cause elevated ADA is more difficult, and hence pleural fluid ADA always needs to be interpreted in the clinical context.

Low pleural fluid ADA (<40 IU/L) does not completely rule out a TPE. In the correct clinical context, finding of granulomas on pleural biopsy and exclusion of other causes of granulomas will confirm the diagnosis of TPE even if fluid ADA is low. Pleural fluid ADA can be low in patients with TPE who are elderly, critically ill or have multi-organ failure.

ADA has two iso-enzymes, ADA 1 and ADA 2. ADA 2 is elevated in TPE, whereas ADA 1 is elevated in MPE/PPE and other inflammatory disorders. However, due to poor discriminatory potential, this isoenzyme analysis is not routinely clinically utilized. To further improve the diagnostic ability of ADA levels, several ratios have been proposed and tested. These include the age/PF ADA level ratio, the cancer ratio (serum LDH/PF ADA level) and

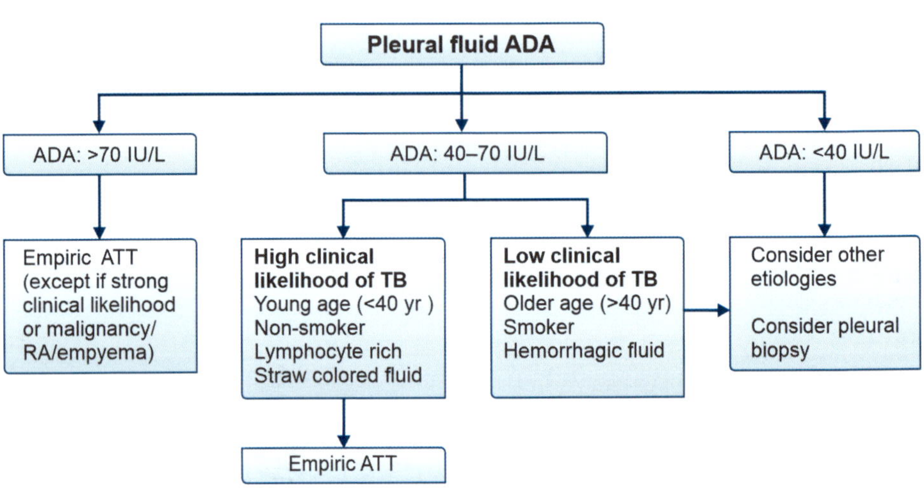

Fig. 11.3: Algorithm showing the approach to an exudative pleural effusion based on pleural fluid adenosine deaminase (ADA) levels.[5]

Table 11.2: Causes of an exudative pleural effusion with elevated ADA level

Disease state	*Pleural fluid cell predominance*
Tubercular pleural effusion	Lymphocyte rich
Empyema/syn-pneumonic effusion	Neutrophil rich
Lymphomas	Lymphocyte rich
Rheumatoid effusions	Variable cell preponderance
Brucellosis effusion	Lymphocyte rich
Q fever related effusions	Lymphocyte rich

cancer ratio plus (cancer ratio/PF lymphocyte count). However, none of these have been consistently shown to be better than PF ADA alone in diagnosing TPE.

Rheumatoid Arthritis Related Pleural Effusion

Rheumatoid arthritis (RA) associated with pleural disease is seen in about 38 to 73% patients but only 5% become symptomatic at any point of time. Pleuritic chest pain, fever and dyspnoea are the common presenting symptoms as the effusion size increases. Effusions usually develop years after the diagnosis of RA (Case vignette 2) but in a quarter of patients, pleurisy can occur before or at the time of development of arthritis (Case vignette 1). Computed tomography can identify any concomitant parenchymal abnormalities, rheumatoid nodules, pneumothorax and bronchopleural fistula. Long standing untreated rheumatoid effusions can also lead to development of a pseudochylothorax, though it is becoming less common in the current era.

Pleural fluid analysis typically reveals an exudative effusion with low pH, low glucose and elevated LDH. White cell count and cell predominance is variable with some cases showing characteristic RA cells/ragocytes (polymorphonuclear phagocytes with intracellular inclusions). Rheumatoid factor levels higher than 1:320 are usually seen. PF rheumatoid factor however has low specificity in confirming the diagnosis of RA related pleural effusion and hence is not often performed. PF rheumatoid factors levels often mirror the serum levels.

ADA levels are elevated mimicking TPE which may require thoracoscopic pleural biopsy to confirm the diagnosis. The parietal pleura is thickened with a gritty granular appearance and histopathology examination shows multinucleated giant cells with foci of fibroblasts and lymphocytes surrounding necrotic centers similar to rheumatoid nodules.

Most rheumatoid effusions are asymptomatic and small and do not require specific treatment. Treatment of the underlying RA usually leads to resolution of associated effusions. Complete resolution of the pleural effusion may occur over a period of months to years. In cases of persistent pleural effusion despite appropriate treatment, pleural decortication may be necessary to prevent pleural fibrosis.

In both the index cases, pleural fluid analysis showed an exudative lymphocyte rich effusion with high ADA levels. Thoracoscopic pleural biopsy in both the cases showed features of chronic fibrinous pleuritis and no granulomas thus ruling out tuberculosis. Diagnosis of rheumatoid arthritis and a diagnosis of rheumatoid arthritis associated pleural effusion was made based on clinical history and examination. Both the patients were started on steroids, hydroxychloroquine and methotrexate. Clinical and radiological resolution was seen in both the patients.

FURTHER READING

1. Sharma SK, Ryan H, Khaparde S, Sachdeva KS, Singh AD, Mohan A, Sarin R, Paramasivan CN, Kumar P, Nischal N, Khatiwada S, Garner P, Tharyan P. Index-TB guidelines: Guidelines on extrapulmonary tuberculosis for India. Indian J Med Res. 2017 Apr;145(4):448–463.
2. Shimoda, M, Hirata, A, Tanaka Y, et al. Characteristics of pleural effusion with a high adenosine deaminase level: a case–control study. BMC Pulm Med 22, 359 (2022).
3. Anthony J. Esposito, Sarah G. Chu, Rachna Madan, Tracy J. Doyle, Paul F. Dellaripa, Thoracic Manifestations of Rheumatoid Arthritis, Clinics in Chest Medicine, Volume 40, Issue 3, 2019, Pages 545–560, ISSN 0272-5231, ISBN 9780323710367.
4. Aggarwal AN, Agarwal R, Sehgal IS, Dhooria S. Adenosine deaminase for diagnosis of tuberculous pleural effusion: A systematic review and meta-analysis. PloS one. 2019 Mar 26;14(3):e0213728.
5. Maturu VN, Dhooria S, Bal A, Singh N, Aggarwal AN, Gupta D, Behera D, Agarwal R. Role of medical thoracoscopy and closed-blind pleural biopsy in undiagnosed exudative pleural effusions: a single-center experience of 348 patients. J Bronchology Interv Pulmonol. 2015 Apr;22(2):121–9.

Chapter

12

Approach to a Case of Milky White Pleural Effusion

• *Srinivas Rajagopala*

LEARNING POINTS

1. Chylothorax, pseudo-chylothorax and empyema are the differential diagnoses for a milky-appearing pleural fluid.
2. Clinical history, examination and fluid centrifugation can help to easily distinguish these three entities. A diagnosis of chylothorax is made by demonstrating pleural fluid triglyceride >110 mg/dL. Definitive diagnosis requires lipoprotein analysis.
3. Chylothorax can occur in the absence of turbid, milky fluid especially if the patient is fasting.
4. The differential diagnosis of a non-traumatic chylothorax is wide and must be narrowed using history, examination, identification of associated systemic diseases, presence of chylous ascites, mediastinal adenopathy and side of chylothorax.

INTRODUCTION

A milky white pleural effusion, often indicating chylothorax, is a rare finding with various potential causes, including trauma, malignancies, or idiopathic factors. The unique appearance results from the high lipid content, particularly triglycerides, in the chyle. Diagnosing and managing such effusions requires a thorough approach, considering fluid characteristics and underlying causes. This clinical vignette illustrates the diagnostic evaluation of a milky white pleural effusion in a 40-year-old female presenting with a constellation of gastrointestinal and respiratory symptoms. This case underscores the significance of a comprehensive evaluation for milky white pleural effusions, encompassing a broad spectrum of differential diagnoses, and employing pertinent imaging modalities and laboratory analyses to reach a conclusive diagnosis.

CASE VIGNETTE

A 40-year-old woman presented with regurgitation, heartburn, increased frequency of stools, leg swelling, productive cough and breathlessness on exertion for three weeks duration.

The stools were watery, without mucus or blood, and were associated with bloating, anorexia, and unquantified weight loss. She was a homemaker with no exposure to pets, cigarettes, alcohol, or drugs. There was no history of recent chest trauma. The past medical history was unremarkable. Physical examination revealed anasarca, pallor, normal nails, and absent right-sided breath sounds; no shifting dullness, organomegaly, or lymphadenopathy was evident.

Initial investigations (Table 12.1) included a chest radiograph that showed an opaque right hemithorax (Fig. 12.1A) and a massive pleural effusion was confirmed on thoracic ultrasound. Abdominal ultrasound revealed a few splenic cysts, mild ascites, mesenteric thickening, and multiple retroperitoneal and mesenteric cysts with septations. Contrast-enhanced computed tomography (CECT) of the chest and abdomen was performed which revealed a right massive effusion and mild-moderate pericardial effusion (10 mm posteriorly) without any pericardial thickening or mediastinal lymphadenopathy and an associated right sided consolidation. Multiple heterogeneous, hypodense, partly-cystic lesions in mesentery and in the spleen were noted (Fig. 12.2). Blood investigations revealed hypokalemia (serum potassium: 2.46 mEq/L), severe hypoprotenemia (Protein: 3 g/dL), hypoalbuminemia (albumen: 1.4 g/dL) and low serum vitamin D levels. Serum rheumatoid factor was negative

Table 12.1: Summary of relevant pleural fluid investigations in the index patient

Investigation	***Observed value***
Gross appearance	Whitish
Total count	490 cells/µL
Differential count	Neutrophils: 13%, lymphocytes: 80%, macrophages: 7%
Pleural protein	0.6 g/dL
Pleural LDH	46 U/L
Pleural sugar	78 mg/dL
Pleural fluid triglyceride	210 mg/dL
Pleural cholesterol	56 mg/dL
Pleural adenosine deaminase	2.3 U/L

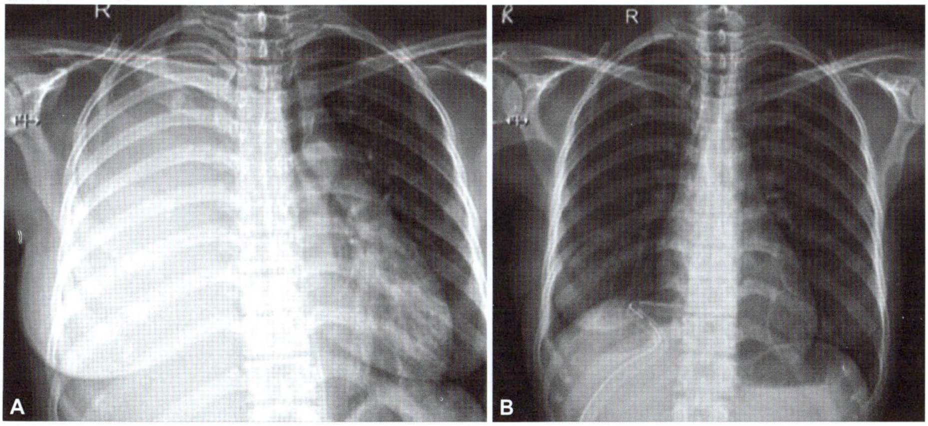

Fig. 12.1: Composite image of the chest radiograph (A) showing right-sided massive pleural effusion and (B) postoperative chest radiograph after successful thoracic duct ligation and pleurodesis

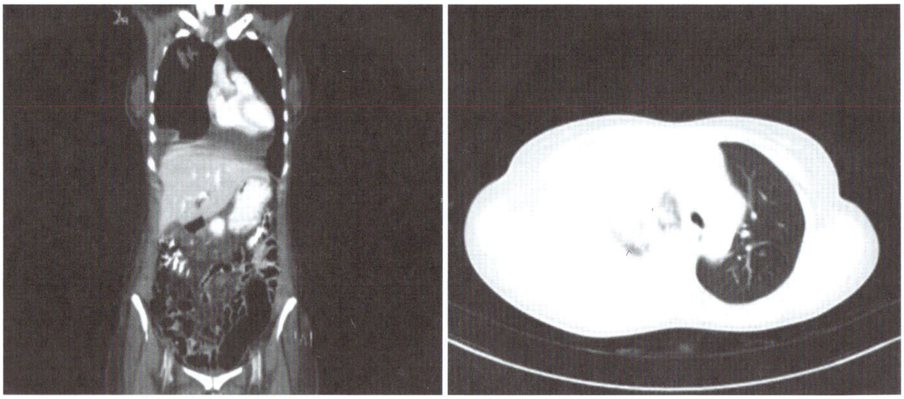

Fig. 12.2: Contrast-enhanced computed tomography (CECT) chest and abdomen showing (left) haziness and thickening along the mesenteric and omental fat planes. Multiple heterogeneous, hypodense, partly-cystic lesions in mesentery and in the spleen and a 33 × 38 mm loculated fluid collection with septations in the hepatorenal pouch were also seen (not shown). Mild ascites was also noted. A right massive effusion was present (right).

at 1:20 by latex agglutination; tests for antinuclear antibodies and antibodies for HIV, hepatitis B, and hepatitis C by ELISA were all negative. Serum complement levels were normal.

Thoracentesis yielded a white, creamy fluid (Fig. 12.3) with characteristics as given in Table 12.1. Ascitic tap confirmed a fluid with similar appearance (not shown). A diagnosis of chylothorax (white colored pleural fluid with elevated pleural fluid triglycerides and a normal pleural fluid cholesterol) was made. Differentials considered for chylothorax aetiology included tuberculosis, constrictive pericarditis, and lymphangiectasia (Table 12.2). Bronchoscopy with bronchoalveolar lavage (BAL) for mycobacterial smears and cultures, and Xpert MTB/RIF from the right lower lobe was performed. BAL isolated *Pseudomonas aeruginosa*, and the patient was administered third generation cephalosporin and quinolone for two weeks resulting in resolution of the cough.

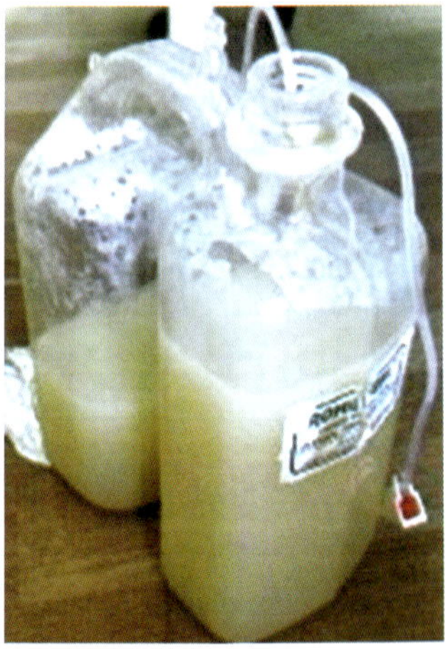

Fig. 12.3: Ultrasound-guided aspirate from the right thoracic cavity showed a white-coloured turbid fluid.

Clinical discussion with a cardiologist and repeat echocardiography showed no features of constrictive pericarditis. Given the anasarca, lymphocytopenia, hypoalbuminemia, hypoglobulinemia, and absence of proteinuria or chronic liver disease, a diagnosis of protein-losing enteropathy with chylous ascites and chylothorax was strongly considered. The presence of cystic splenic, mesenteric, and retroperitoneal hypodense lesions prompted suspicion of abdominal tuberculosis or intestinal lymphangiectasia. Pedal lymphoscintigraphy was attempted but failed to visualise any abdominal leak. Gastroscopy showed edematous mucosa in the second and third parts of the duodenum. Biopsies showed mild villous blunting and large ectatic lymphatic channels in the submucosa and mucosa (Fig. 12.4). Colonoscopy revealed distal ileal nodularity and diffuse edematous colonic mucosal folds. Biopsies from the distal ileum and colon showed ectatic lymphatic channels, consistent with a diagnosis of intestinal lymphangiectasia. A 24-hour faecal α1-antitrypsin test for confirmation of malabsorption

Table 12.2: Etiology of a chylothorax of unclear origin	
Etiology of chylothorax	*Expected frequency in clinical practice*
1. **Traumatic chylothorax**	≈50%
a. Non-Iatrogenic (blunt trauma to chest or vertebra, knife injury to chest/ gunshot injury, childbirth, forceful emesis)	≈12–15%
b. Iatrogenic (thoracic surgeries-oesophagectomy, congenital heart disease, lung/mediastinal resections, head and neck surgery, radiation, pacemaker/ central line insertion/embolisation of arterio-venous malformations)	35–38%
2. **Non-traumatic chylothorax**	≈44%
a. Malignancy (lymphomas, other solid tumors)	≈15–20%
b. Lymphangioleiomyomatosis	–
c. Lymphangiectasia	–
d. Filariasis	–
e. Sarcoidosis	–
f. Amyloidosis	–
g. Tuberculosis	–
h. Superior vena cava obstruction	–
i. Constrictive pericarditis	–
j. Haemangiomatosis (Gorham's disease)/ lymphangiomatosis	–
k. Cardiac failure	–
l. Transdiaphragmatic movement in cirrhosis	–
3. **Idiopathic chylothorax**	≈6%

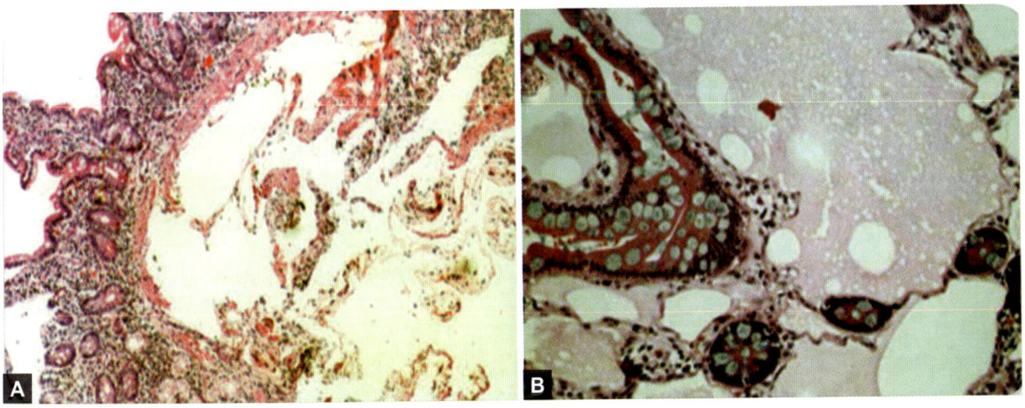

Fig. 12.4A and B: Composite photomicrograph of the low-power view (left, H & E, 10X) of the duodenum showing ectatic lymphatics in the submucosa along with mild villous blunting and high-power view (right, PAS staining, 100X), highlighting the dilated, ectatic submucosal lymphatics.

was not performed. Bone marrow aspirate and trephine biopsy showed normal trilineage hematopoiesis without any evidence of clonal abnormalities.

A final diagnosis of intestinal lymphangiectasia with protein-losing enteropathy and chylothorax was made. She was initiated on vitamin B_{12}, vitamins A, D, K, calcium supplementation, MCT, and high-protein supplementation. Ongoing breathlessness and hypoxemia necessitated tube thoracostomy and subcutaneous octreotide, without significant reduction in drain output. A thoracotomy with thoracic duct ligation, pleural biopsy, and mechanical pleurodesis was performed, resulting in the resolution of the chylothorax (Fig. 12.1B). The pleural biopsy showed chronic non-specific pleuritis without granulomas. She continued to improve on the MCT diet, with resolution of anasarca, weight gain, and a serum albumin level of 3.6 g/dL. She remains asymptomatic at one year of follow-up.

DISCUSSION

Intestinal lymphangiectasia is characterised by abnormal intestinal lymphatic drainage with dilated lymphatic channels due to a variety of causes (Table 12.3). The diagnosis of primary intestinal lymphangiectasia is made by excluding syndromic and secondary causes and confirming the presence of lymphatic abnormalities elsewhere. Most associated causes can be excluded with a thorough clinical examination. Primary intestinal lymphangiectasia (Waldmann's syndrome) is a rare disease, with fewer than 200 cases reported worldwide. It is mostly sporadic but can be associated with characteristic syndromes (Table 12.3). The

Table 12.3: Etiology of intestinal lymphangiectasia	
Primary	Primary intestinal lymphangiectasia (sporadic)
Syndromic congenital malformation of lymphatics	CHAPLE syndrome^ (CD55 biallelic mutations)
	Yellow nail syndrome (lymphedema, yellow nails and pulmonary abnormalities)
	Tuberous sclerosis (TSC2 mutation)
	Turner's syndrome, Noonan's syndrome
	Hennekam syndrome
	Type 1 neurofibromatosis
	Klippel-Trenaunay syndrome
Rare mutations with specific syndromes	
PRG4 mutation	Camptodactyly-arthropathy-coxa varapericarditis syndrome
FGFR3 mutation	Protein-losing enteropathy with intestinal lymphangiectasia and skeletal dysplasia
DGAT1 mutation	Congenital protein-losing enteropathy with errors in lipid metabolism
PLVAP mutation	Plasmalemma vesicle-associated protein deficiency
Secondary intestinal lymphangiectasia	Right heart failure (heart failure, constrictive pericarditis, congenital heart disease, Fontan procedure)
	Thoracic duct obstruction
	Retroperitoneal lymphadenopathy (tuberculosis, sarcoidosis, lymphoma)
	Cirrhosis and portal hypertensive gastroenteropathy
	Hepatic venous outflow obstruction
	Mesenteric venous thrombosis
	Sclerosing mesenteritis, retroperitoneal fibrosis
	Chronic pancreatitis with pseudocysts
	Crohn's disease, Whipple's disease
	Enteric-lymphatic fistula

^Hyperactivation of complement, angiopathic thrombosis and protein losing enteropathy mean age of onset is 11 years, but it can present later in life. The association of chylothorax with this condition is unusual but has been reported and is believed to be due to abnormal pleural lymphatics.

Management of protein-losing enteropathy includes a low-fat, high-protein, medium-chain triglyceride (MCT) diet. MCTs bypass the enteric lymphatics and enter the portal system directly, reducing lymphatic flow and exudation. The diet should also provide adequate polyunsaturated fatty acids, fat-soluble vitamins, and 1.5–3.0 g/kg of protein intake for adults. Monitoring serum albumin, transferrin, and immunoglobulin levels can help assess improvement. The use of octreotide is anecdotal, and surgery is seldom feasible due to the disease's diffuse nature.

Approach to a Patient with white Color Pleural Fluid

When pleural fluid appears visibly turbid upon thoracentesis, it could be due to high cellular content or high cholesterol or triglyceride content. The first step is to observe the supernatant after centrifugation of the pleural fluid. If the turbidity clears, it is likely due to a pleural infection, which can be confirmed by pleural fluid biochemical analysis (leucocyte counts, pH, glucose) and Gram stain and bacterial cultures. If the turbidity persists after centrifugation, it could be due to chylothorax or pseudochylothorax. These can be differentiated by history, pleural fluid analysis for cholesterol/triglycerides, cholesterol crystals, and lipoprotein analysis.

- **Chylothorax:** Often acute in development, diagnosed when pleural fluid triglyceride is ≥110 mg/dL, pleural fluid cholesterol is <200 mg/dL, or pleural/serum cholesterol ratio is <1.
- **Pseudochylothorax:** Develops in long-standing pleural fluid accumulations, characterised by pleural thickening, high cholesterol or lecithin-globulin complexes, low triglycerides, and presence of cholesterol crystals in the fluid.

The distinction between these two is crucial as their causes and management are very different (Table 12.4). A flowchart detailing the utilisation of triglyceride, cholesterol levels and chylomicron analysis is provided to facilitate the diagnosis of chylothorax (Fig. 12.5).

In chylothorax, it is important to identify the underlying cause of the effusion, such as malignancy or syndromic disorders and treat them appropriately. It is also important to understand the potential immunocompromised state that will arise due to the loss of protein, fat, and lymphocytes from significant pleural drainage.

For traumatic/postoperative chylothorax, the initial management involves fasting the patient and providing parenteral nutrition. Chyle leaks typically resolve spontaneously within 10 days in 55–86.4% of cases, as collateral channels develop. This variance in resolution rates may be attributed to the type of surgery/trauma causing the chylothorax and differences between pediatric and adult patient populations. If drainage persists, treatment options include starting octreotide and considering percutaneous thoracic duct embolisation (via a transabdominal approach) or thoracoscopic duct ligation, depending on local resources. Pleuro-peritoneal shunts are an option but are not commonly used.

Pseudochylothoraces occur due to cholesterol accumulation in a long-standing effusion with pleural thickening. The most frequent causes are tuberculosis or, less commonly, chronic bacterial empyema that is partially treated or rheumatoid arthritis related pleural effusion. Treatment focuses on addressing the underlying cause and performing decortication to relieve any functional impairment.

Table 12.4: Differences between chylothorax and pseudochylothorax

	Chylothorax	***Pseudochylothorax (cholesterol pleural effusion)***
Frequency	Uncommon	Rare
Clinical presentation	Acute to sub-acute	Chronic
CT characteristics	Normal pleura	Thickened pleura with or without volume loss
Pleural fluid characteristics		
Triglycerides	>110 mg/dL	<50 mg/dL
Cholesterol	< 200 mg/dL	>200 mg/dL
Chylomicrons (Lipid electrophoresis)	Present	Absent
Cholesterol crystals	Absent	Often present
PF/Serum cholesterol	<1	>1
Predominant cell type	Lymphocytes	Neutrophils
Ether clearance test*	Dissolves the lipid component (triglycerides) and clears the turbidity of the supernatant	Addition of ether does not clear the turbidity of the supernatant
Causes	Trauma, Malignancy, Idiopathic and miscellaneous	Post tuberculous effusion, rheumatoid effusion

PF: Pleural fluid

*Ether clearance test (a bedside test) to distinguish chyle from pseudochyle is no longer considered a reliable test for confirmation of chylothorax.

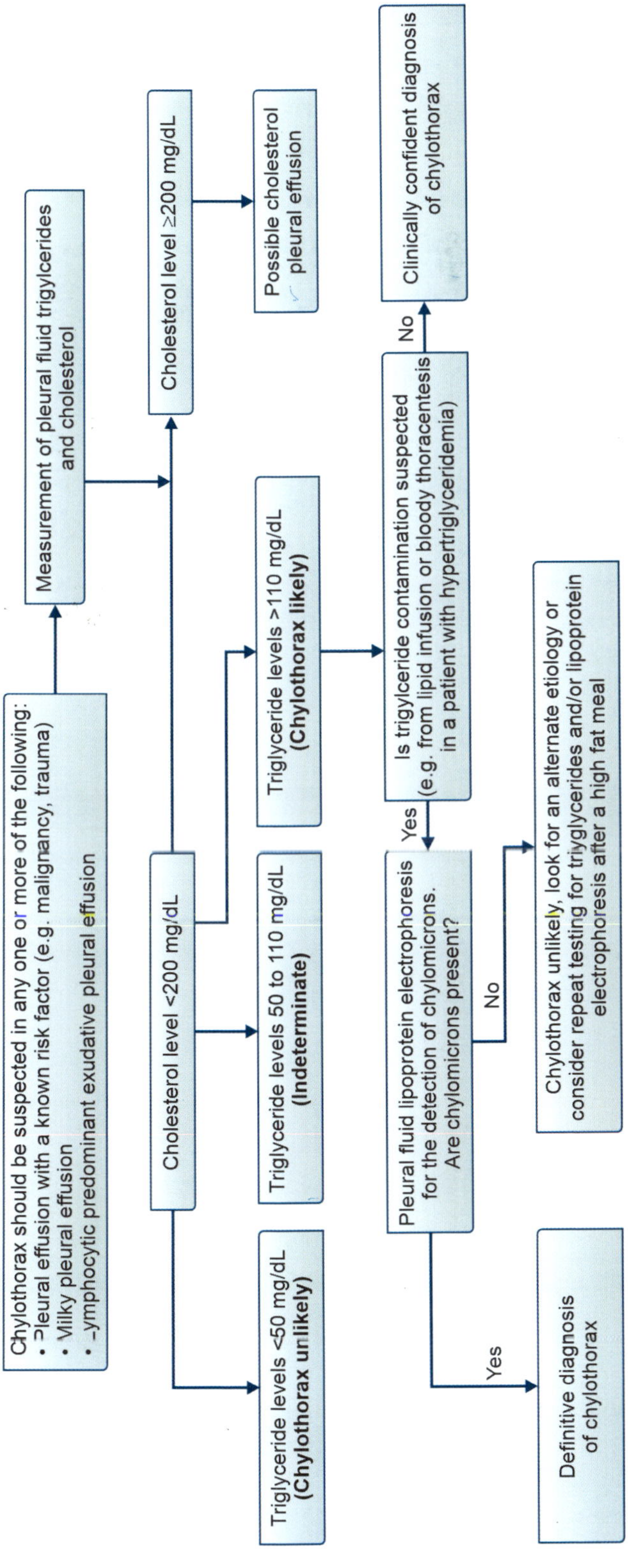

Fig. 12.5: Flowchart for diagnosis of chylothorax.

FURTHER READING

1. Ur Rehman K, Sivakumar P. Non-traumatic chylothorax: diagnostic and therapeutic strategies. Breathe 2022; 18: 210163.

2. Agrawal A, Chaddha U, Kaul V, Desai A, Gillaspie E, Maldonado F. Multidisciplinary Management of Chylothorax. Chest. 2022 Dec 1;162(6):1402–12.

3. McGrath EE, Blades Z, Anderson PB. Chylothorax: aetiology, diagnosis and therapeutic options. Respir Med. 2010 Jan;104(1):1–8.

4. Riley LE, Ataya A. Clinical approach and review of causes of a chylothorax. Respir Med. 2019 Oct;157:7–13.

5. Vignes S, Bellanger J: Primary intestinal lymphangiectasia (waldmann's disease). Orphanet J Rare Dis 2008;3:5.

Chapter 13

Approach to Management of Malignant Pleural Effusion

• *Radhika Banka* • *Ashwini Chawhan*

LEARNING POINTS

1. There are several strategies to optimally palliate dyspnea in a case of malignant pleural effusion (MPE). The options include repeated thoracentesis, chest drain and pleurodesis, or an indwelling pleural catheter (IPC) placement.
2. Decision regarding any procedure should be made on an individual case by case basis, taking into account the patient's preference and social support, performance status, predicted responsiveness to antitumor therapy, expected survival, effusion characteristics such as trapped lung or septated effusion, financial resources and local expertise.
3. More data is needed from our country to assess the cost effectiveness of tube thoracostomy and pleurodesis versus IPC for MPE management.

INTRODUCTION

Malignant pleural effusion (MPE) is the second most common cause of an exudative pleural effusion and is commonly encountered in clinical practice. MPE is seen in about 15% of cancer patients, the majority of which are secondary to lung cancer, breast cancer, lymphoma, gynecological malignancies and malignant mesothelioma. It is usually seen at an advanced stage of cancer and hence MPE is associated with poor prognosis with a median survival of 6–12 months from diagnosis. The treatment is primarily palliative and aimed at relieving symptoms. The treatment options include repeated thoracentesis, chest drain insertion and pleurodesis or indwelling pleural catheters (IPC). The best treatment option for any given case is dependent on the patient's preference and the available resources.

CASE VIGNETTE

A 58-year old lady presented with symptoms of gradually progressive dyspnoea on exertion, dull left sided chest pain, weight loss of 5 kg and reduced appetite for 2 months. Past medical history included hypertension and hypothyroidism. The occupational and family history were unremarkable. On examination, she was hemodynamically stable and respiratory system examination revealed reduced movements of the entire left hemithorax with a dull percussion note and absent breath sounds.

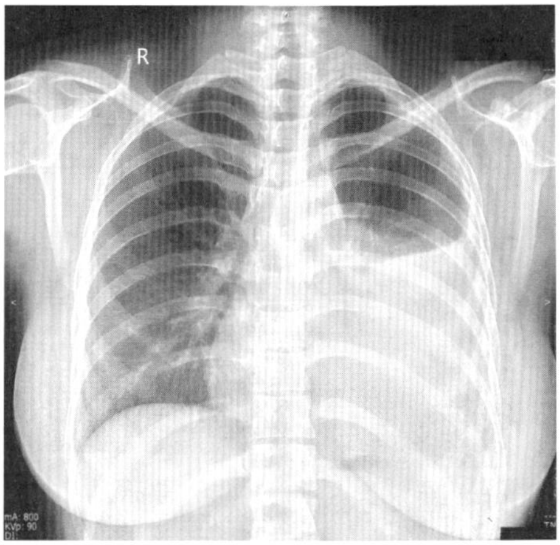

Fig. 13.1: Chest radiograph showing large left pleural effusion.

Initial chest radiograph revealed homogeneous opacification of the left middle and lower zones with blunting of the costo-phrenic angle (Fig. 13.1). Thoracic ultrasound confirmed a large left pleural effusion with echogenic swirls and diaphragmatic irregularity (Fig. 13.2A). One liter of hemorrhagic fluid was aspirated from the left hemithorax and pleural fluid analysis revealed an exudative (protein 5.3 g/L), lymphocytic fluid (80% lymphocytes) with a normal adenosine deaminase (ADA) level . Pleural fluid cytology showed atypical cells and pleural fluid cell block histological examination confirmed metastatic lung adenocarcinoma with exon 19 deletion epidermal growth factor receptor (EGFR) mutation. A contrast enhanced computed tomography of the chest revealed a left sided pleural effusion with a left hilar mass and enlarged mediastinal lymph nodes.

A diagnosis of primary lung adenocarcinoma with metastatic pleural effusion was made and she was referred to the oncologist for therapy. In view of persistent breathlessness, a chest radiograph was repeated which revealed re-accumulation of the pleural fluid within two weeks of initial thoracentesis.

Therapeutic options of chest drain insertion and pleurodesis, or placement of an IPC were discussed with the patient. The patient preferred to undergo an in hospital chest drain insertion and pleurodesis as she was not comfortable with the idea of frequent drainage via an IPC. A 20 Fr chest drain was inserted and over 72 hours, two litres of hemorrhagic pleural fluid was drained. Once minimal fluid was appreciated on ultrasound, pleurodesis was performed with 4 gm talc slurry via the chest drain. The chest drain was removed after three days when drainage was less than 100 ml over 24 hours.

The patient remained asymptomatic for two months, and presented again with shortness of breath and a chest radiograph showed a moderate left pleural effusion. A thoracic ultrasound showed presence of a moderate left pleural effusion with multiple septations (Fig. 13.2B). The white blood cell count and inflammatory markers were normal. Pleural fluid aspiration revealed hemorrhagic fluid. Gram stain was negative and pleural fluid culture was sterile.

Following further informed discussion an IPC was inserted and the drainage technique was taught to the patient and her husband. Symptom directed drainage with vacuum suction bottles was initially performed; however, after two weeks, no drainage was seen from the IPC. A repeat thoracic ultrasound showed presence of a loculated effusion (Fig. 13.2C). As the patient was symptomatic, we performed intrapleural fibrinolysis with urokinase in an attempt to completely drain the MPE. Three doses of 100,000 UI urokinase was instilled through the IPC at 12 hourly intervals. Following the first dose of urokinase the IPC, a total of 800 ml of hemorrhagic fluid was drained. Forty-eight hours following the initial administration of urokinase, an additional 500 ml of hemorrhagic fluid was drained, yielding a total of 1300 ml. There was significant improvement in dyspnea and the chest radiograph showed radiological improvement. IPC drainage was continued weekly and approximately

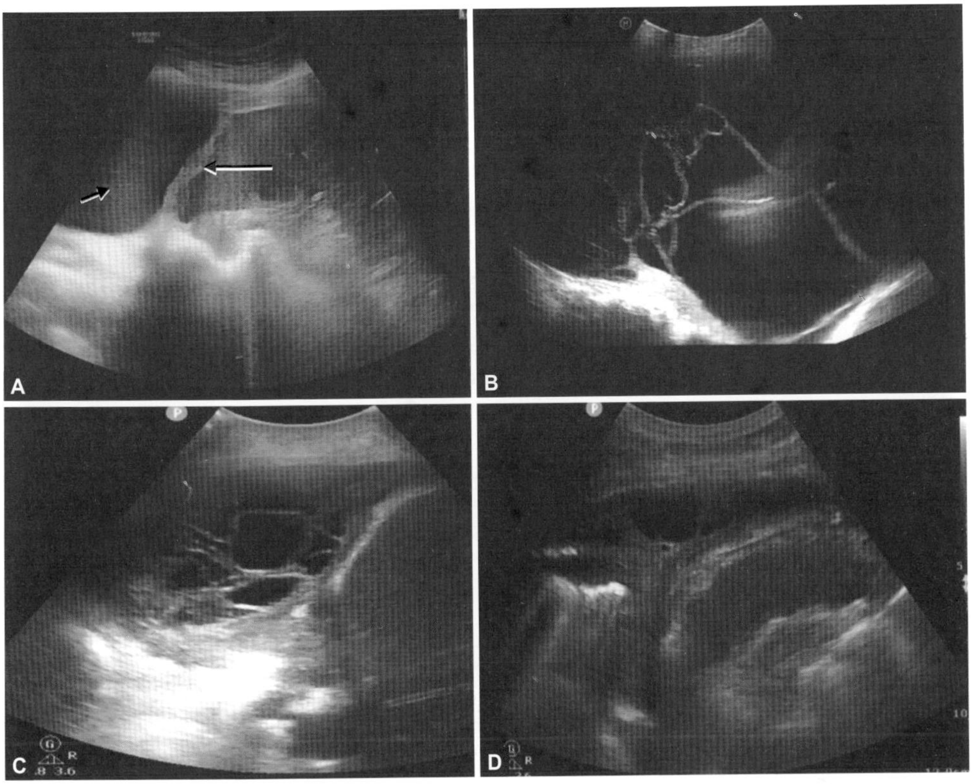

Fig. 13.2: (A) Ultrasound image showing irregular diaphragm (red arrow) along with echogenic pleural fluid (blue arrow); (B) Ultrasound image showing thin septae in left pleural effusion. (C) Ultrasound image showing presence of multiple thin and dense septae within the left pleural effusion. (D) Ultrasound image showing small organized pleural effusion with septae.

400 ml fluid was drained on each occasion. After four weeks, there was gradual decline in IPC drainage and over the following two weeks, each drainage was less than 100 ml. Thoracic ultrasound showed a small loculated pleural effusion (Fig. 13.2D) and lung sliding was absent in the mid-axillary and posterior axillary line, suggesting autopleurodesis, following which the IPC was removed.

DISCUSSION

Malignant pleural effusion represents an advanced stage of cancer. Approximately, 15% of all cancers develop a MPE, and with an increasing trend of global cancer prevalence, it is only expected that the burden of MPE will rise in the future. Currently, there is no cure for MPE and treatment is primarily palliative based on symptom control with the aim of achieving early and successful pleural symphysis.

Treatment options include repeated thoracentesis, insertion of chest drain and indwelling pleural catheters (IPCs) (Table 13.1). Of these, chest drain and indwelling pleural catheters remain choices for 'definitive' management of MPE as pleurodesis can be attempted (Table 13.2). While the former often requires a three to five-day hospital admission, the latter is usually inserted as a day care procedure. With the advent of IPCs, there has been a shift of treatment towards outpatient care to minimise the time spent in hospital.

Table 13.1: Treatment strategies for management of a malignant pleural effusion

Sl.No.	Therapeutic strategy	Indication
1.	Wait and watch strategy	In patients who are asymptomatic/minimally symptomatic
2.	Repeated therapeutic thoracentesis	An option in patients with a very limited life expectancy (< 4 weeks) or when other definitive options for therapy are unavailable. Requires frequent health care visits and not usually a preferred option.
3.	Chest drain placement followed by chemical pleurodesis	One of the preferred options for palliation. It however, necessitates an in-hospital stay for a few days.
4.	Indwelling pleural catheter placement	One of the preferred options for palliation. Can be performed as a day-care procedure. Needs trained and motivated care-givers at home.

Table 13.2: Comparing the strategies-Indwelling pleural catheter versus chest drain and chemical pleurodesis, for managing malignant pleural effusion.

	Chest drain and chemical pleurodesis	Indwelling pleural catheter
Length of in-hospital stay	Longer (3 to 5 days)	Shorter (can be performed as an outpatient procedure)
Availability of equipment	Available in most centers (chest drains and pleurodesis agents-talc, iodopovidone)	Not available in remote/rural areas of the country
Cost of procedure	Lower (may be cost effective in centers where the hospital stay costs are not prohibitive)	Higher cost of catheter and the drainage bottles
Physician expertise	Easy to perform procedure (placement of a chest drain and talc slurry). No extra training needed to manage.	Extra training needed to learn the technique of IPC placement, management of complications and removal of IPC.
Patient/Caregiver training and motivation	Not essential	Need trained caregivers/nurses to take proper care of the IPC.
Utility in the presence of a trapped lung	Cannot be performed	Preferred treatment of choice in the presence of a trapped lung.
Pleural/insertion site infection	Lesser	Higher rate of infectious complications

Chemical Pleurodesis

Pleurodesis, defined as parietal and visceral pleural adhesion with obliteration of the pleural space can be achieved chemically by instillation of a pleurodesis agent or mechanically by surgical abrasion or pleurectomy. For MPE management, chemical pleurodesis can be performed either via an intercostal chest drain or an indwelling pleural catheter. Various pleurodesis agents that have been tried and tested include chemicals (talc, tetracycline, bleomycin and others), bacterial products (*Corynebacterium parvum*, *Streptococcus pyogenes*) and autologous blood patch. In a network meta-analysis, talc was estimated to be the most efficacious agent. It can be administered as a slurry (where talc is mixed with sterile fluid and administered through a chest tube at the bedside), or as a poudrage (performed during medical or surgical thoracoscopy, where it is aerosolised into the pleural cavity as a powder). There is randomised controlled data to show that talc slurry and poudrage are equally effective for pleurodesis and hence a patient should not be subjected to thoracoscopy only for performing pleurodesis. Pleurodesis success with talc (either via slurry or poudrage) has been measured at 70–80% in different clinical trials. However, this may be lower in day to day practice and currently there are no factors to predict pleurodesis success or failure.

Pleurodesis via chest drain should only be performed in the presence of a completely expanded lung. Based on the TIME-1 trial, NSAIDS can be liberally used post pleurodesis as its anti-inflammatory action does not impede pleurodesis, and small (<16 Fr) drains should be avoided for pleurodesis.

Indwelling Pleural Catheters

Since their approval by the US FDA in 1999, IPCs have revolutionised MPE management. Inserted on a daycare basis, these catheters are tunnelled subcutaneously which allows them to remain *in situ* for months. Using vacuum bottles with a one-way valve, IPC drainage flow and volume can be controlled. TIME-2 and AMPLE were RCTs comparing chest drain and pleurodesis versus IPC. The results were re-assuring as both interventions improved dyspnea with no difference in the mean visual analogue scale (VAS) for dyspnea at 30 or 42 days after intervention with hospital stay being less in the IPC arm. IPCs have been associated with 'auto-pleurodesis', simply due to having an IPC *in situ*. The mechanism is unclear, but may be attributed to the presence of a foreign body in the pleural cavity causing low grade pleural irritation. Large randomised trials of IPC with autopleurodesis as the primary outcome have shown success rates of 11–24%.

IPCs are typically drained three times a week or based on symptoms. The ASAP and AMPLE-2 trials showed that aggressive drainage (daily drainage) increased rates of auto-pleurodesis (from 24 to 47% in ASAP at 3 months and 11 to 37% in AMPLE-2 at 2 months). AMPLE-2 also showed that if IPC insertion is only for palliative purposes then drainage when the patient is only symptomatic should suffice.

For IPCs, the concept of either auto-pleurodesis or chemical pleurodesis is very attractive as it facilitates removal of the catheter. Chemical pleurodesis via the IPC was tested in the IPC-Plus trial. In this single blind multicentre RCT, 154 patients were randomised to receive either 4 g of talc slurry or placebo at day 10 via the IPC, after four drainages since insertion and a chest radiograph showing at least three quarters pleural apposition. At day 35, 43% patients in the talc group had successful pleurodesis as compared to 23% in the placebo group, representing an almost two-fold increase

IPCs are also associated with high rates of complications—particularly pleural infection. In a large multi-center study of 1021 patients, pleural infection rates were 4.9%. However, this data is entirely from studies in the west. There is a hypothetical possibility of higher IPC related pleural infection rates in our country possibly due to variable hygiene practices, lack of community nurse support for IPC drainage and lack of physician training for IPC insertion and management of complications. However, no robust data is available yet.

IPCs remain the treatment of choice for non-expandable or trapped lung, defined as the inability of the lung to expand to the chest wall preventing visceral and parietal pleura apposition. Unexpanded lung can be due to either visceral pleural disease, endobronchial obstruction or chronic atelectasis, and is seen in approximately 30% of patients with MPE.

Management of a Loculated Malignant Pleural Effusion

Septations within a MPE can be a challenging situation for clinicians as seen in our patient. Pleural fluid septations develop due to activation of the coagulation cascade, resulting in deposition of fibrin to form fibrin sheets and are associated with higher levels of systemic inflammation and pleural fluid metabolic activity. Septations may be thin which do not form barriers to drainage or may be thick and dense which impede pleural fluid drainage. Septations can be seen in 15% of patients with MPE which hinders drainage and are associated with a poorer prognosis.

The Multicenter Intrapleural Sepsis Trial (MIST2 Trial) demonstrated the benefit of the use of intrapleural fibrinolytics (t-PA and DNase) in patients with infected complex pleural effusions. However, this benefit is not established in patients with septated MPEs. Since then, few studies have evaluated the use of intrapleural fibrinolytics (urokinase or streptokinase) in the management of septated or complex MPE, with variable success results. There is no data to suggest timing of fibrinolytic therapy in septated MPE, but our clinical practice demonstrates that thin freely flowing septa respond better than thick matured adhesions and hence use of fibrinolytics should be decided on a case by case basis depending on patient symptoms and the ultrasound appearance.

Management Algorithm for Malignant Pleural Effusion

In the current era there are various management options for MPE and in our setting we need to develop our own low cost indigenous way of MPE management (Fig. 13.3). It may not be possible to replicate the Western model given our heterogeneous healthcare model and sociocultural and economic differences. Various factors including patient preference, financial constraints, resources and the availability of the appropriate expertise need to be taken into consideration.

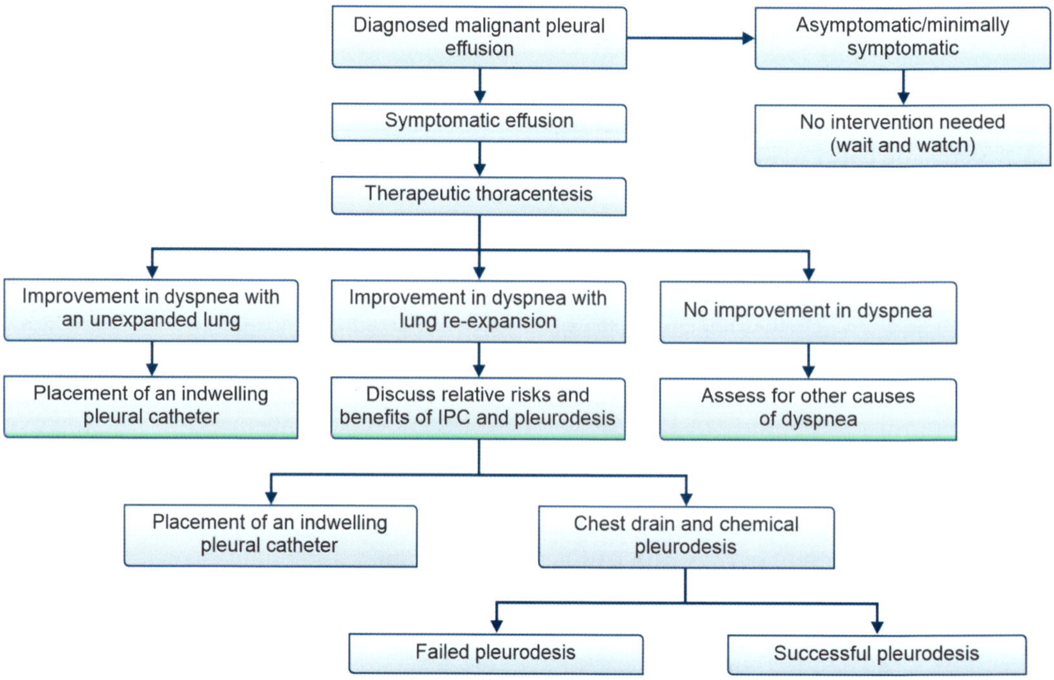

Fig. 13.3: Proposed management algorithm for management of malignant pleural effusions.

While IPCs remain the treatment of choice in patients with a trapped lung, in the absence of one, patients should be given the option of chest drain and pleurodesis versus IPC as patients may find the latter restrictive in their lifestyle with a plastic tube attached to their chest wall and frequent drainages. Pros and cons of each of the interventions should be discussed in depth and the patient should be allowed to then make an informed decision. In our setting it is imperative that patients and their families are taught IPC care and aseptic drainage strategies as any shortcomings in these can lead to disastrous complications of pleural infection. Attempts should be made to remove the IPC early to prevent complications and this can be facilitated by initial aggressive drainage with possible combination of chemical pleurodesis via the IPC. A cost effectiveness analysis is much needed to assess feasibility of IPCs for MPE management in our country. It is also important for physicians who are dealing with IPCs to be well trained not only with insertion, but should also be able to troubleshoot other aspects such as blockage, management of pleural infection and septated collections, and removal of the IPC.

FURTHER READING

1. Rahman NM, Pepperell J, Rehal S, Saba T, Tang A, Ali N, et al. Effect of Opioids vs NSAIDs and Larger vs Smaller Chest Tube Size on Pain Control and Pleurodesis Efficacy Among Patients With Malignant Pleural Effusion: The TIME1 Randomized Clinical Trial. JAMA. 2015;314(24):2641–53.
2. Davies HE, Mishra EK, Kahan BC, Wrightson JM, Stanton AE, Guhan A, et al. Effect of an indwelling pleural catheter vs chest tube and talc pleurodesis for relieving dyspnea in patients with malignant pleural effusion: the TIME2 randomized controlled trial. JAMA. 2012;307(22):2383–9.
3. Banka R, Terrington D, Mishra EK. Management of Septated Malignant Pleural Effusions. Curr Pulmonol Rep. 2018;7(1):1–5.
4. Mishra EK, Clive AO, Wills GH, Davies HE, Stanton AE, Al-Aloul M, et al. Randomized Controlled Trial of Urokinase versus Placebo for Nondraining Malignant Pleural Effusion. Am J Respir Crit Care Med. 2018;197(4):502–8.
5. Roberts ME, Rahman NM, Maskell NA, et al. British Thoracic Society Guideline for pleural disease. Thorax. 2023;78(Suppl 3):s1-s42.

Chapter 14

Approach to a Case with Persistent Air Leak

• *Arvindran Alaga* • *Chan Tha A Hing*

LEARNING POINTS

1. An air leak which persists beyond 5 days is considered a persistent air leak (PAL).
2. Persistent air leaks can be classified either as alveolar-pleural fistulae (APF) or broncho-pleural fistulae (BPF) based on the level at which the airways communicate with the pleural space.
3. Conservative management can be used for most APF air leaks. An ambulatory drain can reduce hospital stay while waiting for spontaneous resolution or surgical intervention, thereby potentially reducing healthcare costs.
4. There are several non-surgical approaches via bronchoscopy or thoracoscopy for closure of PAL with variable success rates.

INTRODUCTION

A persistent air leak (PAL) is defined as an air leak that persists for more than 5 days. An alveolar-pleural fistula creates a communication between the alveoli and the pleural space, leading to the development of pneumothorax as air escapes the lung into the pleural cavity. If this connection persists, there will be a continuous flow of air from the lung parenchyma to the pleural space, worsening the pneumothorax. The presence of an air leak is indicated by air bubbling into the chest drainage system once a chest tube is inserted. This airflow through the fistulous tract into the pleural space delays healing and inhibits lung expansion. Although the majority of air leaks resolve spontaneously with thoracostomy tube drainage, many continue to remain for days after the lung injury.

CASE VIGNETTE

A 50-year-old man with end-stage renal disease (ESRD) on regular dialysis via a brachiocephalic fistula (BCF) presented with complaints of feeling unwell for 1 month with a worsening cough and a fever for 5 days. He visited the emergency department as his dyspnea worsened. The chest radiograph revealed a hydropneumothorax (Fig. 14.1). A 24 Fr chest tube was inserted, and the patient was treated for a complicated parapneumonic effusion with pneumothorax.

Pleural fluid investigation revealed an exudative effusion, and pleural fluid culture grew *Klebsiella pneumoniae*. The recovery was complicated by a persistent air leak (PAL), and a computed tomography (CT) scan of the thorax revealed thick enhancing pleura, a hydropneumothorax and suspicion of a bronchopleural fistula (Fig. 14.2).

A cardiothoracic (CTC) referral was made and in the meantime the patient was fitted with a P-Eggy drain and discharged with oral antibiotics for 4 weeks. The P-Eggy is an innovative device that simplifies the management of spontaneous pneumothorax and persistent air leaks (Fig. 14.3). The P-Eggy Drain can be directly connected to any chest catheter, providing a safe and cost-effective outcome. It allows drainage of air, and also prevents air from returning to the patient via

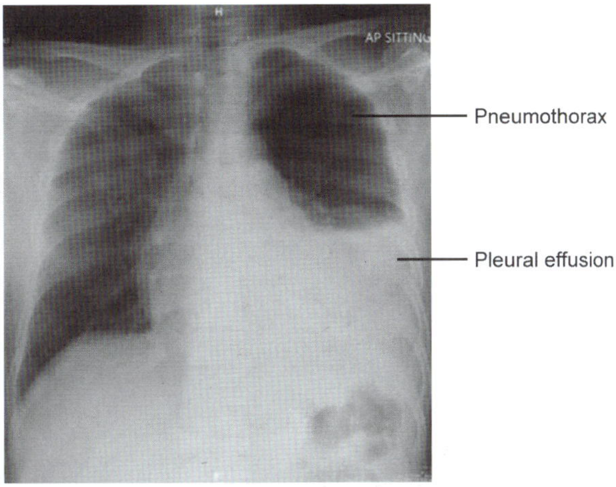

Fig. 14.1: Chest radiograph (CXR) on admission showing the presence of a hydropneumothorax

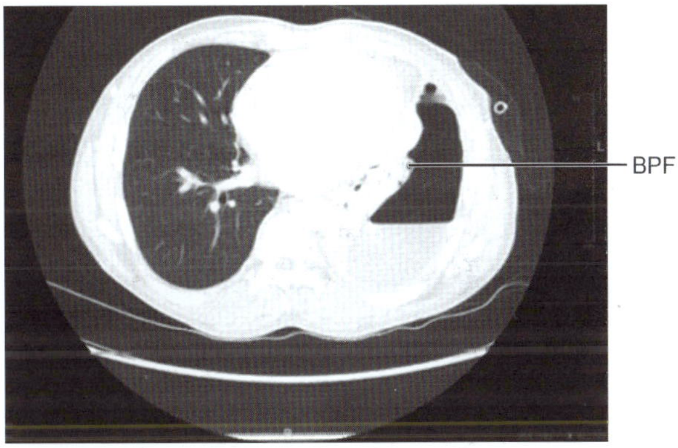

Fig. 14.2: Image of the computed tomography of thorax showing left hydropneumothorax with a bronchopleural fistula (BPF)

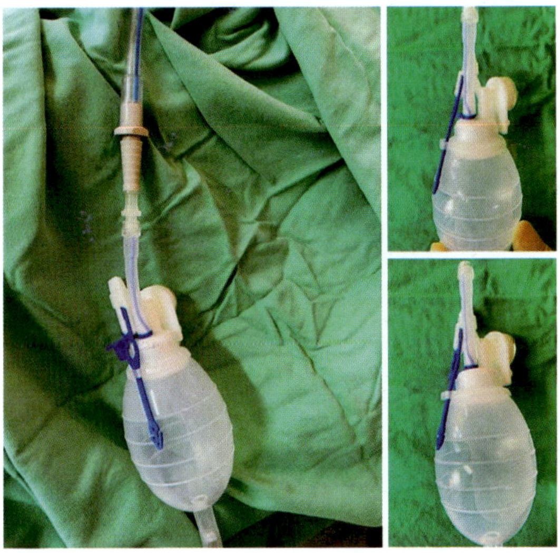

Fig. 14.3: P-Eggy drain (works on the principle of a Heimlich valve)

a one-way valve mechanism This provides a solution for outpatient management in such scenarios. Upon review by the CTC team, the patient opted for conservative management. The PAL resolved after 2 weeks of the P-Eggy drain use.

DISCUSSION

Definition and Causes

In 2001, the American College of Chest Physicians recommended observation with a chest tube for 5 days for the spontaneous closure of air leak/fistulas. Air leaks which fail to spontaneously close by 5 days are considered as persistent air leaks (PALs).

Air leaks are further classified as alveolar pleural fistulae (APF) or bronchopleural fistulae (BPF). It is important to understand the differences between APF and BPF as the management strategy differs (Table 14.1). Most BPFs arise after surgical resection, do not heal spontaneously and would require a surgical or a bronchoscopic intervention to close the fistula. On the other hand APFs occur due to surgical and non-surgical causes, majority heal conservatively and an intervention to close the air leak would be required only in a subset of non-responding leaks.

Quantification of Air Leak

It is important to quantify an air leak, both to monitor its intensity over days, and to predict if it is likely to heal conservatively or will require an intervention to close the leak. There are several ways to quantify/grade an air leak.

1. Qualitative assessment: The simplest way to classify and grade PAL is to use the Cerfolio classification (Table 14.2). A forced expiratory (FE) leak is a smaller leak when compared to an Expiratory (E) leak, which is a smaller leak when compared to a continuous (C) leak.

Table 14.1: Differences between alveolar pleural fistula and bronchopleural fistula

	Alveolar pleural fistula (APF)	*Broncho pleural fistula (BPF)*
Definition	A pathologic communication between lung parenchyma distal to segmental bronchus and the pleural space	A pathologic communication between the main stem, lobar or segmental bronchus and the pleural space.
Common causes	Secondary spontaneous pneumothorax in cases with emphysema or a fibrotic lung disease. Post-surgical (lung volume reduction surgeries/ wedge resections) Post-thoracic trauma Necrotizing pneumonias	Post-lung resection surgeries (pneumonectomy, lobectomy, segmentectomy) Necrotizing pneumonias Malignancy associated BPF
Quantification of air leak	Usually mild (Cerfolio FE or E grade)	Can be mild or severe
Spontaneous closure of the air leak	Most cases resolve spontaneously with time.	Spontaneous closure is unlikely. Most cases will need an intervention (surgical or bronchoscopic closure)

FE: Forced expiratory; *E:* Expiratory

Table 14.2: Cerfolio classification of air leaks		
Grade	*Type of air leak*	*Description/characteristics*
Grade 1	FE (forced expiration)	Air leak occurs during forced expiration only, often when the patient is asked to cough.
Grade 2	E (expiratory only)	Air leak is present during expiration.
Grade 3	I (inspiratory only)	Air leak occurs only during inspiration. This pattern is seen when the PAL occurs in patients on mechanical positive pressure ventilation
Grade 4	C (continuous)	Continuous bubbling in the air leak chamber during both inspiration and expiration. This is also common in patients on positive-pressure ventilation.

2. **Semi-quantitative assessment:** Several commercial chest drainage systems (e.g: Sinapi chest drain, Atrium chest drain) are available which can measure air leak on a scale from 1 to 7. The higher the number, the greater the leak.
3. **Quantitative assessment:** Several digital chest drainage systems (e.g: Thopaz device by Medela) are available which will quantify the flow of air as mL/min. They work by applying negative suction to maintain a steady intrapleural pressure within 0.1 cm H_2O. These drains can be removed once the air leak flow is less than 20 mL/min for at least six hours.

Management Strategy for PAL

Three major factors to consider when initially evaluating an air leak are the volume, duration, and trend of the leak. For example, a larger air leak that has been present for a longer time without any improvement has a low likelihood of resolution, whereas a smaller air leak that is improving daily is more likely to resolve spontaneously. In the absence of a bronchopleural fistula, when the underlying cause of the air leak is treated, most air leaks (up to 80%) will resolve over time, even if that time spans weeks.

The treatment options for managing a PAL due to an alveolo pleural fistula include (A) Conservative approach; (B) Bronchoscopic intervention to identify and close the air leak; (C) Surgical closure of the PAL.

1. **Conservative approach to management of a PAL:** A chest drain is placed for all cases with a PAL. Treatment of the pleural space infection and underlying pulmonary infection (if any) is essential. In case of a APF, while awaiting the leak to spontaneously close, patients can be discharged with an ambulatory one-way valve device. Several commercial ambulatory devices (Heimlich valve, pneumostat device, P-Eggy device) are available for home-based management of a pneumothorax and air leaks. These will reduce the length of hospital stay.

   Application of negative suction to the chest drain is also widely practiced and there are two differing schools of thought. Some feel that application of low pressure negative suction promotes apposition of visceral and parietal pleura and this aids in closure of fistula. Others feel that application of suction promotes continued patency of the air leak. It is suggested that negative suction should not be applied when there is incomplete lung expansion.

Table 14.3: Anecdotal approaches to bronchoscopic closure of a persistent air leak.

Method	*Type of Study/No. of Patients*	*Air Leak Improved or Resolved*	*Complications*
Fibrin sealant (bronchoscopy)	3 case reports (1 patient each)	3 of 3	None reported
Fibrin sealant (thoracoscopy)	Case series (12 patients)	11 of 12	None reported
Platelet gel	Case report (1 patient)	1 of 1	None reported
Ethanolamine	2 case series (15 and 5 patients)	12 of 15, 5 of 5	First series: Fever, chest pain, pulmonary infiltrates, hydropneumothorax; Second series: None reported
Metal coils	Case series (5 patients)	4 of 5	None reported
Watanabe spigots	Case series (60 patients)	58 of 60	Pneumonia, dyspnea, fever
Laser	Case series (13 patients)	11 of 13	None reported
Synthetic hydrogel	Case series (22 patients)	19 of 22	Hydrogel expectoration, hypoxia

Please note that the complications for ethanolamine were specific to the first case series (fever, chest pain, pulmonary infiltrates, hydropneumothorax) with none reported in the second series.

Adapted from: Dugan et al, Management of persistent air leaks. Chest. 2017 Aug 1;152(2):417–23.

2. **Bronchoscopic closure of a PAL:** Bronchoscopic closure of APF/BPF can be considered in centers with experience in performing these procedures. The first step is to localise the air leak to a segment(s) using sequential balloon occlusion of the airways. Decrease in air leak by >50% when an occlusion balloon is applied is an indicator for the presence of air leak from that segment. Another technique to localise the air leak is to instil methylene blue dye into the chest drain while simultaneously visualizing the airways using a bronchoscope. In case of a BPF, direct opening of the fistulous bronchial opening can be identified by using thin bronchoscopes. Once the target segment/fistulous site is identified, the opening can be sealed using several approaches. Commonly used blocking devices include commercially available Watanabe endobronchial spigots, customised spigots using silicone stents, one-way endobronchial valves, amplatzer devices (for larger BPF), and others (Table 14.3).
3. **Surgical closure of a PAL:** All patients with a PAL that persists beyond 5 days should be evaluated for surgery to close the air leak, followed by pleurodesis to prevent recurrence. Surgical closure is the treatment of choice for closure of BPF. For APF, surgical intervention is performed when conservative approach fails. Surgical techniques for closure of APF include stapling of parenchymal lesions and application of sealants/fibrin mesh.

Other techniques which have been tried for closure of PAL include autologous blood patch pleurodesis and chemical pleurodesis. In the presence of an air leak, chemical pleurodesis with talc slurry or doxycycline is generally not recommended due to the parenchymal toxicity of sclerosing agents.

FURTHER READING

1. Roberts ME, Rahman NM, Maskell NA, Bibby AC, Blyth KG, Corcoran JP, Edey A, Evison M, de Fonseka D, Hallifax R, Harden S. British Thoracic Society guideline for pleural disease. Thorax. 2023 Aug 8.
2. Dugan KC, Laxmanan B, Murgu S, Hogarth DK. Management of persistent air leaks. Chest. 2017 Aug 1;152(2):417–23.
3. Sakata KK, Reisenauer JS, Kern RM, Mullon JJ. Persistent air leak - review. Respir Med. 2018 Apr;137: 213–218.
4. Lazarus DR, Casal RF. Persistent air leaks: a review with an emphasis on bronchoscopic management. J Thorac Dis. 2017 Nov;9(11):4660–4670.
5. Duron G, Backer E, Feller-Kopman D. Evaluation and management of persistent air leak. Expert Rev Respir Med. 2023 Jul-Dec;17(10):865–872.

SECTION IV

Critical Care Medicine

Chapter

15

Approach to a Patient with Hypoxia and a Normal Chest Radiograph

• *Naresh Chandra* • *Venkat Raman Kola* • *V Nagarjuna Maturu*

LEARNING POINTS

1. Several disease states can lead to respiratory failure but have a normal chest radiograph (CXR). Diseases of pulmonary vasculature /airways or interstitium may not have abnormal findings on a chest radiograph.
2. Presence of a normal CXR does not rule out significant pulmonary pathology.
3. Arterial blood gas analysis, 2D echocardiography and a high-resolution computer tomography (HRCT) chest help in identifying the correct etiology when there is respiratory failure and a normal chest radiograph.
4. Failure of supplemental oxygen to improve oxygen levels indicate the presence of right to left shunt or an abnormal hemoglobin.
5. Presence of a saturation gap (>5%) is a clue to the presence of abnormal hemoglobins.

INTRODUCTION

Hypoxia and hypoxemia are terms often used interchangeably in clinical practice, yet they describe distinct physiological conditions. Hypoxia refers to reduced oxygen availability or utilization by body tissues, regardless of the cause. Hypoxemia, on the other hand, specifically denotes a decrease in the oxygen content of the blood.

Managing hypoxemia may involve interventions such as oxygen therapy or ventilatory support. However, addressing hypoxia effectively requires a thorough understanding of its etiology and pathophysiology. This is especially challenging in cases where hypoxia presents with normal lung parenchyma on chest radiograph, necessitating a comprehensive and detailed evaluation to determine the underlying causes. Here we discuss two clinical scenarios with hypoxemia and normal chest imaging.

CASE VIGNETTE 1

A 58-year-old female patient presented with a sudden onset of breathlessness and desaturation, which progressively worsened over hours, necessitating mechanical ventilation. She had tachycardia (pulse rate of 124 per minute) and a normal blood pressure. The patient's medical history was significant for polytrauma, including a right-sided mid-shaft femur fracture, which had been surgically fixed one week prior to presentation.

Upon physical examination, normal vesicular breath sounds were noted in all lung fields. A chest X-ray was performed at admission which did not reveal any abnormality. However, a 2D echocardiogram revealed right ventricular dilatation and pulmonary hypertension (PH). Given the clinical history, and hypoxemia with a normal CXR, a possibility of pulmonary embolism (PE) was considered. An urgent CT pulmonary angiography (CTPA) was performed (Fig. 15.1), which confirmed the presence of a large saddle pulmonary embolism.

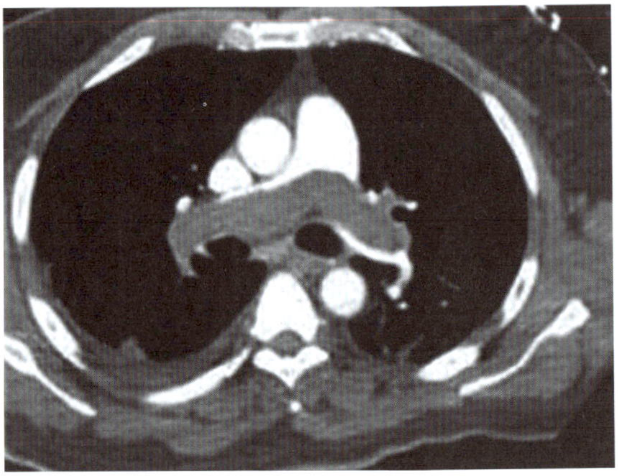

Fig. 15.1: Axial section of CT pulmonary angiogram showing a large saddle thrombus in the main pulmonary artery.

She then underwent catheter-directed embolectomy, supplemented by catheter guided fibrinolytic therapy. This approach was chosen as there was a high possibility of bleeding due to systemic thrombolysis (in consideration of the patient's recent history of polytrauma and surgical interventions). Subsequently, systemic anticoagulation was initiated using low-molecular-weight heparin (LMWH). Her respiratory failure gradually improved over the next 48 hours. She was weaned off the ventilator and was discharged home on oral anticoagulants.

CASE VIGNETTE 2

An 18-year-old girl was scheduled for an elective hemorrhoidectomy to treat thrombosed hemorrhoids. The procedure was planned under saddle block anesthesia. Upon arrival in the operating room, the patient was connected to standard monitoring equipment. Baseline vital signs, including heart rate and blood pressure, were within normal limits. However, pulse oximetry revealed an oxygen saturation of only 85%, despite the patient being asymptomatic with a respiratory rate of 18/min.

Initial attempts to increase oxygen saturation through supplemental oxygen were unsuccessful, even with gradual increases in oxygen flow. Consequently, the decision was made to defer the surgery and initiate further diagnostic investigations due to persisting desaturation.

Arterial blood gas (ABG) analysis, performed while the patient was receiving 4 liters of oxygen, showed a pO_2 of 294 mm Hg, a pCO_2 of 39 mm Hg and oxygen saturation of 99%. pH, bicarbonate, and lactate levels were within normal ranges. At the time ABG was performed, saturation on pulse oximeter was showing as 85% (saturation gap of 14%). A comprehensive review of the pre-operative evaluation revealed no new clinical findings. Additional tests, including a 2D-echocardiogram, electrocardiogram (ECG), and chest X-ray, were conducted, all of which did not indicate any obvious infective or non-infectious etiologies.

Given the findings of low oxygen saturation with a normal CXR, pulmonary thromboembolism was considered as a differential diagnosis. D-dimer levels were elevated;

however, this was deemed unreliable due to the presence of thrombosed hemorrhoids. A CT pulmonary angiogram was subsequently performed, which did not show any features of pulmonary embolism. It also confirmed normal lung parenchyma. The patient's desaturation persisted without accompanying symptoms.

In view of the fact that the supplemental oxygen did not improve oxygen levels, a high index of suspicion led to the consideration of an alternative diagnosis: Methemoglobinemia. Testing for serum methemoglobin levels revealed a significantly elevated methemoglobin level of 18%. As there was no preceding infection or drug exposure and the fact that there were no clinical symptoms, she was diagnosed as having congenital Methemoglobinemia. She was counselled appropriately and was sent home with a rescheduled date for elective surgery.

DISCUSSION

The two cases described above illustrate two causes of respiratory failure where the individual has low oxygen saturations but a normal chest radiograph (CXR). Approach to a case where there is hypoxemia and a normal CXR needs a systematic approach. There are several diseases which can lead to respiratory failure but with a normal appearing CXR (Table 15.1). Investigations which help in confirming the cause include:

A. Arterial blood gas (ABG) analysis with (A-a)D O_2 assessment
B. High resolution CT chest (with or without contrast)
C. 2D-echo (with bubble contrast)
D. Co-oximetry
E. Ability of supplemental oxygen to improve oxygen levels
F. Spirometry (when feasible)

A brief description of the disease states which can lead to hypoxemia in the presence of a normal CXR is given below.

A. Vascular Causes of Hypoxemia

Pulmonary vascular disease can lead to hypoxemia in the presence of normal CXR. Acute onset hypoxemia in the presence of a normal CXR should always raise the suspicion of a pulmonary thromboembolism. ABG shows type 1 respiratory failure. A 2D-echocardiogram and a contrast CT scan help in confirmation of pulmonary thromboembolism as the cause of respiratory failure.

B. Right to Left Shunts

Right to left shunts cause hypoxemia due to blood bypassing the pulmonary capillary bed. The right to left shunt can be intrapulmonary (pulmonary AV malformations, hepato-pulmonary syndrome) or intracardiac (atrial septal defect, patent foramen ovale with right to left shunt). These are also one of the causes of hypoxemia with a normal CXR. Initial clue to the presence of a vascular shunt is the inability of supplemental oxygen to improve the oxygen saturation. When the shunts are in basal regions of the lung, patients may also have platypnea-orthodeoxia syndrome.

A right to left shunt is confirmed by a bubble contrast 2D-echocardiography, 99mTc macro-aggregated albumin (MAA) labelled nuclear scan or a pulmonary angiogram. Appearance of bubbles in the left heart within 3 cycles (intracardiac shunt) or after 3 cycles (intrapulmonary shunt) on bubble contrast 2D-echo confirms the presence of a right to left shunt.

Table 15.1: Causes of hypoxemia with a normal lung parenchyma on a chest radiograph

Cause	*Diseases*	*Clues/tests to diagnose*
Pulmonary vascular cause of hypoxemia	• Pulmonary thromboembolism • Pulmonary arterial hypertension • Pulmonary A-V fistulae	• Careful examination for features of pulmonary hypertension on a CXR • 2D-echo will identify elevated right heart pressures • When in doubt, perform a CT pulmonary angiogram
Right to left shunt physiology	• Pulmonary arteriovenous malformations • Intracardiac right to left shunt	• Failure of supplemental oxygen to improve oxygen saturation should raise the suspicion of a shunt physiology • A bubble contrast 2D-echo will aid in identification of a right to left shunt
Interstitial diseases with predominant ground glass opacities	• *Pneumocystis jirovecii* pneumonia • Viral pneumonia (H1N1, COVID) • NSIP pattern ILD	• A HRCT chest will identify ground glass opacities which may be missed on a CXR, and will help in diagnosing the cause
Neuromuscular/ central causes of respiratory failure	• Morbid obesity • Neuromuscular diseases leading to respiratory muscle involvement (myasthenic crisis, neuroparalytic snake bite, GBS) • Central suppression of respiratory drive (drug overdose, CO_2 narcosis)	• Presence of type 2 respiratory failure (elevated $PaCO_2$) with a normal (A-a)DO_2 should raise the suspicion of a neuromuscular or a central cause of respiratory failure
Airway obstruction leading to respiratory failure	• Central airway obstruction • Diseases causing peripheral airway obstruction (asthma/ bronchiolitis)	• Presence of type 2 respiratory failure with an elevated (A-a) DO_2 • Careful examination of CXR can show features of hyperinflated lung fields • Spirometry and a biphasic HRCT chest (inspiratory and expiratory) help in confirming obstruction
Presence of abnormal hemoglobins	• Methemoglobinemia • Sulfhemoglobinemia • Carboxyhemoglobinemia	• Presence of oxygen saturation gap • Inability of supplemental oxygen to improve oxygen saturation • Co-oximetry will help in identifying the abnormal hemoglobin

C. Interstitial Causes of Hypoxemia

Acute interstitial lung diseases and viral infections cause ground glass opacities (GGO) on a HRCT chest which are not seen on a CXR. When the GGOs are diffuse, there can be respiratory failure. However, as the GGOs are not seen on a CXR, the CXR will appear normal. Hence when a person has type 1 respiratory failure with a normal CXR, a possibility of acute interstitial lung disease (infective or non-infective) needs to be considered and a HRCT chest needs to be performed. It is also widely believed that in a HIV positive individual if there is subacute history of fever and respiratory failure with a normal CXR, a possibility of *Pneumocystis jirovecii* pneumonia needs to be considered.

D. Neuromuscular/Central Cause of Respiratory Failure

These are another group of diseases where there is respiratory failure with a normal CXR. When there is a neuromuscular or a central cause of respiratory failure, it is usually a Type 2 respiratory failure (T2RF)-elevated $PaCO_2$ and a low PaO_2. Another important differentiating feature for this group of diseases from intrinsic lung parenchymal/airway/vascular and interstitial diseases is the presence of a normal alveolar-arterial oxygen gradient (P(A-a) DO_2).

P(A-a) DO_2, which indicates the difference between the partial pressures of oxygen in alveolar gas and arterial blood, is a crucial tool for differentiating between the various causes of type 2 respiratory failure. An airway cause of T2RF has an elevated p(A-a) DO_2, whereas a neuromuscular cause of T2RF will have a normal p(A-a) DO_2.

E. Obstructive Airway Causes of Respiratory Failure

Presence of a central airway obstruction or an extensive small airway disease also can lead to respiratory failure with a normal CXR. These diseases also lead to T2RF but with an elevated p(A-a) DO_2. Presence of wheeze/stridor on auscultation and an obstructive physiology on spirometry will help in diagnosis. A biphasic (inspiratory and an expiratory) HRCT chest can identify otherwise occult small airway disease, and also help in identifying diseases of central airways which may not be otherwise visible on a CXR.

F. Presence of Abnormal Hemoglobin

Presence of high levels of less common hemoglobin variants like methemoglobin, sulfhemoglobin and carboxy hemoglobin can also show a low SpO_2 and with a normal CXR. In the presence of methemoglobin and sulfhemoglobin, a normal pulse oximeter will show a low SpO_2. However, when an ABG is performed the oxygen saturation (SaO_2) is normal. Presence of this **saturation gap** (low SpO_2 and a higher/normal SaO_2) greater than 5% is a clue to identifying the presence of such abnormal hemoglobins. Another clue to identifying these abnormal hemoglobins is the inability of supplemental oxygen to improve SpO_2. These diseases lower the oxygen carrying capacity of blood and lead to anemic hypoxia (Table 15.2) A high index of suspicion is needed to diagnose these conditions.

Methemoglobinemia

Normally, a minute quantity of methemoglobin is constantly formed during normal oxygenation and deoxygenation of hemoglobin. Methemoglobin is incapable of carrying oxygen because oxidized ferric iron cannot bind to it. NADH cytochrome b5 reductase 3 (NADH-methemoglobin reductase) pathway normally limits its accumulation to only 1% of the entire hemoglobin. Any amplification in methemoglobin level will result in obtunded delivery of oxygen to the tissues.

Individuals with methemoglobin levels less than 25% are by and for the most part asymptomatic. If the methemoglobin level increases to more than 30% of total hemoglobin, cyanosis (bluish discoloration of skin and mucous membranes) and symptoms of hypoxia

Table 15.2: Types of hypoxia and the causes

	Definition	*Possible causes*
Hypoxic hypoxia	Tissue hypoxia due to impaired oxygenation of blood (low PaO_2 and SpO_2).	• Any disease leading to pulmonary airway/interstitial/vascular/ neuromuscular cause of respiratory failure
Anemic hypoxia	Tissue hypoxia due to low oxygen carrying capacity of blood	• Anemia • Carbon monoxide poisoning • Sickle cell anemia • Met and Sulfhemoglobinemia
Histotoxic hypoxia	Tissue hypoxia due to impaired ability of tissues to utilize the delivered oxygen	• Cyanide poisoning • Beri beri disease
Stagnant/Ischemic hypoxia	Tissue hypoxia due to poor blood flow to the tissue and not due to low oxygen content of the blood	• Cardiogenic shock • Hemorrhagic shock • Septic shock

(dyspnea, headache, vertigo, change in mental status) occur. Levels of methemoglobin beyond 50% can lead to coma and death. With high levels of methemoglobin, the blood takes on a chocolate brown color and does not revert back to normal red color after oxygen contact.

Methemoglobinemia can be acquired or hereditary. The acquired form, also called toxic methemoglobinemia, occurs in normal individuals after exposure to an exogenous oxidant, such as nitrites, primaquine, dapsone or benzocaine. As the oxidant exhausts the hemoglobin reduction systems, the concentration of methemoglobin steeply rises and the patient may exhibit cyanosis and symptoms of hypoxia. Withdrawal of the offending oxidant is adequate for recovery in most of the cases, but if the level of methemoglobin increases to 30% or more of total hemoglobin, intravenous methylene blue (1–2 mg/kg) is administered, and repeated as necessary with due monitoring. Methylene blue acts by reducing methemoglobin ferric iron to the ferrous state. In life-threatening cases however, the options will be limited to exchange transfusion.

Co-oximeter: Co-oximetry is the diagnostic tool of choice to identify the presence of abnormal hemoglobins. Methemoglobin shows a peak absorption at 630 nm. Co-oximeter analyzers quantify hemoglobin oxygen saturation in a blood sample. A Co-oximeter uses between four and eight different wavelengths of light, the majority between 475 nm and 600 nm, to quantify the fractions of all relevant species of hemoglobin. Values usually reported comprise total hemoglobin (tHb), oxyhemoglobin (O_2Hb), deoxyhemoglobin (HHb), methemoglobin (MetHb), and carboxyhemoglobin (COHb).

Most co-oximeters do not recognize sulfhemoglobin. If sulfhemoglobinemia is suspected due to applicable toxin ingestion, care should be taken when interpreting values provided by co-oximetry. Sulfhemoglobinemia can cause a falsely elevated result for methemoglobin and a falsely decreased result for carboxyhemoglobin.

Co-oximeter estimates the hematocrit (HCT) based on the electricity transmitted through the sample. The co-oximeter then uses a standard calculation to determine the tHb from the

HCT. Once the co-oximeter has determined tHb, the percentages of tHb that are oxy-, de-, carboxy-, and methemoglobins are calculated. The co-oximeter directly measures each of the species' concentrations via spectrometric means and then reports them in percentages of tHb. For example, carboxyhemoglobin percentage would be calculated as:

$$COHb,\% = (COHb/tHb) \times 100$$

Many co-oximeters are combined with basic analyzers that also provide blood gas values, metabolites, and electrolytes. Some also report calculated values such as the alveolar-arterial oxygen gradient, bicarbonate concentration, and base deficit, which makes these machines good all-purpose analyzers for an intensive care setting or emergency department.

Approach to an Individual with Respiratory Failure and a Normal CXR

Figure 15.2 shows a simple algorithm to narrow down the differentials when a person presents with low SpO_2 in the presence of a normal CXR. Subtle clues on a CXR will help in pointing towards a possible etiology (Table 15.3). A good understanding of the physiology of oxygen diffusion and delivery is important when we interpret the tests in the correct clinical context.

Interventions have to be tailored to the case history and case scenario. Inability to anticipate or identify causes of hypoxia would either delay the appropriate treatment or worse still lead to false diagnosis and misdirected investigations and unfruitful treatments eventually leading to delay in time sensitive treatment options.

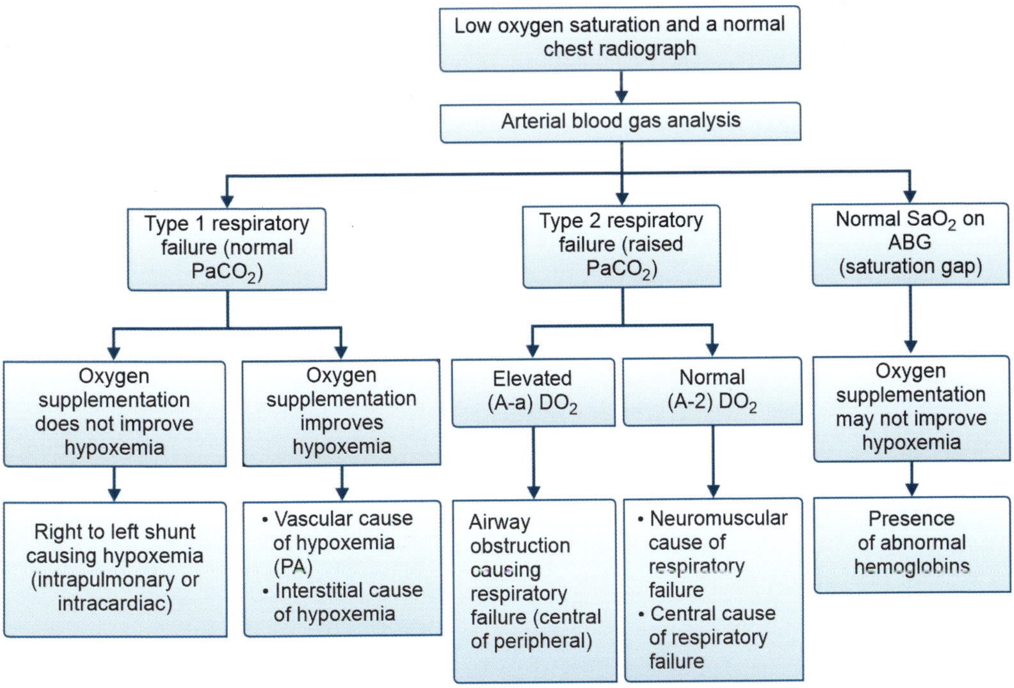

Fig. 15.2: An algorithm to approach a patient with low oxygen saturation and a normal chest radiograph

Table 15.3: Subtle clues on a chest radiograph which help in identifying the cause of hypoxemia

Chest radiographic finding	*Description*	*Clinical implication*
Prominent right descending pulmonary artery (RDPA)	RDPA >14 mm in females and >16 mm in males is suggestive of dilated RDPA	Pulmonary hypertension
Prominent hilum and a straight left heart border	Hilar prominence with a positive hilum convergence sign is an indicator of vascular cause of hilar enlargement	Pulmonary hypertension
Flattened diaphragmatic contour	On a frontal chest radiograph, the normal dome of each hemi-diaphragm should rise at least 1.5 cm above a line connecting the costophrenic and cardiophrenic angles. If it is <1.5 mm, diaphragm is said to be flattened	Obstructive airway disease
Hyper-inflated lung fields	Presence of more than 6 anterior or 10 posterior ribs above the diaphragm level on the midclavicular line (OR) horizontalization of ribs on frontal CXR	Obstructive airway disease
Shrunken lung fields	Four or less anterior ribs seen above the diaphragm on a frontal CXR	Bilateral diaphragmatic paresis/interstitial lung disease
Reduced tracheal lumen diameter/intraluminal lesion	A careful examination of central airways will help in identifying focal narrowings on a CXR	Central airway obstruction

FURTHER READING

1. Tarbox AK, Swaroop M. Pulmonary embolism. Int J Crit Illn Inj Sci. 2013 Jan;3(1):69–72.
2. Chua MT, Sim TB, Ibrahim I. Not all unexplained hypoxia is pulmonary embolism. Singapore Med J. 2015 Feb;56(2):e32–5.
3. Hammond S, Phillips JA. Carbon Monoxide Poisoning. Work Heal Saf. 2019;67(1):47–8.
4. Mack E. Focus on Diagnosis: Co-oximetry. Pediatr Rev. 2007;28(2):73–4.
5. Al-Mobeireek AF, Babatin MA. A patient with hypoxemia and a normal chest radiograph. Saudi Med J. 2001 Oct;22(10):924–7.

Chapter 16

Approach to a Patient with Hemoptysis and Diffuse Alveolar Opacities

• *Shamil PK* • *Nitesh Gupta*

LEARNING POINTS

1. Cases of diffuse alveolar hemorrhage (DAH) require a systematic and thorough evaluation of clinical, radiological, and serological findings to arrive at a specific etiological diagnosis.
2. The possibility of underlying celiac disease should be considered in patients with unexplained DAH, even in the absence of typical gastrointestinal manifestations.
3. Timely introduction of a gluten-free diet can improve the quality of life for patients with Celiac disease/Lane-Hamilton syndrome and helps prevent or reduce the progression of organ damage. Diet modification may itself be sufficient, potentially avoiding the need for pharmacotherapy and the associated adverse effects of systemic steroids and immunosuppressants.

INTRODUCTION

Diffuse alveolar hemorrhage (DAH) is an alarming clinical condition characterised by hemoptysis, alveolar opacities, and varying degrees of hypoxemia. Evaluating DAH requires a systematic analysis of clinical, radiological, and laboratory parameters to identify a specific etiology. Idiopathic pulmonary hemosiderosis (IPH) is a rare disorder characterised by recurrent episodes of diffuse alveolar hemorrhage without any apparent cause, leading to permanent lung damage. We present a case of a young male with a long-standing history of hemoptysis, dyspnea, and abdominal symptoms, ultimately diagnosed with DAH associated with celiac disease and cardiomyopathy

CASE VIGNETTE

An 18-year-old male college student, a never-smoker, presented with a history of dyspnea since five years and hemoptysis since two years. The dyspnea was persistent without any diurnal or seasonal variation, progressing from grade 1 to grade 3 mMRC, and worsened over the last few months to grade 4. He also had a history of daily hemoptysis for the last 2 years, about one teaspoonful occurring 1 to 3 times a day, not associated with chest pain or expectoration of purulent sputum. Additionally, he reported fatigue and occasional palpitations, but no history of wheeze, ankle edema, or allergic symptoms. There was no history of other bleeding manifestations, fever, loss of appetite, joint symptoms, redness of the eye, nasal/paranasal sinus symptoms, skin rash, numbness or weakness of limbs, oral ulcers, Raynaud's symptoms, hematuria, or frothing.

His diet was mixed, with a history of mild bloating after meals and occasional constipation. There was no similar illness in his family. He had previously received empirical anti-tuberculosis therapy for these symptoms but without any symptomatic benefit and had multiple blood transfusions in the past for anemia.

On physical examination, he was tachypneic at rest and pale, poorly built with a body mass index of 17 kg/m^2, pulse rate of 98/minute, blood pressure of 94/54 mmHg, respiratory rate of 24 breaths per minute, and oxygen saturation of 93% while breathing room air. General physical examination was normal. Respiratory system examination revealed bilateral mid to late inspiratory crackles. Cardiac examination showed normal heart sounds with a systolic murmur at the apex. The abdomen was soft and nontender. Neurological examination was unremarkable.

Investigations revealed hemoglobin to be low at 6.6 gm/dL, with a total leukocyte count of 8400 cells per microliter and normal differential counts. Peripheral blood smear examination showed microcytic hypochromic red cells with aniso-poikilocytosis, without any immature cells or parasites. Serum iron study revealed iron deficiency anemia. Platelet count, activated partial thromboplastin time, and prothrombin time test with International Normalised Ratio (INR) were within normal limits. Serum electrolytes, blood sugar, liver, renal, and thyroid functions were within normal limits. Urine routine examination was negative for dysmorphic red cells, casts, or any crystals. Serum tests for hepatitis and HIV infections were negative. Arterial blood gas (ABG) analysis showed pH 7.44, PaO_2 73 mmHg, pCO_2 31 mmHg, bicarbonate of 21 mmol/L, and a P(A-a) DO_2 of 38.8 mmHg.

Chest radiograph (Fig. 16.1) showed bilateral predominantly peri-hilar reticulonodular opacities, and cardiomegaly. Computed tomogram (CT) of the chest showed patchy areas

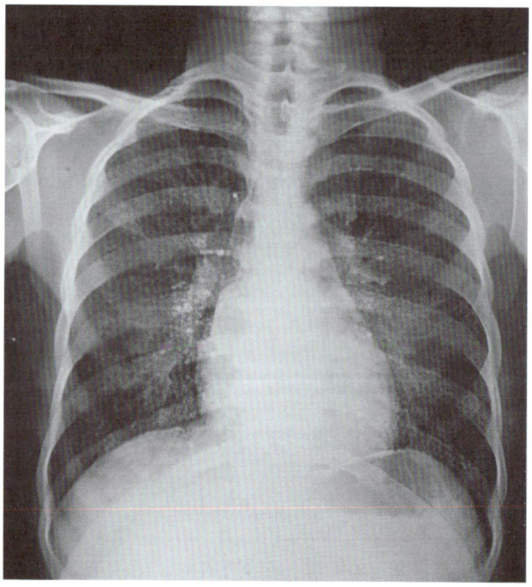

Fig. 16.1: Chest radiograph showing bilateral reticulonodular shadows distributed predominantly centrally with preserved lung volume and normal costophrenic angle.

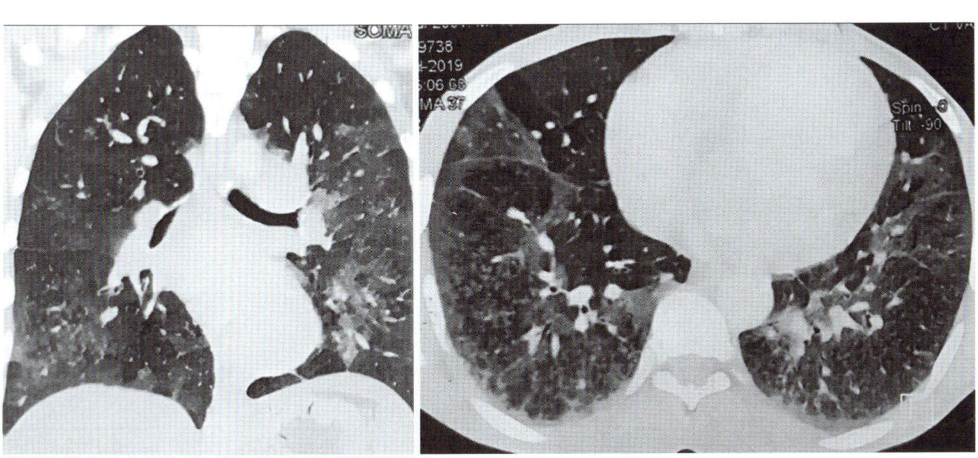

Fig. 16.2: Coronal (panel A) and cross-sectional (panel B) views of CT chest showing ground glass opacities distributed in the bilateral lung field with a mosaic pattern. Centrilobular nodules are visible predominantly in the lower lobe.

of ground glass opacities in the bilateral lung parenchyma (Fig. 16.2), and associated centrilobular nodules in bilateral lower lobes. The pulmonary trunk (with a diameter of 30 mm) and its branches were dilated. No significant mediastinal lymphadenopathy was observed. In view of hemoptysis, anemia, hypoxemia and bilateral lung infiltrates, a diagnosis of diffuse alveolar hemorrhage was established.

A 12-lead electrocardiogram showed normal sinus rhythm with the left bundle branch block. 2D echocardiography showed a dilated and globally hypokinetic left ventricle with severely reduced systolic function and an ejection fraction of 25–30%. Cardiac valves were normal, and there was no pericardial effusion.

Antinuclear antibody (ANA) testing by indirect immunofluorescence showed moderate homogeneous positivity, but the ANA profile by ELISA was negative. Cytoplasmic-anti neutrophil cytoplasmic antibody (ANCA) and perinuclear-ANCA were also negative, as were rheumatoid factor and anti-cyclic citrullinated peptide (CCP) antibodies. C3 and C4 complement levels were within normal limits. Serum anti-glomerular basement membrane (GBM) antibody by ELISA was negative.

Ophthalmological examination of the fundus and nail bed capillaroscopy were normal. Bronchoscopy showed a normal tracheobronchial tree without any signs of inflammation. Bronchoalveolar lavage (BAL) from the right middle lobe was progressively bloody in appearance, and cytological examination showed hemosiderin-laden macrophages consistent with alveolar hemorrhage. BAL fluid microbiology testing for Gram stain, acid-fast stain, CB-NAAT for tuberculosis, bacterial and fungal cultures, and cytology for malignant cells were negative. Lung biopsy could not be performed as the patient did not provide consent for a biopsy.

Stool examination was negative for occult blood, ova, parasites, or any cysts. Since this young male had dilated cardiomyopathy with evidence of alveolar hemorrhage and nonspecific gastrointestinal symptoms, analysis for serum anti-tissue transglutaminase (tTG-IgA) level was done, which was found to be more than 200 unit/ml (normal range 4–10 unit/ml). Following this, he underwent an upper gastrointestinal endoscopy and biopsy from the second part of the duodenum, which revealed focal blunting of villous architecture with increased intraepithelial lymphocytes and lymphoplasmacytic inflammatory infiltrates in the lamina propria. A diagnosis of Lane Hamilton syndrome (celiac disease with idiopathic pulmonary hemosiderosis) with dilated cardiomyopathy was made.

The patient was initiated on a strict gluten-free diet and medical therapy for cardiac failure. He began to improve symptomatically after the diet modification. His abdominal symptoms reduced, and his bowel habits normalized. Hemoptysis gradually decreased and eventually stopped. There was radiological improvement with a reduction in pulmonary parenchymal opacities. The dyspnea also reduced in intensity, and he resumed his studies. A follow-up echocardiogram after 6 months of diet modification showed a marginal improvement in left ventricular systolic function. At 3 years of follow-up, he is totally free of hemoptysis and doing well in his studies.

DISCUSSION

Diagnosis of Diffuse Alveolar Hemorrhage

Diffuse alveolar hemorrhage should be suspected when patients present with a triad of hemoptysis, bilateral lung infiltrates and anemia (classic triad). Associated respiratory failure or hypoxemia may or may not be present. The classic triad of DAH is, however, seen in only 50–60% of cases with DAH. In up to one third of the cases hemoptysis may be absent at clinical presentation. DAH may also be suspected when there is a clinical triad of bilateral lung infiltrates, hypoxemia and anemia (in the absence of overt hemoptysis).

When in doubt, a BAL can help in establishing the diagnosis of DAH. Sequential BAL showing progressively increasing hemorrhagic return is a characteristic finding in DAH. Initial aliquot collects the fluid return from the distal airways and further aliquots collect the true alveolar sample. Hence the return is less bloody in the first aliquot and progressively becomes more bloody in the second and third aliquot. Sequential BAL is performed by wedging the bronchoscope in a sub-segmental bronchus and instilling and retrieving three aliquots of 50–60 ml sterile saline. The return is collected in separate containers and examined visually. A progressive increase in the hemorrhagic discoloration or a lack of decrease in the bloody discoloration in the sequential aliquots suggests DAH (Table 16.1). Identification of

Table 16.1: Interpretation of Sequential BAL examination

Visual inspection findings of the three sequential aliquots of bronchoalveolar lavage	*Interpretation*
Progressively increasing bloody return	Confirms diffuse alveolar hemorrhage in the correct clinical scenario (first aliquot which represents a distal airway return is less bloody when compared to later aliquots which represent alveolar sample)
Uniform bloody discolouration	Likely diffuse alveolar hemorrhage (when a significant bleed happens, all aliquots may show a bloody return)
Progressively decreasing bloody return	Likely bleed due to airway trauma from the bronchoscope. No alveolar hemorrhage (the initial return which collects the airway return is bloody and not the later returns which collect the alveolar sample)
Uniformly non-bloody return	Unlikely to be diffuse alveolar hemorrhage. (however, if Prussian blue stain identifies significant siderophages, a DAH may be confirmed even if the return is macroscopically non-bloody)

hemosiderin laden macrophages (siderophages) in BAL fluid by prussian blue staining is another characteristic of DAH. Siderophages can be seen if the bleed occurs between 2 days and 2 weeks prior to the procedure. Presence of >20% siderophages on a BAL differential cell count suggests DAH.

In individuals who are stable enough to perform pulmonary function testing, increase in DLCO above 100% predicted is a sensitive test for presence of DAH. This happens due to increased availability of extravascular hemoglobin in the alveoli which can bind to carbon monoxide. It is important to understand that not all patients need a BAL or a DLCO to establish a diagnosis of DAH. They need to be performed when the diagnosis is in doubt and if the patient is stable enough to undergo the procedure.

The diagnosis of DAH can also be confirmed pathologically by demonstration of the presence of hemosiderin laden macrophages in the alveoli, with or without fibrosis. Absence of capillaritis favors a diagnosis of idiopathic DAH.

Causes of DAH and Etiologic Evaluation

Diffuse alveolar hemorrhage (DAH) can be caused by a variety of etiological factors (Tables 16.2 and 16.3). The causes of DAH can be classified as per the three histopathological patterns of DAH: Pulmonary capillaritis, bland hemorrhage, and diffuse alveolar damage (DAD). It is important for the clinician to ascertain the accurate cause for DAH as the treatment approach and prognosis for each cause is different.

The diagnostic workup of DAH requires a systematic analysis of detailed clinical history, signs and symptoms, radiological appearance, pulmonary function tests, bronchoscopy with alveolar lavage, lung biopsy, and serological tests for connective tissue disorders and vasculitis. An algorithmic approach to DAH is shown in Fig 16.3. Investigations that need to be performed in cases where the cause is not evident by clinical history are shown in Table 16.4.

Coeliac Disease and DAH

Idiopathic pulmonary hemosiderosis (IPH) is a rare condition characterised by recurrent episodes of diffuse alveolar hemorrhage without any apparent underlying etiology. Different hypotheses that may lead to IPH include immune-mediated injury, structural defect in alveolar capillaries, hypersensitivity reaction, and free radical-mediated injury due to a disorder of iron metabolism. Long-standing disease can eventually progress to lung fibrosis, leading to significant long-term morbidity and mortality.

Table 16.2: Causes of diffuse alveolar hemorrhage (DAH) syndrome (stratified as per the histopathologic pattern)

Bland hemorrhage	*Capillaritis*	*Diffuse Alveolar Damage*	*Others*
• Drugs-anticoagulant • Platelet dysfunction • Mitral stenosis/ pulmonary vein stenosis • Goodpasture disease* • Systemic lupus erythematosis*	• Systemic vasculitides • Connective tissue diseases • Drugs-carbimazole, hydralazine • Acute lung transplant rejection	• Infection • Rheumatic-SLE, PM • Toxins • Drugs-isocyanate • Radiation therapy	• Angiosarcoma • PVOD/PCH

*Both bland hemorrhage and capillaritis may be seen in these diseases.

Table 16.3: Causes of diffuse alveolar hemorrhage (stratified based on etiology)	
Autoimmune causes of DAH	***Drugs associated with DAH***
Primary pauci-immune vasculitis (granulomatosis with polyangiitis (GPA), microscopic polyangiitis, eosinophilic GPA)	Drugs causing Coagulopathy (Anticoagulants/ Antiplatelet/ thrombolytics)
Primary immune complex vasculitis (Goodpasture's syndrome, Henoch-Schönlein purpura)	Drugs causing Diffuse alveolar damage (Amiodarone, Nitrofurantoin, Propylthiouracil, Cytotoxic drugs, isocyanates, crack cocaine)
Secondary vasculitis in connective tissue diseases (SLE, RA, MCTD, APLA syndrome)	Drugs causing capillaritis (Carbimizole, propylthiouracil, retinoic acid, TNF alpha antagonists)
Behçet's disease	
Essential cryoglobulinemia	**Coagulopathy associated DAH**
	Any cause leading to a systemic coagulopathy
Isolated pulmonary capillaritis	
Idiopathic pulmonary hemosiderosis	**Miscellaneous causes of DAH**
	Raised pulmonary venous pressure (Mitral stenosis, Pulmonary vein stenosis, PVOD, PCH)
Infections associated with DAH	Malignancy associated DAH (angiosarcoma, choriocarcinoma, epithelioid hemangio epithelioma, metastatic RCC)
Severe viral pneumoniae (COVID, H1N1 influenza, dengue hemorrhagic fever, hantavirus, CMV pneumonia)	Post-autologous stem cell transplantation
Bacterial infections (leptospirosis–more common, Tuberculosis–less common)	Acute lung transplant rejection
Sepsis due to any cause with disseminated intravascular coagulation	Coeliac disease with DAH (Lane-Hamilton syndrome)

APLA: Anti phospholipid antibody syndrome; *CMV:* Cytomegalovirus; *DAH:* Diffuse alveolar hemorrhage; *MCTD:* Mixed connective tissue disorder; *PVOD:* Pulmonary veno-occlusive disease; *PCH:* Pulmonary capillary hemangiomatosis; *RA:* Rheumatoid arthritis; *RCC:* Renal cell carcinoma; *SLE:* Systemic lupus erythematosus; *TNF:* Tumor necrosis factor.

Celiac disease (CD) or gluten-sensitive enteropathy is a genetic disorder characterised by immune-mediated inflammation of the small intestine due to sensitivity to gluten and related proteins in the diet. Adult patients often present with atypical symptoms of variable severity, in contrast to life-threatening malabsorption seen in the pediatric population. Gastrointestinal symptoms may range from mild bloating, flatulence, and steatorrhea to more severe diarrhea and metabolic abnormalities.

Extra-gastrointestinal manifestations and associated conditions of CD include dermatitis herpetiformis, secondary hyperparathyroidism, iron deficiency anemia, and various neuropsychiatric manifestations. CD has been associated with as many as 5% of cases of autoimmune myocarditis and idiopathic dilated cardiomyopathy. Pulmonary manifestations associated with CD include diffuse pulmonary nodules, lymphocytic bronchoalveolitis, bronchiectasis, emphysema, and interstitial fibrosis. Idiopathic pulmonary hemosiderosis coexisting with CD is known as Lane-Hamilton syndrome. DJ Lane and WS Hamilton first reported this association of IPH with idiopathic steatorrhea in 1971.

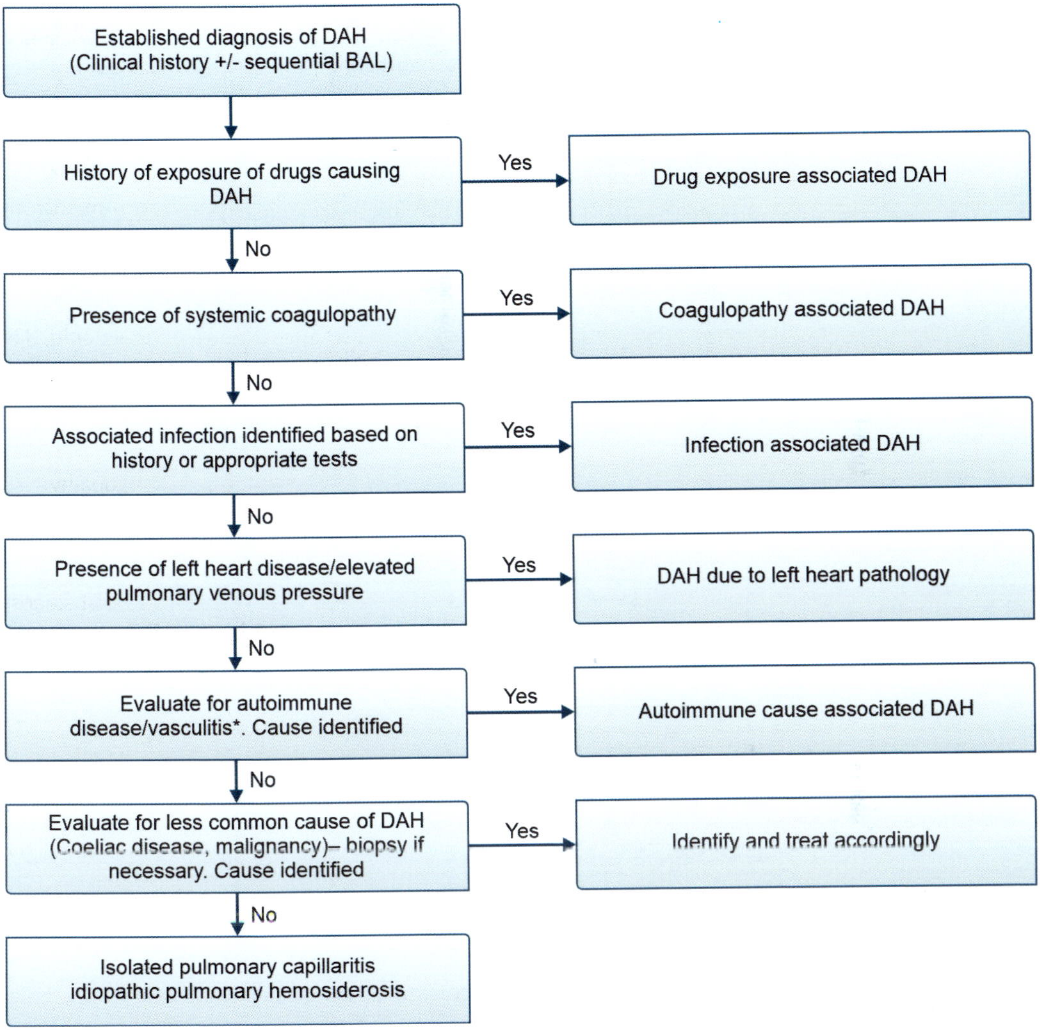

Fig. 16.3: Algorithmic approach to diagnosis of diffuse alveolar hemorrhage.

*Tests needed for diagnosis: ANA by IF, ANCA by ELISA, anti-GBM antibody, ANA profile, RA factor, anti-CCP antibody, serum cryoglobulin levels, C3, C4 level, APLA workup.

Hypotheses for this association include the deposition of circulating immune complexes involving food allergens on the basal membrane of alveolar capillaries, cross-reaction between anti-reticulin antibodies and alveolar basal membrane antigens, and the effect of adenovirus 12, a possible cause of CD, on the lungs.

The mainstay of treatment for Lane Hamilton syndrome is diet modification with complete avoidance of dietary gluten. A gluten-free diet alone has been shown to ameliorate pulmonary symptoms like hemoptysis and dyspnea, improve lung function, and reduce the need for blood transfusions. Systemic glucocorticoids have been used to reduce morbidity and mortality secondary to acute episodes of alveolar hemorrhage in IPH. A second immunosuppressant may be used along with steroid pulse therapy in life-threatening cases with respiratory failure. Anecdotal reports suggest the benefit of long-term oral steroids in

Table 16.4: Investigations for a case of diffuse alveolar hemorrhage	
Investigations to assess the severity of DAH	
• Radiology (chest X-ray, HRCT chest)	Presence of bilateral opacities on chest X-ray. HRCT shows bilateral ground glass opacities or a crazy paving appearance
• Hemoglobin/CBC	To confirm the presence of anemia
• Sequential BAL examination	When in doubt, sequential BAL examination will help in establishing the diagnosis of DAH
• DLCO	Optional and less often performed as most patients will not be able to perform the test in the acute presentation
• Hemoglobin/CBC	
• Pulse oximetry/ABG	
Investigations to ascertain the cause of DAH	
• Platelet count, INR, aPTT	To assess for systemic bleeding diathesis
• 2D ECHO, NT Pro BNP level	To assess for presence of left heart pathology/ associated pulmonary hypertension
• CUE, creatinine	To diagnose associated renal involvement /pulmo-renal syndromes (Goodpasture's syndrome, SLE and primary vasculitis)
• ANCA by ELISA	Positive ANCA in the clinical context will confirm the diagnosis of primary systemic vasculitis
• Anti-GBM antibody	Test for diagnosing Goodpasture syndrome
• ANA (IF), anti-dsDNA, C3, C4 level	Tests for diagnosing SLE
• Anti-cardiolipin Ab, LAC, anti β2GP Ab	Tests for diagnosing APLA syndrome
• Anti tTG Ig A antibody, serum Ig A level	Test for diagnosing coeliac disease
• RA factor, anti-CCP antibody	Tests for diagnosing RA vasculitis
• Serology for leptospira/dengue • BAL for cytology and microbiology • Throat swab for viral infections	Tests for identifying an infectious cause of DAH
• Transbronchial lung biopsy	To ascertain the histologic type of DAH. Not necessary when a diagnosis can be established by less invasive investigations

ABG: Arterial blood gas; *ANA:* Antinuclear antibody; *ANCA:* Anti-neutrophil cytoplasmic antibody; *APLA:* Anti-phospholipid antibody syndrome; *BAL:* Bronchoalveolar lavage; *CBC:* Complete blood count; *CCP:* Cyclic citrullinated peptide; *CUE:* Complete urine examination; *DAH:* Diffuse alveolar hemorrhage; *DLCO:* Diffusion capacity of lung for carbon monoxide; *GBM:* Glomerular, basement membrane; *HRCT:* High resolution Computed tomogram; *INR:* International normalized ratio; *LAC:* Lupus anticoagulant; *RA:* Rheumatoid arthritis; *SLE:* Systemic lupus erythematosus.

reducing the frequency of alveolar hemorrhage, thereby delaying or halting lung fibrosis. However, formal studies on such pharmacotherapies for Lane-Hamilton syndrome are lacking due to the rarity of the condition.

FURTHER READING

1. Loachimescu OC, Sieber S, Kotch A. Idiopathic pulmonary hemosiderosis revisited. Eur Respir J. 2004;24:162–70.

2. Saha BK, Datar P, Aiman A, Bonnier A, Saha S, Milman NT. Comparative Analysis of Adult Patients with Idiopathic Pulmonary Hemosiderosis and Lane-Hamilton syndrome: A Systematic Review of the Literature in the Period 1971-2022. Cureus. 2022 Mar 25;14(3):e23482.

3. BSB, SK, Elilarasi S, SS. Respiratory Symptoms as Atypical Manifestation of Celiac Disease. Pediatr Oncall J. 2016;13:46-47.

4. Lara AR, Schwarz MI. Diffuse alveolar hemorrhage. Chest. 2010 May;137(5):1164-71.

5. Loachimescu OC, Stoller JK. Diffuse alveolar hemorrhage: diagnosing it and finding the cause. Cleve Clin J Med. 2008 Apr;75(4):258,260,264–5.

Chapter

17

Approach to a Case of Acute Respiratory Distress Syndrome

• *Sricharan G* • *Venkat Raman Kola*

LEARNING POINTS

1. Acute respiratory distress syndrome is a potentially fatal respiratory emergency characterized by an acute onset (<7 days) bilateral lung infiltrates and respiratory failure in the absence of pulmonary edema.
2. The causes of ARDS are many. It is important to identify the cause and initiate treatment for the primary cause of ARDS as soon as possible.
3. The crux of supportive care in managing ARDS is the ventilatory strategy. It is important to maintain oxygenation, reduce the work of breathing and prevent ventilator induced lung injury.
4. Ways to maintain oxygenation include HFNC and NIV in mild-moderate ARDS; and invasive mechanical ventilation and VV-ECMO in severe-refractory cases of ARDS.

INTRODUCTION

Acute respiratory distress syndrome (ARDS) is an acute ($\leq$7 days) clinical syndrome characterized by acute hypoxemic respiratory failure and bilateral pulmonary infiltrates on chest imaging. ARDS is broadly categorized into pulmonary (direct) and extrapulmonary (indirect) ARDS. ARDS can be caused by both infectious and non-infectious etiologies. Despite the diversity in its causes, the management approach for ARDS is notably consistent. It is essential to address the underlying cause of ARDS, with a focus on meticulous ventilatory management. This involves optimizing patient oxygenation while simultaneously preventing ventilator-induced lung injury. We present a case of a young male diagnosed with viral infection leading to ARDS.

CASE VIGNETTE

A 28-year-old male, with no prior medical history, presented to the emergency department with a five-day history of fever, cough, and shortness of breath. On arrival, he had hypoxia (room air pulse oximetry oxygen saturation of 70%) and tachycardia (heart rate: 120 beats per minute) with a respiratory rate of 35 breaths per minute. Clinical examination revealed pronounced respiratory distress, including the use of accessory muscles for breathing. His sensorium was normal. Chest auscultation revealed bilateral basal decreased breath sounds with associated coarse crackles and normal heart sounds were noted on auscultation. He received immediate oxygen support via a venturi oxygen mask at 15 L/min. Arterial blood gas (ABG) analysis showed a PaO_2 of 55 mmHg on oxygen supplementation.

A chest X-ray confirmed bilateral pneumonia (Fig. 17.1). He was started empirically on broad-spectrum antibiotics and oseltamivir. Despite initial interventions, the patient's condition progressively worsened, evidenced by decreasing SpO_2 (88%) and a persistent high respiratory rate (35/min). High-flow nasal cannula (HFNC) therapy was initiated at a rate of 60 L/min with an FiO_2 of 0.6. A follow-up ABG showed an improved PaO_2 of 90 mmHg, with SpO_2 rising to 97%. CT scan of the chest was done which showed bilateral dense consolidations (Fig. 17.2).

However, within the next few hours, his PaO_2 decreased to 80 mmHg despite an increased FiO_2 of 0.8, and his respiratory rate escalated to 40/min and ROX index was found to be 3.06. The patient also exhibited signs of decompensation with minimal activity. Subsequently, non-invasive ventilation (NIV) was started with a positive end-expiratory pressure (PEEP) of 8 cm H_2O, a pressure support (PS) of 14 cm H_2O, and an FiO_2 of 0.8. This intervention initially improved his condition (SpO_2 96%, PaO_2 110 mmHg). However, his respiratory status rapidly deteriorated and his HACOR score was found to be 10, necessitating intubation and mechanical ventilation.

Endotracheal (ET) secretions of the patient tested positive for H1N1 infection. A diagnosis of H1N1 related severe ARDS was thus established. Investigations did not show any evidence of secondary bacterial infection.

In parallel, lung protective ventilation strategies were employed, adhering to tidal volumes set at 6 ml/kg of the patient's ideal body weight (IBW). Despite these measures, the patient's PaO_2/FiO_2 (PF) ratios persisted around 110, indicative of ongoing hypoxia. As a result, prone ventilation was implemented for 16 hours daily.

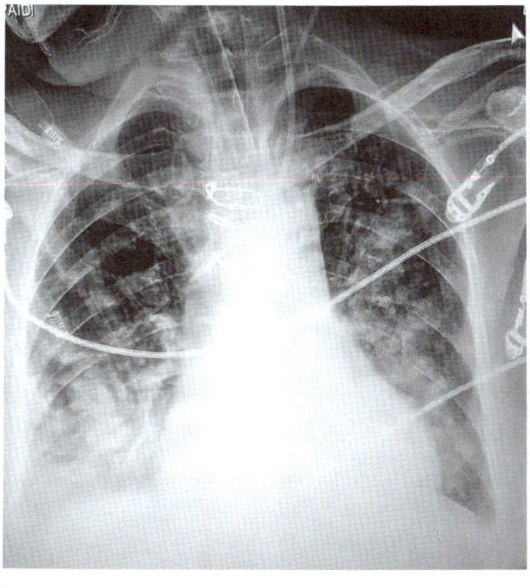

Fig. 17.1: Chest X-ray (AP view) reveals presence of bilateral mid and lower zone inhomogenous opacities

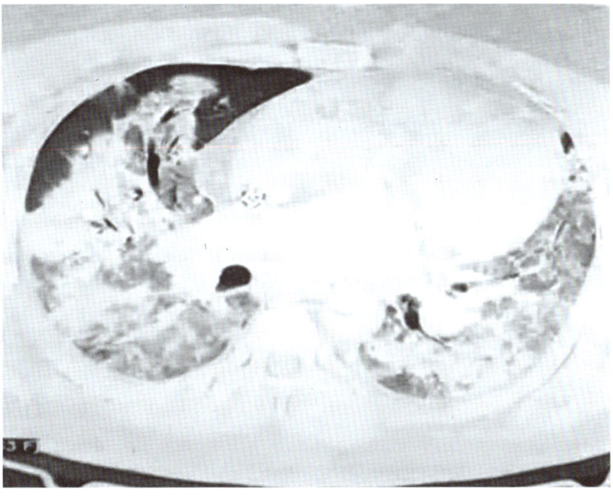

Fig. 17.2: HRCT chest axial cut reveals presence of extensive bilateral lower lobe consolidation

After completing six cycles of prone ventilation, a notable improvement in the patient's PF ratios was observed. This improvement allowed the discontinuation of prone sessions once the PF ratios exceeded 150. The patient's PF ratios continued to show an upward trend. Subsequently, he successfully completed a spontaneous breathing trial. On the 8th day of mechanical ventilation, the patient was extubated. He showed stable respiratory function and was eventually discharged home on day 12, no longer requiring oxygen support.

DISCUSSION

Definition of ARDS

ARDS is a severe, inflammatory lung condition characterized by the rapid onset of widespread inflammation in the lungs. It is caused by various etiologies and leads to significant respiratory distress and hypoxemia. The Berlin definition, a widely used criterion for diagnosing ARDS, is illustrated in Table 17.1. Recent guidelines suggest alternative/additional approaches to Berlins criteria:

- **Use of lung ultrasound:** Lung ultrasound, when performed by an experienced operator, can be used as an alternative to chest X-ray for detecting bilateral chest infiltrates.
- **Definition of mild ARDS:** It can be defined with PF ratios between 200 and 300, either with a minimum PEEP of 5 cm H_2O or with HFNC support at flows greater than 30 L/min.
- **Inclusion of SpO_2/FiO_2 ratios:** The SpO_2/FiO_2 (SF) ratio is increasingly used alongside PF ratios for defining hypoxia in ARDS. An SF ratio of less than 315 indicates ARDS.

Causes of ARDS

ARDS can be caused by a variety of factors leading to either direct or indirect lung injury (Table 17.2).

Treating ARDS

Treating ARDS involves a combination of treating the primary cause of ARDS, advanced ventilation strategies, supportive care, fluid management, and pharmacotherapy. The primary goal is to ensure adequate oxygenation while minimizing the risk of ventilator-induced lung injury (VILI) and other complications. The key elements of ARDS management are as follows.

1. Fluid Management

In ARDS management, a restrictive fluid strategy, though weakly recommended due to limited evidence, is favored for increasing ventilator-free days and reducing hypoxia, despite lacking a clear mortality benefit.

Table 17.1: Berlin's definition of acute respiratory distress syndrome (ARDS)

Category	*Criteria*
Timing	Within 1 week of known insult or worsening respiratory symptoms
Imaging	Bilateral chest infiltrates as demonstrated by chest X-ray
Cause of Edema	Respiratory failure not explained by pulmonary edema or intravascular fluid overload
Oxygenation	Classified based on PF ratios with a minimum PEEP of 5 cm H_2O: Mild: PF ratio of 200–300 Moderate: PF ratio of 100–200 Severe: PF ratio of <100

Table 17.2: Etiology of acute respiratory distress syndrome (ARDS)

Type of Lung Injury	*Causes of ARDS*
Direct lung injury	• Pneumonia (bacterial, viral, etc.) • Aspiration • Lung contusion • Air, fat embolism • Drowning • Toxic inhalation • Seat belt injuries
Indirect lung injury	• Sepsis • Pancreatitis • Cardiopulmonary bypass • Poly trauma • Drug toxicity • Transfusion-related acute lung injury

2. Ventilation Strategies

A. High Flow Nasal Cannulae (HFNC)

HFNC therapy is an advanced form of oxygen delivery that is increasingly being used in the management of patients with respiratory distress, including those with ARDS.

Mechanism of Action

- HFNC delivers heated and humidified oxygen at high flow rates (up to 60 L/min), which can improve patient comfort and compliance compared to conventional oxygen therapy.
- It reduces the work of breathing by providing a constant flow of air that flushes out carbon dioxide from the dead space in the upper airways.
- The high flow rate also creates a mild positive pressure in the airways, which can improve alveolar recruitment.

ROX Index: The ROX index is a useful tool to assess the efficacy of HFNC in patients. It is calculated using the formula: (SpO_2/FiO_2)/Respiratory rate. A ROX index of <3.85 is considered an indicator of HFNC failure at 1, 4 and 6 hours. This suggests that the patient might not be responding adequately to HFNC and may require escalation of care, such as mechanical ventilation.

Role in ARDS: HFNC is now recognized in the ARDS defining criteria due to its effectiveness in improving oxygenation. It can be particularly useful in early stages of ARDS or in milder forms of the syndrome. When using HFNC, close monitoring of the patient's respiratory status, oxygenation, and the ROX index is essential to assess the response to therapy. While HFNC can delay the need for intubation in some cases, it is crucial to monitor patients closely to ensure timely intubation if their condition deteriorates.

B. Non-invasive Ventilation

NIV can be beneficial in mild-moderate ARDS cases by providing ventilatory support and PEEP, which can improve oxygenation and reduce the work of breathing. However, the use of NIV in ARDS is limited and somewhat controversial, mainly because of the risk of delayed intubation. Delayed intubation in deteriorating patients can lead to increased mortality.

HACOR score: To evaluate the effectiveness of NIV and predict potential failure, scoring systems such as the HACOR score are employed. The HACOR score takes into account heart rate (HR), acidosis, consciousness, oxygenation (PF ratio), and respiratory rate (Table 17.3). A HACOR score above 5 is indicative of a high risk of NIV failure. This scoring system helps clinicians in making timely decisions about the escalation of care, including the transition to invasive mechanical ventilation if necessary. Various modalities of non-invasive ventilation are compared in Figs 17.3 and 17.4.

C. Mechanical Ventilation

Mechanical ventilation is indeed the cornerstone of management for patients with ARDS. The primary aim is to support adequate oxygenation and ventilation while minimizing

Table 17.3: HACOR score for monitoring on non-invasive ventilation

Parameter	***Score***	***Value***
Heart rate	0 1	<120 >120
Acidosis (pH)	0 2 3 4	>7.35 7.30–7.34 7.25–7.29 <7.25
Consciousness (GCS)	0 2 5 10	15 13–14 11–12 <10
Oxygenation (PaO_2/FiO_2 ratio)	0 2 3 4 5 6	>200 175–200 150–175 125–150 100–125 <100
Respiratory rate	0 1 2 3 4	<30 30–35 35–40 40–45 >46

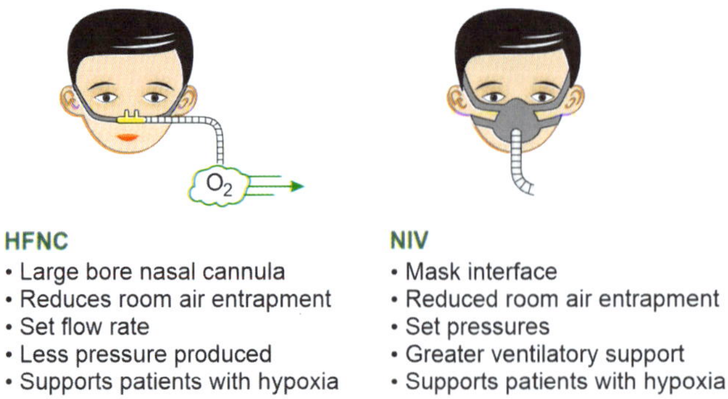

Fig. 17.3: Comparison between HFNC and NIV (non-invasive ventilatory modalities)

Non-invasive respiratory support for acute hypoxemic respiratory failure

Non-invasive ventilation: CPAP and pressure support ventilation (PSV)

High flow nasal oxygen	Facemask	Helmet
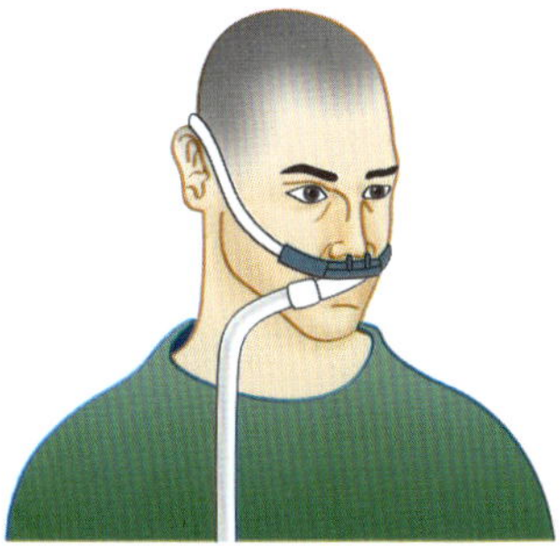	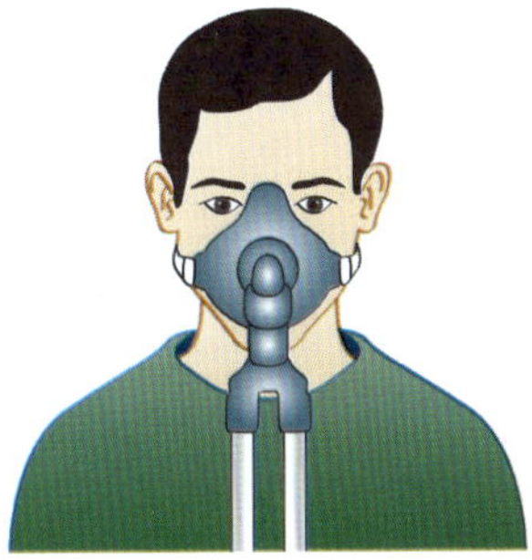	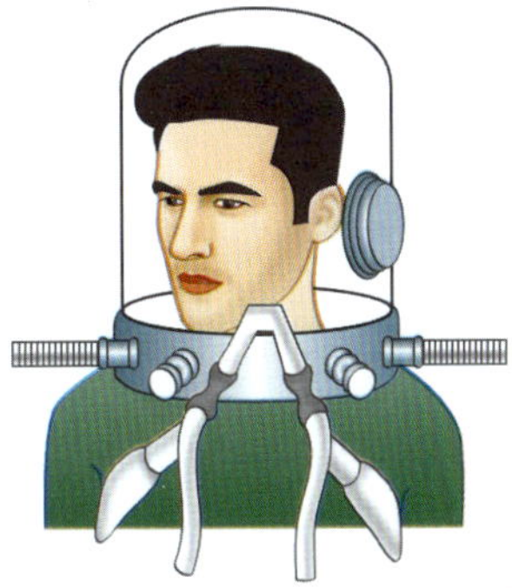
Settings • FiO_2: 0.21–1 • Gas flow: 40–60 lpm • Temperature: 31–37°C	**Settings** PSV-requires a ventilator • FiO_2: 0.21–1 • PEEP: 5–8 cmH_2O • PS: 7–10 cmH_2O CPAP • Continuous flow (>30 L/min) or CPAP mode on the ventilator • PEEP: 5–8 cmH_2O Use of HME is advisable	**Settings** PSV-requires a ventilator • FiO_2: 0.21–1 • PEEP: 10–12 cmH_2O • PS: 10–12 cmH_2O • No humidification needed • Fastest pressurization time CPAP-requires a flow generator • Continuous flow (>60 L/min) • PEEP valve: 10–12 cmH_2O • Active humidification possible
Benefits • Matches inspiratory flow • Delivers set FiO_2 • Delivers fully conditioned gas • Enhances comfort • Provides positive airway pressure (up to 4 cmH_2O) • Washout of nasopharyngeal dead space • Reduces inspiratory effort	**Benefits** • Delivers set FiO_2 • Delivers fully conditioned gas • Provides PEEP to allow alveolar recruitment • Provides PS (only for PSV) to unload inspiratory muscles • Allows to monitor tidal volume (only PSV)	**Benefits** • Delivers set FiO_2 • Provides high PEEP to allow alveolar recruitment and enhance ventilator homogeneity • Continuous treatments with good tolerability • Provides PS (only for PSV) to reduce inspiratory effort • Asynchronous PS may prevent positive P_L swings
Pitfalls Small amount of PEEP delivered	**Pitfalls** • Skin ulcer • Air leaks, difficult delivery of high PEEP • Full inspiratory synchronization may increase P_L swings and tidal volume • Poor tolerability: need for treatment interruptions	**Pitfalls** • Impossibility to measure tidal volume • Upper limbs edema, with possible vasal thrombosis

Fig. 17.4: Illustration of benefits and pitfalls of various non-invasive ventilation modalities

Adapted from: Grieco DL, et al. Non-invasive ventilatory support and high-flow nasal oxygen as first-line treatment of acute hypoxemic respiratory failure and ARDS.

Table 17.4: Mechanical ventilation parameters and recommendations	
Parameter	*Recommendation*
Mode of ventilator	Volume control ventilation (VCV), pressure control ventilation (PCV), airway pressure release ventilation (APRV)
Tidal volumes	6 ml/kg of Predicted Body Weight (PBW)
PEEP	Moderate PEEP; as per PEEP/FiO_2 table
Plateau pressures	<30 cm H_2O
Driving pressures	<16 cm H_2O
Transpulmonary pressures	<30 cm H_2O
Recruitment maneuvers	Not recommended
Prone ventilation	For a minimum of 16 hours a day if PF ratio remains <150

VILI through lung-protective strategies. Various recommendations for ARDS are enlisted in Table 17.4. A positive end expiratory pressure is applied to prevent alveolar collapse and improve oxygenation, but it should be carefully titrated to avoid over-distention of the lungs. Techniques to titrate PEEP are beyond the scope of this chapter.

For severe ARDS, prone positioning can significantly improve oxygenation by redistributing lung perfusion and ventilation.

D. Venovenous Extracorporeal Membrane Oxygenation (ECMO)

Venovenous extracorporeal membrane oxygenation (VV-ECMO) is a critical intervention used in severe cases of ARDS where conventional mechanical ventilation strategies remain inadequate.

Indications for VV-ECMO

1. PF ratios less than 80 despite maximal conventional mechanical ventilation following a trial of prone ventilation.
2. Hypercapnic respiratory failure (pH <7.25) despite optimized ventilator management with a respiratory rate of 35/min or higher.
3. As a bridge to lung transplantation in selected cases.

Mechanism: VV-ECMO involves draining venous blood, oxygenating it externally, and then returning the oxygenated blood to the right atrium. This process allows the patient's lungs to rest while ensuring adequate gas exchange.

Complications: Potential complications include bleeding, consumptive coagulopathy, infections, and acute kidney injury (AKI).

RESP Score: The RESP score is used to assess the probability of success with VV-ECMO. Factors considered in the RESP score include age, BMI, immunocompromised status, duration of mechanical ventilation pre-ECMO, sequential organ failure assessment (SOFA) score, use of prone positioning, PEEP, and peak inspiratory pressures. A RESP score greater than 6 is associated with a good survival rate (greater than 92%), while a score less than–6 correlates with poor survival (less than 18%).

A step by step approach to ventilatory management of ARDS is depicted in Fig. 17.5.

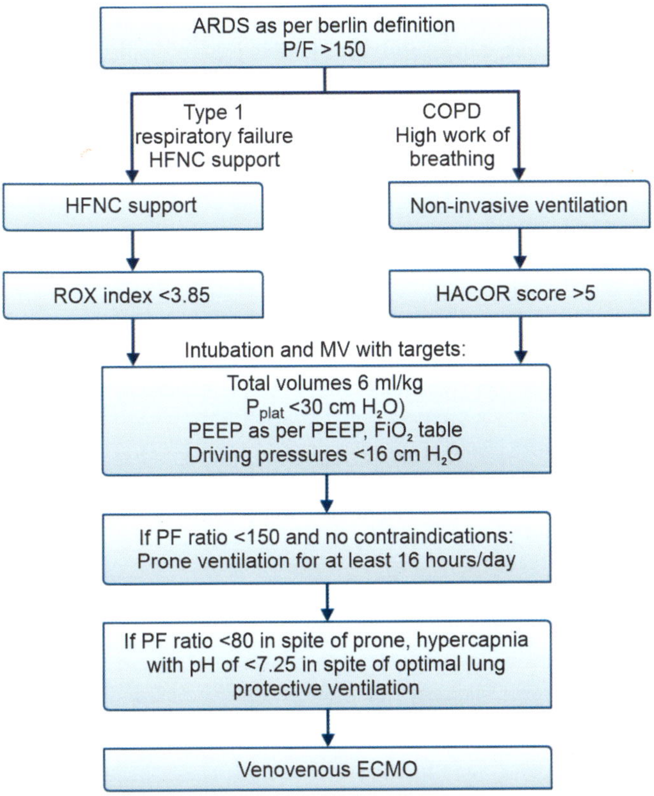

Fig. 17.5: Step by step ventilatory management of ARDS

3. Pharmacotherapy for ARDS

In addition to use of pharmacotherapy for treating the primary cause of ARDS, certain medicines have been tested to improve the outcomes in ARDS.

A. Glucocorticoids

May be used to reduce lung inflammation, although their use remains controversial and should be carefully considered on a case-by-case basis.

B. Neuromuscular Blockers

In cases of severe ARDS, especially with high oxygen requirements and poor lung compliance, neuromuscular blocking agents can be used to improve oxygenation and reduce VILI.

C. Inhaled Pulmonary Vasodilators

These can be used to reduce pulmonary artery pressure and improve ventilation-perfusion matching in the lungs, though their long-term benefits are still under investigation.

4. Supportive Therapies

Supportive care is essential to manage ARDS and reduce complications. This includes nutritional support, prophylaxis for deep vein thrombosis and gastric ulcers, antibiotics for ongoing infection (if any) and management of comorbidities.

Monitoring and Adjustment: Continuous monitoring of oxygenation, lung mechanics, and hemodynamics is essential. Treatment strategies should be adjusted based on the patient's evolving clinical status.

FURTHER READING

1. Grasselli G, Calfee CS, Camporota L, et al. ESICM guidelines on acute respiratory distress syndrome: definition, phenotyping and respiratory support strategies. Intensive Care Med. 2023 Jul;49(7):727–59.
2. Hancı P, Uysal A, Yüksel B, İnal V. Rox Index Dynamics According to High Flow Nasal Cannula Success in Intensive Care Unit Patients with COVID-19-Related Acute Respiratory Failure. Balkan Med J. 2023 Mar 8;40(2):111–16.
3. Duan J, Han X, Bai L, Zhou L, Huang S. Assessment of heart rate, acidosis, consciousness, oxygenation, and respiratory rate to predict noninvasive ventilation failure in hypoxemic patients. Intensive Care Med. 2017 Feb;43(2):192–99.
4. Villar J, Ferrando C, Martínez D, Ambrós A, Muñoz T, Soler JA, Conesa LA (2020). Dexamethasone treatment for the acute respiratory distress syndrome: a multicentre, randomised controlled trial. The Lancet Respiratory Medicine.
5. Grieco DL, Maggiore SM, Roca O, Spinelli E, Patel BK, Thille AW, Barbas CS, de Acilu MG, Cutuli SL, Bongiovanni F, Amato M. Non-invasive ventilatory support and high-flow nasal oxygen as first-line treatment of acute hypoxemic respiratory failure and ARDS. Intensive care medicine. 2021 Aug;47:851–66.
6. Tonna, Joseph E, Abrams, Darryl, Brodie, Daniel, et al. Management of Adult Patients Supported with Venovenous Extracorporeal Membrane Oxygenation (VV ECMO): Guideline from the Extracorporeal Life Support Organization (ELSO). ASAIO Journal. 2021 Jun 1;67(6):601–10.

Chapter 18

Approach to a Case with Extensive Surgical Emphysema

• *Arvindran Alaga* • *Chan Tha A Hing*

LEARNING POINTS

1. Subcutaneous emphysema (SE) associated with pneumothorax is often self-limiting and usually does not require intervention.
2. Extensive SE can significantly increase morbidity and may necessitate early intervention.
3. This case illustrates the effectiveness of using a subcutaneous drain with additional fenestrations as an intervention for extensive SE.

INTRODUCTION

Subcutaneous emphysema (SE), also known as surgical emphysema, occurs when air becomes trapped in the subcutaneous space beneath the skin. This condition can result from both penetrating and blunt trauma to the respiratory and gastrointestinal tracts. SE is often associated with pneumothorax, occurring in up to 20% of patients who undergo intercostal drainage for pneumothorax. Approximately 7% of patients develop SE following medical thoracoscopy as well.

Radiographically, SE presents as radiolucent striations across muscle and subcutaneous tissues. It usually follows a benign, self-limiting course, often requiring only conservative treatment. However, in some cases, SE can be extensive and life-threatening, necessitating more aggressive intervention.

CASE VIGNETTE

A patient in his twenties, newly diagnosed with human immunodeficiency (HIV) infection was admitted with prolonged cough and reduced effort tolerance. He was recently treated for *Pneumocystis jerovicii* pneumonia (PJP) based on chest X-ray findings and clinical presentation. On the 10th day of hospitalization, the patient's dyspnea worsened. Repeat chest X-rays revealed a left-sided pneumothorax, necessitating the insertion of a 24 Fr intercostal chest tube (Fig. 18.1A). This procedure, however, was complicated by the development of SE, which rapidly expanded to cover the thorax, neck, face, abdomen, and bilateral upper limbs

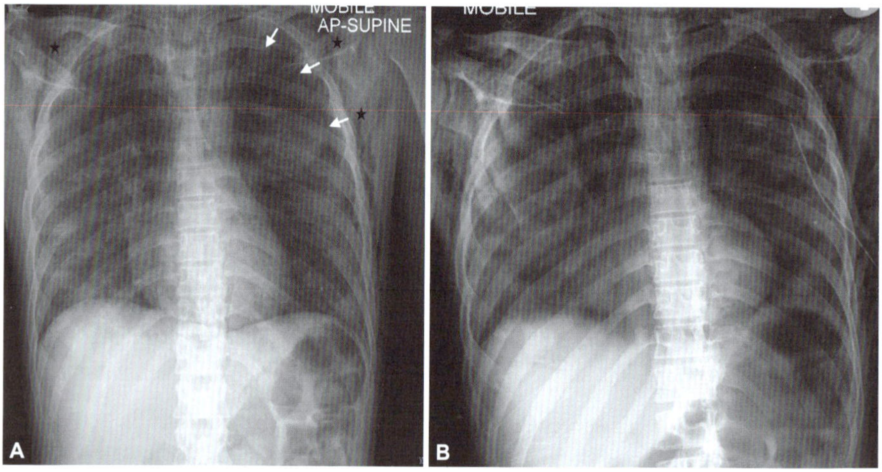

Fig. 18.1: (A) Left sided Pneumothorax (white arrows) with minimal subcutaneous emphysema (black stars); (B) Chest radiograph showing worsening of subcutaneous emphysema despite on chest tube.

(Fig. 18.1B). The patient's oxygen needs increased significantly, prompting a referral to the respiratory team due to the worsening surgical emphysema.

In an attempt to halt the progression of SE, a low-pressure suction (20 cm H_2O) was applied to the existing chest tube. Despite this, the SE worsened, and the patient required intubation and mechanical ventilation. To address the SE, a modified 20 Fr chest tube was inserted as a subcutaneous drain in the right hemi-thorax.

Steps of Placement of a Subcutaneous Drain

1. The right hemi-thorax area was cleaned and draped.
2. Following local anaesthesia, a 1 cm transverse skin incision was made in the anterior axillary line at the 5th–6th intercostal space.
3. A caudo-cranial oriented subcutaneous tract about 10 cm long was created superficial to the pectoral fascia using blunt dissection.
4. Additional fenestrations were made on the 20 Fr chest tube to enhance SE drainage (Fig. 18.2A).

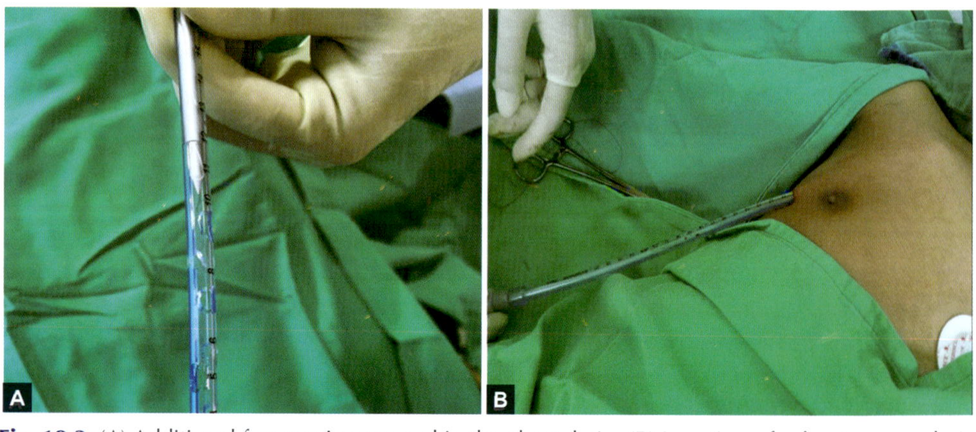

Fig. 18.2: (A) Additional fenestration created in the chest drain; (B) Insertion of subcutaneous drain

5. The chest tube was inserted into the tract, sutured in place, and connected to an underwater seal drainage system set at a low suction of 5 cm H_2O (Fig. 18.2B).
6. Rapid decompression was achieved on the same day, allowing ventilator settings to be reduced to a FiO_2 of 0.6, with subsequent extubation three days later.

Once the patient's oxygen requirement decreased to nasal prong 3 L and the near complete resolution of SE, the subcutaneous drain was removed.

DISCUSSION

Surgical emphysema, also known as subcutaneous emphysema (SE), is characterized by the presence of air beneath the skin. Common signs and symptoms include swelling around the neck with accompanying chest pain, neck pain, dysphagia (difficulty swallowing), dyspnea (shortness of breath), and wheezing. Diagnosis is typically made through palpable crepitation upon physical examination and imaging studies that reveal air in the affected areas.

SE is graded by the level of its extent (Fig. 18.3). Massive subcutaneous emphysema is defined as SE extending beyond the torso to include the neck and head (grades IV and V).

Pathophysiology: Air from the lungs can cause SE through several mechanisms:

1. Direct passage of air into the chest wall and subcutaneous tissues when the parietal pleura is punctured, often seen with pneumothorax.
2. The 'Macklin-effect' describes a process where alveolar rupture leads to air leakage into the connective tissue around the pulmonary vasculature. This air then travels along the bronchovascular sheath to the mediastinum and eventually into the soft tissues.
3. Migration or inadequate anchorage of an intercostal drain can also contribute to SE.

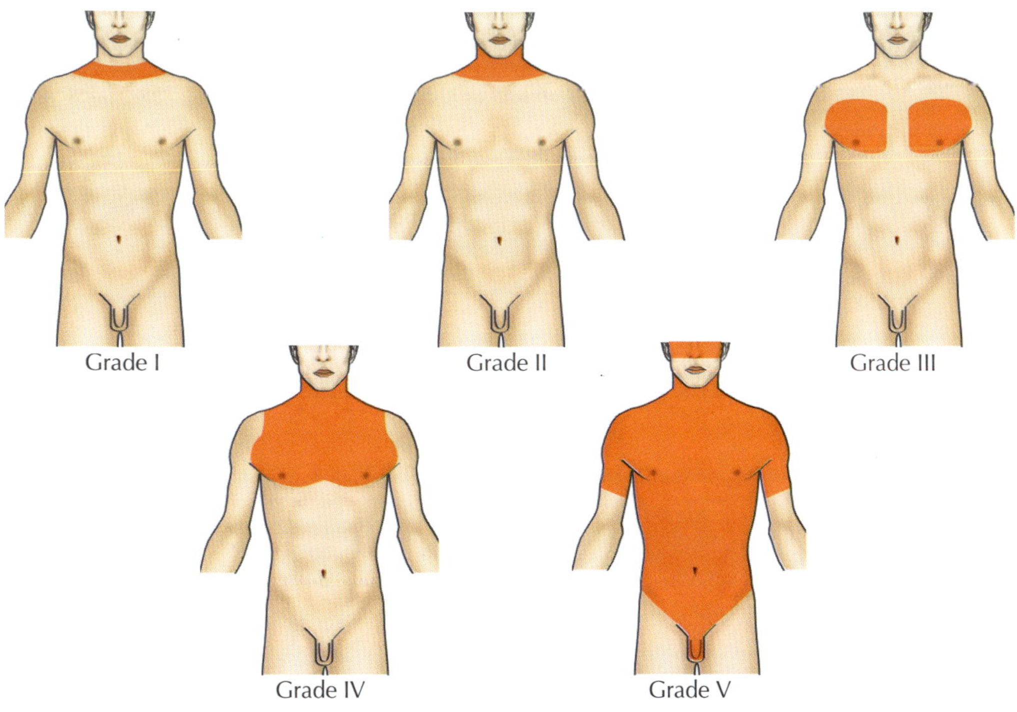

Fig. 18.3: Grading of subcutaneous emphysema

Aghajanzadeh M et al. Classification and management of subcutaneous emphysema: A 10-year experience. Indian J Surg. 2015 Dec;77(Suppl 2):673–7.

Initial Management

After initial patient assessment, in cases with symptomatic SE, it is advisable to administer supplemental high FiO_2 oxygen. Similar to its effect in resolution of a pneumothorax, administration of high FiO_2 oxygen hastens the resorption of SE. Imaging studies, such as a chest X-ray or CT thorax may be obtained. Various approaches to management of patients with severe and symptomatic SE are outlined in Table 18.1, and an algorithm is proposed for the management of SE (Fig. 18.4).

Table 18.1: Various approaches to manage subcutaneous emphysema

Approach	*Purpose*
Placing existing intercostal drain on suction	• Increase flow into the chest drain and reduce flow into subcutaneous tissue. • Pressure can be applied up to 20 cm H_2O. • May cause discomfort for patients.
Placing wider bore intercostal drain	• Allow a greater total flow rate of air. • Applicable for SE that persists after applying suction.
'Blow-holes'	• Create unilateral or bilateral incisions in the skin to drain the SE. • Incisions 2–4 cm in length, deep to external thoracic fascia. • Risk of wound infection.
Subcutaneous fenestrated angio-catheters insertion	• Create additional fenestrations on the sides of a large bore IV cannula. • One or multiple such catheters are inserted into the subcutaneous plane and secured with a stitch, and may be connected to an underwater drain. • Compressive massage of the SE may be done to accelerate the resorption of SE.
Subcutaneous drain insertion	• Create a subcutaneous tract superficial to the pectoral fascia using blunt dissection. • Additional fenestration can be created in the chest tube to facilitate drainage of SE efficiently. • Apply low-pressure suction to the subcutaneous drain. • Mean resolution of SE is approximately 3.7 days based on available literature.
Surgical management	• Potential definitive solution for SE resulting from a pneumothorax due to bronchopleural fistula.

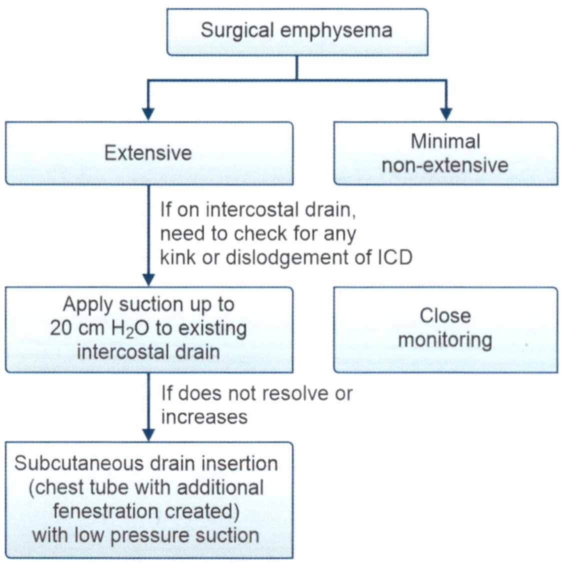

Fig. 18.4: Algorithm for management of subcutaneous emphysema

FURTHER READING

1. Tran Q, Mizumoto R, Mehanna D. Management of extensive surgical emphysema with subcutaneous drain: A case report. Int J Surg Case Rep. 2018;44:126–130.

2. O'Reilly P, Chen HK, Wiseman R. Management of extensive subcutaneous emphysema with a subcutaneous drain. Respirol Case Rep. 2013 Dec;1(2):28–30.

3. Melhorn, J., Davies, H.E. The Management of Subcutaneous Emphysema in Pneumothorax: A Literature Review. Curr Pulmonol Rep 10, 92–97 (2021).

4. Aghajanzadeh M, Dehnadi A, Ebrahimi H, Fallah Karkan M, Khajeh Jahromi S, Amir Maafi A, Aghajanzadeh G. Classification and Management of Subcutaneous Emphysema: a 10-Year Experience. Indian J Surg. 2015 Dec;77(Suppl 2):673–7.

Chapter 19

Approach to a Case of Obesity with Type 2 Respiratory Failure

• Amrutha P • Shikha KC • Arjun P

LEARNING POINTS

1. Always suspect obesity hypoventilation syndrome (OHS) in morbidly obese patients.
2. Suspect OHS in obese patients who present with awake hypoxia.
3. A polysomnography is essential to distinguish between those who have apneas and those who have pure hypoventilation.
4. Treatment of OHS is by a combination of weight reduction and a positive airway pressure (PAP) device.

INTRODUCTION

Obesity is one of the world's most rapidly increasing and often neglected public health problems. Obesity alters the pulmonary mechanics directly and affects other organs such as the cardiovascular system, leading to secondary pulmonary complications. Obesity can lead to various pulmonary disorders leading to respiratory failure such as restrictive lung disease, obesity-related asthma, sleep-disordered breathing, and hypoventilation syndromes. Here, we describe a patient with obesity and respiratory failure.

CASE VIGNETTE

A fifty-five-year-old gentleman, a teacher by profession, presented to us with excessive tiredness and increased daytime sleepiness. He also had complaints of loud snoring and frequent awakenings at night. These complaints started more than two years back, but he presented to us when he could not do his day-to-day activities due to excessive tiredness. He denied cough, breathlessness or symptoms suggestive of neuromuscular weakness.

He was on regular medications for systemic hypertension and diabetes mellitus. On clinical examination, his weight was 96 kg and height was 153 cm. His body mass index (BMI) was 41 kg/m^2 and neck circumference was 46 cm with a modified Mallampatti score of class IV. His heart rate was 84/min and BP 160/100 mm Hg. His respiratory rate was 18/minute.

His room air saturation (SpO_2) was 88%. On auscultation of the chest, normal breath sounds were heard bilaterally. On cardiovascular system examination, a loud second heart sound was heard, and no murmurs were appreciable.

A clinical diagnosis of OSA and obesity hypoventilation syndrome (OHS) was considered as he was an obese patient with resting awake room air saturation of less than 94%. On further evaluation, he was found to have polycythemia (hemoglobin: 18.2 g%). His serum electrolytes, liver, renal, and thyroid function tests were normal. Arterial blood gas (ABG) showed $paCO_2$ of 54 mmHg, pO_2 of 50 mmHg, HCO_3 27 mEq/L and a pH of 7.38. Spirometry revealed normal FEV_1/FVC ratio with reduced FEV_1 and FVC which was suggestive of apparent restriction probably due to his obesity. Chest radiograph showed cardiomegaly (Fig. 19.1), and a 2D echocardiography showed right atrial and ventricular dilatation, moderate pulmonary hypertension, and normal left ventricular function.

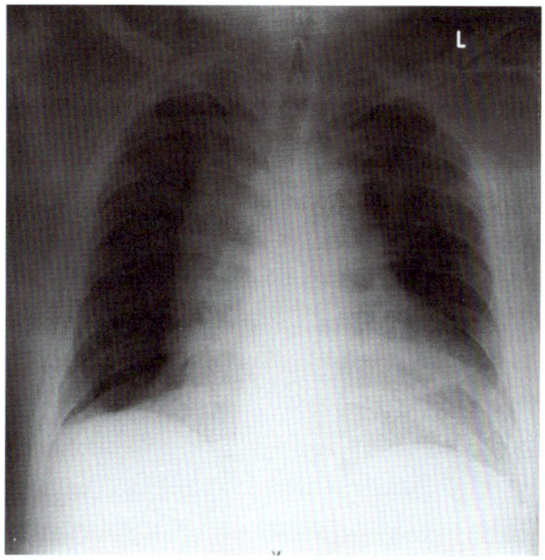

Fig. 19.1: Chest X-ray PA view showing apparent cardiomegaly

A full night, level one polysomnography (PSG) showed an apnea-hypopnea index (AHI) of 75 events/hour and a rapid eye movement (REM) AHI of 120 events/hour. The lowest oxygen saturation recorded was 60%. With these, a diagnosis of obesity hypoventilation syndrome with obstructive sleep apnea (OSA-OHS) was established. A manual positive airway pressure (PAP) titration study was performed and he was advised to use continuous positive airway pressure (CPAP) therapy during sleep with 14 cm of H_2O.

He was started on CPAP with a pressure of 14 cm H_2O during sleep and was advised to lose weight, which he strictly adhered to. At follow-up after four weeks, his $paCO_2$ was within normal limits, and he had no complaints of excessive daytime sleepiness and snoring.

DISCUSSION

Obesity hypoventilation syndrome (OHS) is diagnosed when there is a triad of obesity (body mass index >30 kg/m^2), chronic alveolar hypoventilation associated with daytime hypercapnia (awake $paCO_2 \geq 45$ mm Hg), and sleep-related breathing disorder. There should not be any other cause of hypoventilation. It is also called Pickwickian syndrome, named after the popular character Joe in posthumous papers of *Pickwick Club* by Charles Dickens.

The mechanism by which obesity leads to hypoventilation is not completely understood. There is an interaction between:

1. Abnormal mechanics of respiratory system leading to an increased work of breathing due to obesity (reduced chest wall respiratory system compliance, reduced respiratory muscle efficiency, raised airway resistance, expiratory flow limitation).
2. Sleep-related breathing disorder.
3. Blunted central hypercapnic and hypoxic ventilatory drive (central hypothalamic resistance to leptin).

Up to 90% of OHS patients have an associated obstructive sleep apnea (OSA), and nearly 70% have severe OSA (AHI>30 events/hour). In the remaining 10% patients, OHS is not associated with OSA. In these indivdiuals, the sleep related breathing disorder is purely non-obstructive sleep hypoventilation which is characterized by sustained hypoxia and increase in $paCO_2$ by 10 mmHg above wakefulness level. This becomes very important from the treatment point of view, especially regarding the choice of PAP device that needs to be used. Typical symptoms of OSA are also reported by OHS patients. In addition, they also can have symptoms of hypercapnia like morning headaches. Excessive daytime sleepiness despite adequate control of OSA may be present. Dyspnea occurs more often than in eucapnic OSA patients. Pulmonary hypertension, corpulmonale and polycythemia also occur more commonly in patients with OHS compared with patients with OSA alone.

Physical examination findings of OHS include facial plethora, injected sclera, a prominent pulmonic component of the second heart sound, and other signs of right heart failure such as pedal edema. Awake hypoxemia is not common in eucapnic OSA patients, and a pulse oximetry recording of <94% in patients with OSA should prompt consideration of ABG analysis.

The diagnosis of OHS relies on demonstration of awake hypercapnia, and hence an arterial blood gas in room air is essential. In the absence of an elevated $PaCO_2$ on ABG, chronic hypercapnia may be suggested by an elevated serum bicarbonate. A serum bicarbonate ≥ 27 mEq/L has been shown to be highly sensitive (92%) but not specific (50%) for chronic hypercapnia (Box 19.1).

OHS is a diagnosis of exclusion. Other disorders which cause chronic hypoventilation such as significant pulmonary disease, chest wall disorders, neuromuscular disorders, hypothyroidism and other central hypoventilation syndromes must be excluded before an individual is labelled as OHS. Based on clinical history and physical examination, diagnostic testing may include pulmonary function testing, lung imaging, electrocardiography, thyroid function testing and a sleep study (Table 19.1).

Treatment of Obesity Hypoventilation Syndrome

First line therapy for management of OHS is a combination of non-invasive positive pressure ventilation and weight loss. It is important to stress that positive airway pressure (PAP) therapy should not be delayed while the patient tries to lose weight.

Non-invasive PAP in the Treatment of OHS

- **Continuous positive airway pressure (CPAP):** Patient should be titrated first with CPAP and if apneas or hypopneas are not abolished with maximal pressures of CPAP, patients can be titrated with bi-level PAP.
- **Bi-level positive airway pressure (BiPAP):** Apart from above written indication, BiPAP-S/T mode is used for OHS patients without OSA.

Box 19.1: Clinical scenarios where OHS should be suspected
Obese patients with suspected/known severe OSA (AHI > 30 events/hour)
Obese patients with or without OSA with • Unexplained awake room air SpO_2 ≤ 94% • Unexplained dyspnea on exertion • Symptoms and signs of pulmonary hypertension and/or right heart failure • Facial plethora (polycythemia) • Increased serum bicarbonate level (> 27 mEq/L)

Table 19.1: Investigations and likely abnormalities in patients suspected with OHS		
Lab investigation	***Likely abnormality***	***Comments***
Arterial blood gas analysis	• Elevated $PaCO_2$ (>45 mmHg) • Low PaO_2 (< 80 mmHg) • Elevated HCO^{3-}	Essential test for diagnosing obesity hypoventilation syndrome
Serum bicarbonate level	Elevated (>27 mEq/L)	Can be used as a screening test in patients suspected with OHS.
Overnight level 1 lpolysomnography	Obstructive sleep apnea (likely severe), with more severe desaturations during apneic events, and presence of hypoxemia even in non-apneic duration.	Essential test to confirm the presence of associated sleep related breathing disorder and to quantify the severity
2D echocardiogram	Evidence of elevated pulmonary artery pressure and right heart failure	Essential test in all patients of OHS to rule out associated cardiac disease
Chest radiograph	Normal/ cardiomegaly /features of pulmonary hypertension	To rule out other coexisting pulmonary disorders
Pulmonary function testing (spirometry)	Normal/ restriction due to obesity	May be performed to rule out associated pulmonary disorders
Hemogram	Polycythemia	Indirect indicator of chronic daytime hypoxemia

Other Non-invasive Ventilation Modes

1. Average volume assured pressure support (AVAPS) is a novel and a hybrid mode of PAP which has features of standard bilevel positive airway pressure (BPAP) ventilation and volume cycled positive pressure ventilation (VCPPV). In the AVAPS mode, IPAP does not remain constant, and it varies between respiratory cycles to achieve a preset tidal volume, which is usually set at 7 to 10 ml/kg of ideal body weight. It remains an option in patients with OHS when patients cannot be manually titrated in sleep lab.
2. Intelligent volume assured pressure support (IVAPS): A mode similar to AVAPS, in which the machine delivers a preset minute ventilation and not a preset tidal volume. The inspiratory pressure varies between respiratory cycles to ensure the delivery of the present minute ventilation.

Role of Supplemental Oxygen

Patients of OSA-OHS usually do not require oxygen if they are titrated properly in sleep lab. Supplemental oxygen alone without a PAP therapy should not be administered for patients with OHS because this may actually worsen hypercapnia. In situations in which a patient with OHS requires supplemental oxygen (like comorbid COPD, severe nocturnal desaturations unresponsive to non-invasive PAP therapy), it should only be used concurrently with optimally titrated PAP therapy. It is also important to realize that as hypercapnia improves with good adherence to PAP therapy, oxygen requirements may decrease. Hence periodic monitoring to reassess the need for continued supplemental oxygen needs to be performed.

Therapies of Limited Value or Associated with Harm

Respiratory stimulants like progestins and acetazolamide are adjunctive therapies that remain a last resort for patients who continue to have serious alveolar hypoventilation despite optimal PAP therapy and weight loss. When prescribed, it should be done only on a trial basis and only in conjunction with an optimally titrated PAP therapy.

An approach to a case of suspected obesity hypoventilation syndrome is outlined in Fig. 19.2.

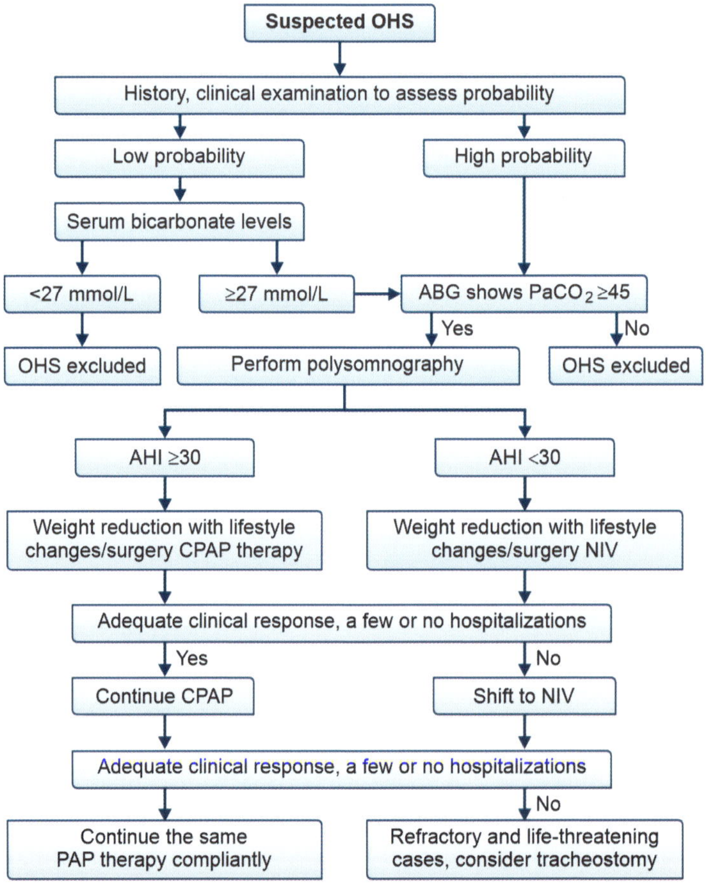

Fig. 19.2: Approach to a case of suspected obesity hypoventilation syndrome

FURTHER READING

1. Masa JF, Corral J, Alonso ML, Ordax E, Troncoso MF, Gonzalez M, et al. Efficacy of Different Treatment Alternatives for Obesity Hypoventilation Syndrome. Pickwick Study. Am J Respir Crit Care Med. 2015 Jul 1;192(1):86–95.
2. Mokhlesi B, Tulaimat A, Faibussowitsch I, Wang Y, Evans AT. Obesity hypoventilation syndrome: prevalence and predictors in patients with obstructive sleep apnea. Sleep Breath Schlaf Atm. 2007 Jun;11(2):117–24.
3. Mokhlesi B. Obesity hypoventilation syndrome: a state-of-the-art review. Respir Care. 2010 Oct;55(10):1347–62; discussion 1363–1365.
4. Utpat K, Desai U, Joshi JM, et al. Obesity Hypoventilation Syndrome: New Insights in Diagnosis and Management. Indian J Sleep Med 2020;15(1):9–14.

SECTION V

Interstitial Lung Diseases

Chapter 20

Approach to a Patient with Diffuse Cystic Lung Disease (Case 1)

• *Hariprasad Kalpakam* • *Madhuri Batyala* • *Pooja Bajaj*

LEARNING POINTS

1. Cysts are defined on radiology as thin-walled air lucencies with well-defined but thin (<2 mm thickness) walls.
2. Major causes of diffuse cystic lung diseases include lymphangioleiomyomatosis (LAM), pulmonary Langerhans cell histiocytosis (PLCH), Birt-Hogg-Dubé syndrome, and lymphocytic interstitial pneumonia (LIP).
3. LAM predominantly affects premenopausal women, and commonly presents as pneumothorax.
4. Typical HRCT features or elevated VEGF levels (>800 pg/ml) or presence of angiomyolipomas negate the need for biopsy.
5. mTOR inhibitors are the drugs of choice for management of LAM.

INTRODUCTION

Diffuse cystic lung diseases (DCLDs) encompass several conditions where multiple air-filled spaces, called cysts, are found in the lungs. Key examples of cystic lung diseases are lymphangioleiomyomatosis (LAM), pulmonary langerhans cell histiocytosis (PLCH), Birt-Hogg-Dube syndrome (BHD), and lymphoid interstitial pneumonia (LIP). Here we present a case of LAM and propose an approach to evaluation of cystic lung diseases.

CASE VIGNETTE

A 33-year-old female with no significant past medical history presented to the emergency department complaining of acute onset left-sided chest pain and breathlessness. These symptoms had been persisting for three days. Notably, she denied any history of cough, fever, wheezing, or trauma preceding the symptom onset.

Upon examination, the patient exhibited signs of dyspnea and tachypnea, with an oxygen saturation of 93% on room air. She was promptly administered supplemental oxygen, and intravenous access was established. Auscultation of the chest revealed an absence of breath sounds on the left side.

An urgent chest X-ray was performed, revealing a large left-sided pneumothorax. Subsequently, a 24-size intercostal tube was inserted at the bedside, leading to a marked improvement in the patient's symptoms and an increase in oxygen saturation to 96% on room air.

A similar history of pneumothorax was present in the patient's mother, who had undergone pleural drainage and pleurodesis a decade earlier. Given this significant family history, a high-resolution computed tomography (HRCT) scan of the thorax was obtained. The scan showed multiple well-defined cysts with normal intervening lung parenchyma, suggestive of a cystic lung disease, and near-complete expansion of the left lung (Fig. 20.1). Abdominal ultrasound was negative for angiolipomatous lesions. Elevated VEGF-D levels in a blood sample confirmed the diagnosis of LAM. The patient underwent chemical pleurodesis with two grams talc slurry prior to the removal of the intercostal tube. Pulmonary function tests performed at a later date indicated mild restriction (Table 20.1).

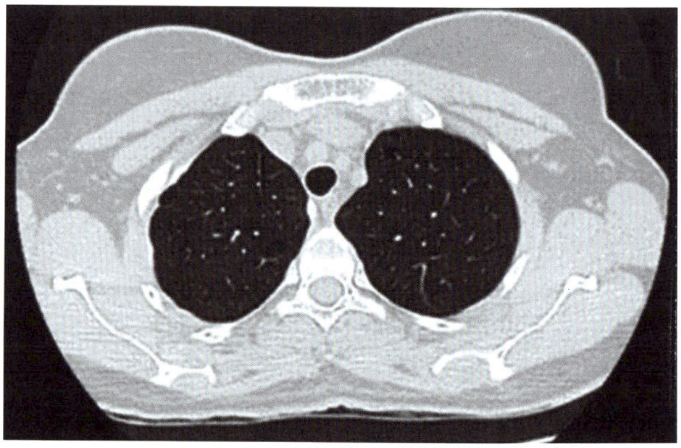

Fig. 20.1: CT thorax axial view showing multiple well-defined, thin-walled cysts of varying sizes.

Table 20.1: Pulmonary function test (spirometry) of the index case

Lung function	*At baseline*	*At 6 months follow-up*	*At 18 months follow-up*
FVC	2.16 (72.7%)	2.23 (76.4%)	2.21 (74.4%)
FEV_1	1.72 (67.2%)	1.82 (72.6%)	1.80 (70.3%)
FEV_1/FVC ratio	0.79	0.81	0.81

*Values of FVC and FEV_1 expressed as litres (% predicted)

Considering the elevated VEGF levels and presence of multiple rounded cysts, and a positive family history, a diagnosis of LAM was confirmed. Treatment with sirolimus (1 mg/day) was initiated, with ongoing monitoring of liver function tests. At an 18-month follow-up, the patient's spirometry remained stable, and no further episodes of pneumothorax were reported.

The patient's mother subsequently underwent a CT thorax, which also was suggestive of LAM. Despite the absence of other features of tuberous sclerosis in both patients, TSC genetic testing was recommended but declined by the patient.

DISCUSSION

Cystic lung diseases, characterized by the presence of air lucencies bordered by a thin wall (cyst), represent a diverse group of disorders. A cyst on radiology is defined as a discrete area of parenchymal lucency surrounded by lung parenchyma and which has a well-defined and a thin wall (<2 mm in diameter). In pathology, a cyst is defined as a rounded air space that is surrounded by an epithelial or a fibrous wall. Cysts are usually air filled but sometimes can

Table 20.2: Fleischner society definitions for various types of air lucencies seen on a HRCT chest (arranged sequentially based on the thickness of the wall)

Lesion	*Wall thickness*	*Definition*
Emphysema	No wall	Discrete areas of low attenuating lung parenchyma which do not have a discrete wall. The distribution can be either subpleural (paraseptal emphysema) or within the lung parenchyma (centri-acinar and pan acinar emphysema)
Bulla	<1 mm	Spherical air lucency, >1 cm in diameter and bounded by a very thin wall (<1 mm). Often accompanied by emphysema in adjacent lung parenchyma (bullous emphysema)
Bleb	<1 mm	A cystic air space with a thin wall (<1 mm) and adjacent to the visceral pleura, usually <1 cm in size. The use of this term is now discouraged as the difference between bleb and bulla is only the size
Cyst	<2 mm	Thin walled (<2 mm) parenchymal lucencies with surrounding lung parenchyma
Honeycomb cyst	<2 mm or sometimes thicker walls	A single or more layers of closely approximated cysts present subpleurally (each ranging in diameter from 3–10 mm). Usually seen in presence of fibrotic interstitial lung diseases
Cavity	>2 mm	Air filled space surrounded by a wall which is thick (>2 mm). Cavities can be within a consolidation, mass or a nodule or can be independently present.

be filled with fluid. It is also important to understand how to differentiate cyst from other air lucencies such as emphysema, cavity, bulla and bleb (Table 20.2).

Pulmonary cysts are classified as either being focal (presence of one more cysts in one lobe(s) of the lung) or diffuse (presence of multiple cysts bilaterally). In this chapter we give the approach to a case with diffuse cystic lung disease which presents a diagnostic challenge to the clinician. It is important to try to ascertain the correct cause for the DCLD as the treatment and prognosis for each of the diseases is different. The list of diseases which can present as a DCLD is shown in Table 20.3.

Approach to a Case with DCLD

When a diffuse cystic lung disease is identified on a HRCT chest, it is important to follow as a stepwise approach to establish the diagnosis. Diagnosis often relies on clinical and radiological features, although biopsies are sometimes necessary for ambiguous cases. We propose the four step approach to a case with DCLD.

STEP 1: History and Examination

Assessment of the clinical presentation is often the first step in the diagnostic approach. When there is development of a rapidly progressive cysts (acute to subacute presentation), possibility of an infection related DCLD or traumatic cysts need to be considered. Presence of fever and other constitutional symptoms also point towards an infectious cause of a DCLD. Most other causes of DCLD have a chronic indolent course or are incidentally picked up while a HRCT chest is performed for some other reason.

Age at presentation is also important in considering the differentials. Lymphangioleiomyomatosis (LAM) generally affects young premenopausal females, while Birt-Hogg-Dube (BHD) is more common in patients over 40 years old. LAM is a disease which

Table 20.3: Causes of diffuse cystic lung disease (DCLD)

Classification	*Diseases*
Genetic/developmental causes of DCLD	• Birt-Hogg-Dube syndrome • Neurofibromatosis • Ehlers-Danlos syndrome • Congenital pulmonary airway malformation
Malignancy associated DCLD	• Lymphangioleiomyomatosis (LAM) • Cystic metastases from primary adenocarcinoma of gut or genitourinary tract • Pulmonary sarcomas (less common)
Interstitial lung disease associated DCLD	• Lymphocytic interstitial pneumonia • Hypersensitivity pneumonitis • Desquamative interstitial pneumonia
Infection associated DCLD	• *Pneumocystis jirovecii* pneumonia • Staphylococcal pneumonia • Recurrent respiratory papillomatosis • Certain endemic mycoses (coccidioidomycosis)
Smoking associated DCLD	• Desquamative interstitial pneumonia • Pulmonary Langerhans cell histiocytosis
Lymphoproliferative diseases associated DCLD	• Lymphocytic interstitial pneumonia • Amyloidosis • Light chain deposition disease
Miscellaneous causes of DCLD	• Fire eaters lung • Post-traumatic pseudocysts

is almost exclusively seen in women, whereas other causes of DCLD do not show much sexual predilection. DCLD such as pulmonary Langerhans cell histiocytosis (PLCH) and respiratory bronchiolitis (RB)/desquamative interstitial pneumonia (DIP) are usually seen in people who smoke nicotine.

A detailed family history for pneumothoraces, skin lesions or renal tumors, or tuberous sclerosis is essential and when present helps in establishing the diagnosis of LAM or BHD syndrome. Patients with LAM may have subtle features of underlying tuberous sclerosis complex (TSC) and thus a thorough history and examination should be performed. DCLD when identified in an immunocompromised host should raise the suspicion for lymphocytic interstitial pneumonia (LIP) or *Pneumocystis jirovecii* pneumonia (PJP).

Presence of associated features also help in narrowing the differentials. Associated characteristic skin lesions (fibrofolliculomas, trichodiscomas, achrochordons in BHD syndrome; ash-leaf macules, shagreen patches and facial angiofibromas in tuberous sclerosis associated LAM) when seen confirm the diagnosis of respective syndromes. Renal tumors may be seen in patients with LAM or BHD syndrome and an abdominal imaging is warranted to look for the same. Particular attention must also be given to identify the symptoms or signs of any associated connective tissue diseases.

STEP 2: Interpretation of Radiology

A careful interpretation of a HRCT chest is of utmost importance. Interpretation of the shape of cysts, distribution of cysts and associated radiologic features help in pointing to an

Table 20.4: Radiologic (HRCT chest) features of diffuse cystic lung diseases

	LAM	*BHD syndrome*	*PLCH*	*LIP*	*Amyloid/LCDD*
Shape of cysts	Uniformly round	Oval/ lentiform	Bizarre/ irregular	Round, variable	Round, variable
Distribution of cysts	Diffuse, no lobe predilection	Bibasal, more in subpleural or para-mediastinal and along vessels	Upper and middle lobes, sparing costo-phrenic angles	Diffuse, often near vessels	Diffuse, no lobe predilection
Size of cysts	2 mm to 2 cm	Usually <1 cm	2 mm to >2 cm	3 mm to 1 cm	Usually >1 cm
Intervening lung parenchymal abnormalities	Normal	Normal	Associated nodules, cavities and reticulations	Associated ground glass opacities, nodules	Associated nodules
Other associated radiologic features	Pleural effusions (chylous)	–	–	–	–

BHD: Birt-Hogg-Dube syndrome; *PLCH:* Pulmonary Langerhans cell histiocytosis; *LIP:* Lymphoid interstitial pneumonia; *LCDD:* Light chain deposition disease; *LAM:* Lymphangioleiomyomatosis.

etiology. In cases where multiple cysts are present with adjacent normal parenchyma, the differential diagnosis typically includes LAM or BHD syndrome. Both conditions can lead to pneumothorax, with LAM also potentially causing chylothorax.

Presence of round-shaped cysts diffusely with an intervening normal lung parenchyma points towards a diagnosis of LAM. Presence of oval shaped cysts in bases predominantly in the paramediastinal or subpleural location, along the pulmonary veins, and with an intervening normal lung parenchyma suggests a diagnosis of BHD syndrome. Presence of bizarre/irregular shaped cysts predominantly in upper lobes suggests a diagnosis of pulmonary langerhan cell histiocytosis. Presence of rounded cysts with intervening lung parenchyma having nodules or ground glass opacities should raise the suspicion of LIP, desquamative interstitial pneumonia (DIP), amyloid, light chain deposition disease (LCDD) or a PJP pneumonia. Table 20.4 summarized the salient HRCT chest finding of some of the major DCLDs.

STEP 3: Genetic and other Non-Invasive Testing

Genetic testing is helpful in confirming the diagnosis of BHD syndrome and tuberous sclerosis LAM syndrome. Identification of pathologic heterozygous mutations in the TSC1 or TSC2 gene confirms the diagnosis of tuberous sclerosis complex. Presence of mutations in the FLCN gene confirm the diagnosis of BHD syndrome. An elevated serum vascular endothelial growth factor (VEGF)-D level of >800 g/ml also confirms the diagnosis of LAM in a patient with typical HRCT findings. In a case of DCLD, when suspecting LIP, it is important to evaluate for associate autoimmune diseases, immune deficiency states and lymphoproliferative diseases by appropriate blood tests.

STEP 4: Biopsy and Histopathologic Examination

When an accurate diagnosis cannot be established by non-invasive means a biopsy will help in confirming the diagnosis. While surgical lung biopsy remains the gold standard, more centres are now resorting to transbronchial lung cryobiopsy to obtain tissue for histopathological examination (HPE).

HPE examination is diagnostic in LAM, PLCH and several other DCLDs. Infiltration of parenchyma, airways, lymphatics and vessels by spindle-shaped smooth muscle cells (LAM cells) is typical in LAM. Similarly, PLCH is characterized by accumulation of Langerhans cells (stain positive by S-100 and CD1a) in bronchiolocentric distribution. Amyloid, LIP, LCDD and other malignancies can also be confirmed on histopathology. It is important to realize that HPE does not help in confirming the diagnosis of BHD syndrome.

An outline of major cystic lung diseases is presented in Table 20.5, and an approach to cystic lung diseases is outlined in Fig. 20.2.

Lymphangioleiomyomatosis

LAM, a rare cystic lung disease, can be sporadic (S-LAM) or inherited (TSC-LAM, associated with tuberous sclerosisc complex). It typically presents with dyspnea, chest pain, persistent cough, and hemoptysis, with pneumothorax and chylous effusions being common. Radiologically, LAM is identified by diffuse, round, thin-walled cysts with spared lung parenchyma. Associated features may include mediastinal adenopathy, pleural effusions, and angiomyolipomas (AMLs), benign renal tumours which are more common in TSC-LAM.

The pathogenesis of LAM involves genetic mutations in the TSC gene, uncontrolled LAM cell proliferation, and estrogen's stimulatory effects. Post-menopause, lung function may stabilise, which previously guided anti-estrogen treatments. Elevated levels of lymphangiogenic proteins, including VEGF-C and VEGF-D, are associated with disease progression and serve as diagnostic and prognostic biomarkers. Typical HRCT findings, TSC features, elevated VEGF levels, presence of angiomyolipoma, or chylous effusion can eliminate the need for a biopsy. VEGF levels above 800 pg/ml when combined with typical

Table 20.5: Salient features of major cystic lung diseases

Lung disease	*Demographics*	*Radiological findings*	*Other features and Genetic testing*
Lymphangioleiomyomatosis (LAM)	Young females	Diffuse, bilateral, round, well-defined cysts. Thin-walled, >10 cysts	Family history, features of TSC, angiomyolipoma, genetic testing for TSC
Pulmonary Langerhans cell histiocytosis (PLCH)	Young adults (20–40 years), Smokers	Bizarre-shaped, upper lobe predominance, CP angle sparing, ill-defined upper lobe nodules	
Birt-Hogg-Dubé syndrome (BHD)	30–40 years of age	Thin-walled, lentiform-shaped, lower lung predominance, subpleural, paramediastinal location	Family history, cutaneous features, renal neoplasms, FLCN gene analysis
Lymphoid pneumonia (LIP)	No age predilection	Few thin-walled cysts with a background of GGO, ill-defined centrilobular or subpleural nodules	Immunodeficiency, connective tissue disease

CP: Costophrenic; *TSC:* Tuberous sclerosis complex; *FLCN:* Folliculin; *GGO:* Ground-glass opacities.

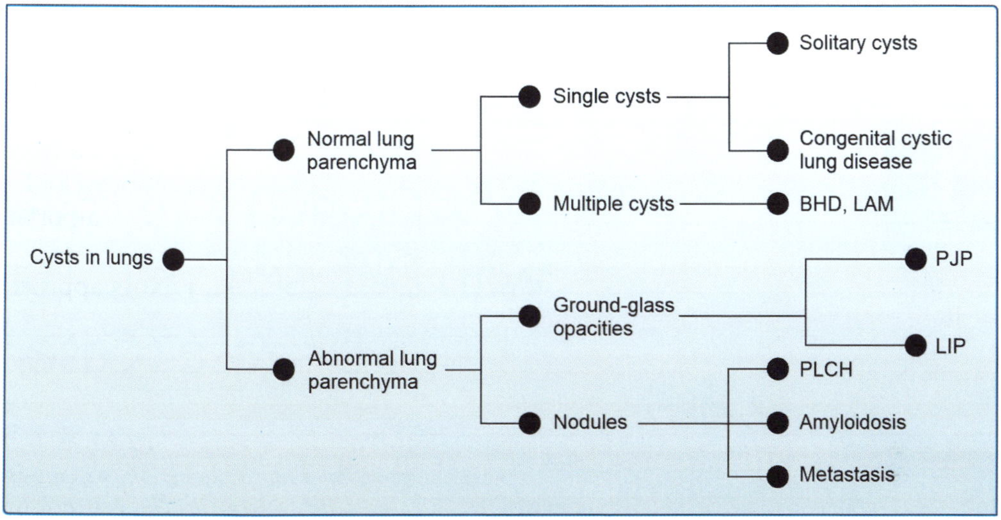

Fig. 20.2: Flowchart for evaluation of cystic lung disease

BHD: Birt-Hogg-Dube syndrome; *LAM:* Lymphangioleiomyomatosis; *LIP:* Lymphocytic interstitial pneumonia; *PJP: Pneumo-cystis jirovecii* pneumonia; *PLCH:* Pulmonary Langerhans cell histiocytosis

radiological findings is highly specific for LAM diagnosis, although testing is limited to advanced laboratories.

Past treatments included hormonal therapies and bronchodilators, but the MILES trial established the efficacy of mTOR inhibitors (Sirolimus and Everolimus) in stabilising lung function and improving quality of life, typically starting at 1–2 mg/day. Lung transplantation is the definitive treatment for progressive respiratory failure, though recurrence post-transplantation is possible.

FURTHER READING

1. Cong CV, Anh TT, Ly TT, Duc NM. Pulmonary lymphangioleiomyomatosis (LAM): A literature overview and case report. Radiology Case Reports. 2022 May 1;17(5):1646–55.
2. O'Mahony AM, Lynn E, Murphy DJ, Fabre A, McCarthy C. Lymphangioleiomyomatosis: a clinical review. Breathe. 2020 Jun 1;16(2).
3. McCormack FX, Inoue Y, Moss J, Singer LG, Strange C, Nakata K, Barker AF, Chapman JT, Brantly ML, Stocks JM, Brown KK. Efficacy and safety of sirolimus in lymphangioleiomyomatosis. *New England Journal of Medicine*. 2011 Apr 28;364(17):1595–606.
4. Gupta N, Finlay GA, Kotloff RM, Strange C, Wilson KC, Young LR, Taveira-DaSilva AM, Johnson SR, Cottin V, Sahn SA, Ryu JH. Lymphangioleiomyomatosis diagnosis and management: high-resolution chest computed tomography, transbronchial lung biopsy, and pleural disease management. An Official American Thoracic Society/Japanese Respiratory Society Clinical Practice Guideline. *American Journal of Respiratory and Critical Care Medicine*. 2017 Nov 15;196(10):1337–48.

Chapter

21

Approach to a Patient with Diffuse Cystic Lung Disease (Case 2)

• *Lekshmipriya Raj* • *Murali Mohan BV* • *Kedar Hibare*

LEARNING POINTS

1. Birt-Hogg-Dube (BHD) syndrome can have varied clinical presentations and can be asymptomatic at presentation. Patients may have normal and stable pulmonary function despite significant lung involvement.
2. Suspected cases of BHD require a multidisciplinary approach to confirm the diagnosis. Once confirmed, follow-up with periodic kidney imaging for early diagnosis of renal cancer is necessary.
3. While evaluating a case with cystic lung disease, genetic testing is recommended when there is a high pretest probability of BHD syndrome.
4. Given the autosomal dominant inheritance of BHD syndrome, screening and genetic counselling for family members is crucial.

INTRODUCTION

Cystic lung diseases often present a diagnostic challenge to the clinician. We present a case of a lady who presented with giddiness and on evaluation had incidental pulmonary cysts. She was confirmed to have Birt-Hogg-Dubé (BHD) sydrome on subsequent germline genetic testing. BHD syndrome is an uncommon autosomal dominant genodermatosis characterised by the presence of benign tumours of the hair follicle, pulmonary cysts with recurrent spontaneous pneumothorax, and increased susceptibility to renal cancers.

CASE VIGNETTE

A female homemaker in her late forties presented with complaints of dizziness lasting two days. She has no known comorbidities. Initial cardiology evaluation was unremarkable; however, a CT coronary angiogram revealed mild coronary artery plaques and incidentally detected multiple pulmonary cysts, prompting a referral to pulmonary medicine for further evaluation. The patient reported no history of fever, cough, palpitations, or breathing difficulties. She had experienced similar episodes of dizziness two years prior, which were not associated with chest pain or breathing difficulty and resolved spontaneously within a few minutes.

She had never smoked and denied exposure to smoke, irritants, fumes, or pets. Additionally, there is no history of allergies, asthma, or pulmonary tuberculosis. On examination, the patient's vitals were normal. General physical examination revealed papular skin lesions on the face, neck, and upper limbs, morphologically resembling fibrofolliculomas (Fig. 21.1); the remainder of the systemic examination was unremarkable. Respiratory system examination showed bilateral equal intensity air entry with no added sounds.

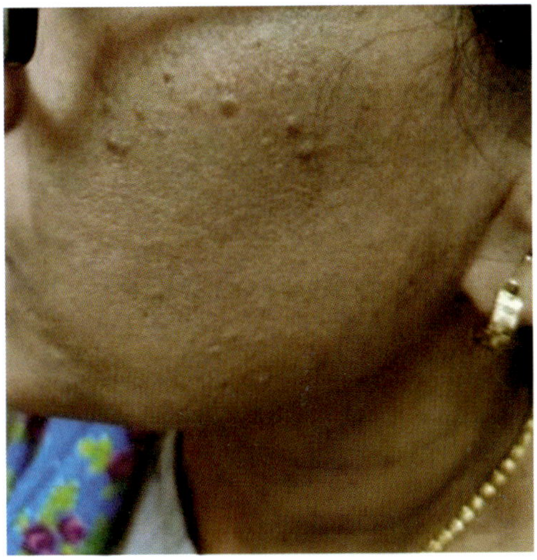

Fig. 21.1: Papular lesions on the face, resembling fibrofolliculomas.

Computed tomogram (CT) of the chest revealed multiple bilateral, well-defined paramediastinal and subpleural cysts in a predominantly basilar medial distribution, with normal intervening parenchyma. The cysts were numerous, oval-shaped, thin-walled, and variable in size (Fig. 21.2). The distribution pattern was suggestive of Birt-Hogg-Dubé syndrome.

There was no personal or family history of renal cancer, thyroid cancer, or spontaneous pneumothorax. Pulmonary function tests showed a normal FEV_1 of 1.63 (82% predicted), normal FVC of 2.19 (94% predicted), an FEV_1/FVC ratio of 0.74, and a normal diffusion study (DLCO 96%). During a six-minute walk test, the patient walked 330 metres without desaturation. An abdominal ultrasound revealed a small intramural fibroid, with normal bilateral kidneys. The skin lesions resembled fibrofolliculomas, but the patient declined a skin biopsy. Genetic testing and whole exome sequencing identified a heterozygous frameshift

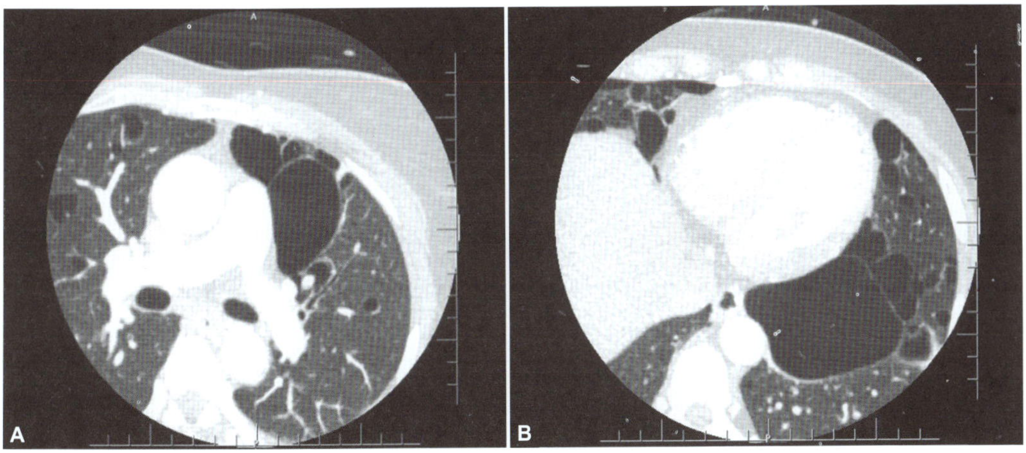

Fig. 21.2: Variable sized and shaped cysts seen predominantly along the paramediastinum region in upper lung zone (A) and in lower lung zone (B).

deletion c.946_947delAG; p.Ser316fs (Chr17:17219133 ACT>A) in the FLCN gene, confirming a diagnosis of Birt-Hogg-Dubé syndrome.

As the patient was asymptomatic, no active intervention was pursued. She received counselling about the disease, and the need for periodic screening, and screening among family members. Recommended screening for BHD syndrome includes annual MRI of the abdomen/pelvis (or CT with contrast if MRI unavailable) for renal tumour detection. If there is a family history of colon cancer, annual colonoscopies after age 40 are advised, or 10 years before the onset age in affected relatives.

DISCUSSION

Approach to a Case with Diffuse Cystic Lung Disease

The earlier chapter on DCLD outlines a four step approach to diagnose a case of DCLD. Two algorithms for diagnosing a case of DCLD are shown in Figs 21.3 and 21.4. Figure 21.3 gives an approach based on interpretation of radiologic findings alone. Figure 21.4 gives an approach incorporating clinical presentation, radiology and other relevant tests.

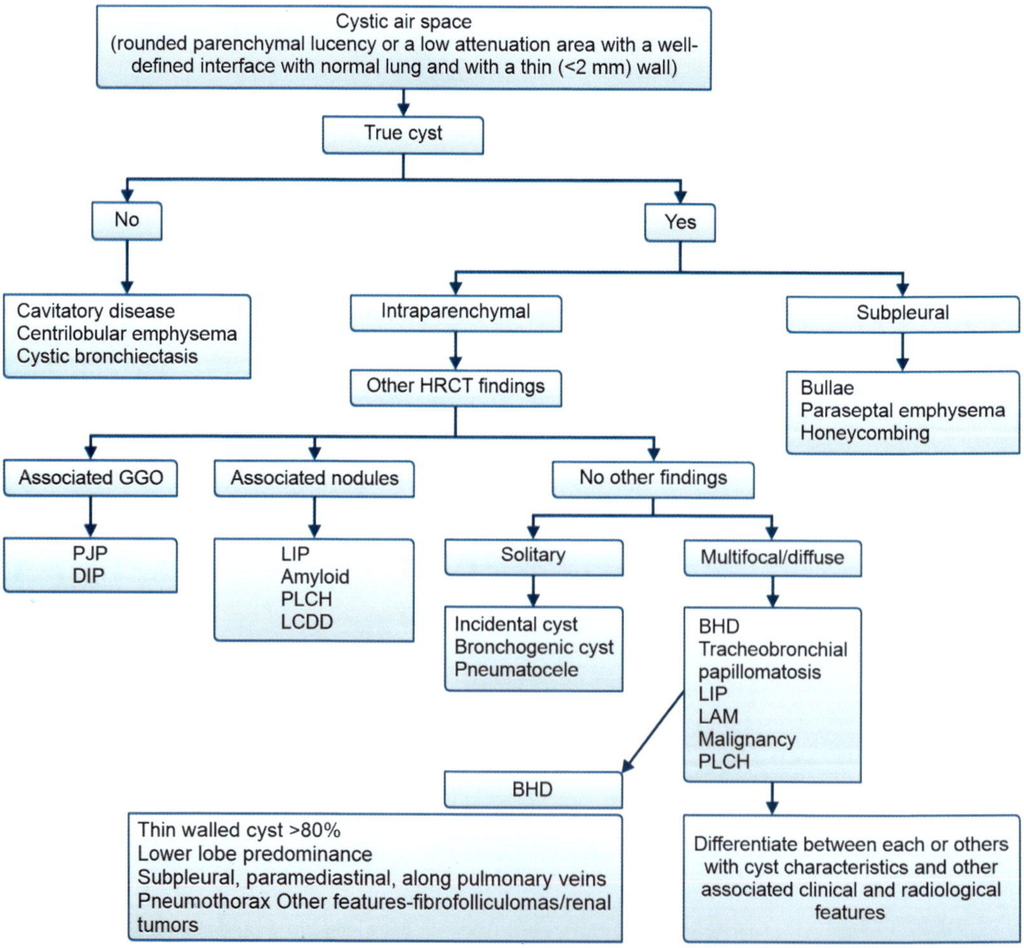

Fig. 21.3: A HRCT chest based algorithmic approach to a cystic lung disease.

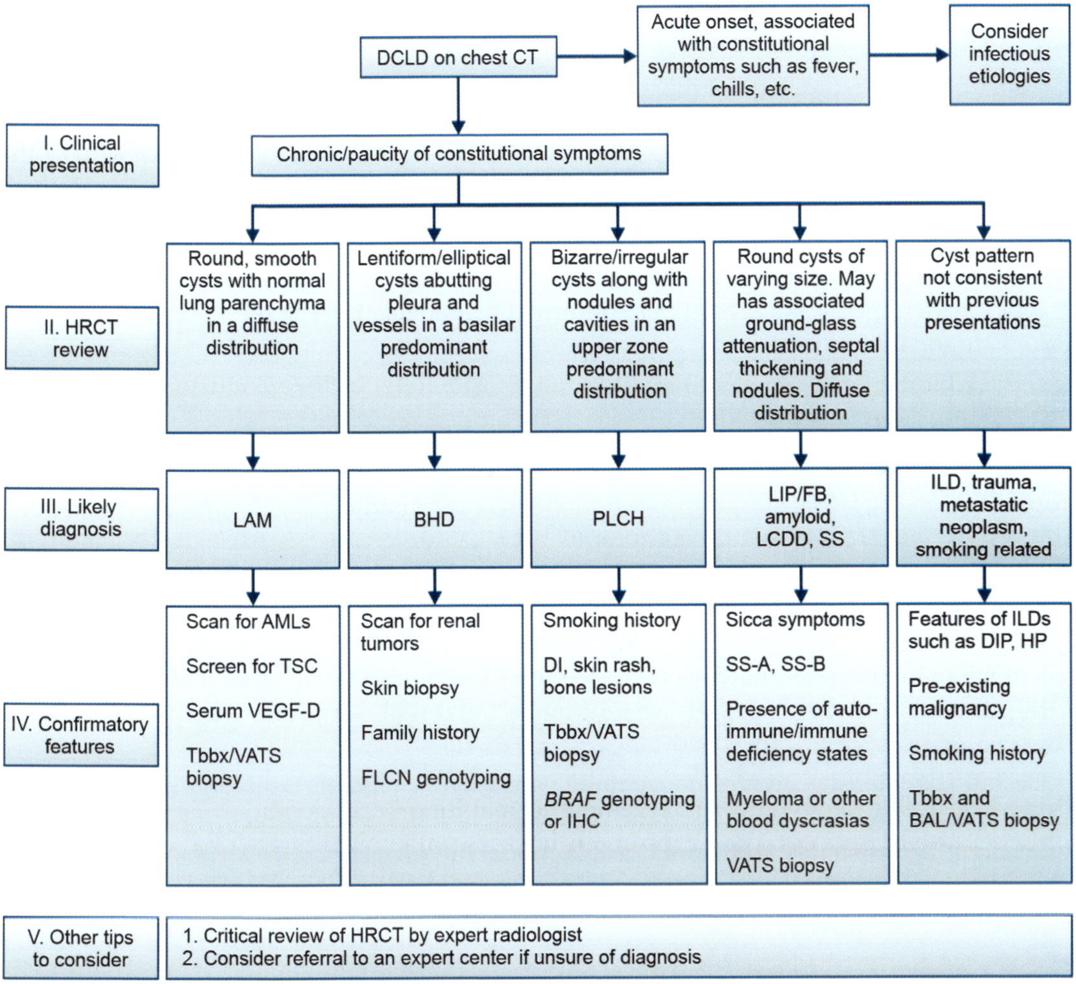

Fig. 21.4: A clinico-radiologic algorithmic approach to a diffuse cystic lung disease.

Footnote: Adapted with permission from Gupta N et al. *Am J Respir Crit Care Med.* 2015 Jul 1;192(1):17–29.

Birt-Hogg-Dubé Syndrome

Birt-Hogg-Dubé (BHD) syndrome is a complex genetic disorder characterized by a range of clinical manifestations primarily involving the skin, lungs, and kidneys. It is an uncommon disease with a prevalence of approximately 1 in 200,000 individuals, and has an autosomal dominant inheritance.

BHD is associated with FLCN gene mutations (chromosome 17). This gene is the sole known genetic factor linked to BHD. More than 200 pathogenic variants, predominantly protein-truncating, have been identified. These often result in the loss of folliculin function. While BHD can be inherited, cases of *de novo* mutations are also reported. The syndrome exhibits high penetrance but with variable expression among individuals and families. Folliculin plays a role in regulating cell growth and proliferation, notably interacting with the mTOR signaling pathway. FLCN acts as a tumour suppressor gene, and its dysfunction can lead to renal cells acquiring somatic mutations or experiencing loss of heterozygosity.

A. Cutaneous Manifestations

Cutaneous involvement in BHD syndrome primarily features skin lesions such as fibrofolliculomas, trichodiscomas, and acrochordons, with a higher prevalence in Caucasians. These lesions typically are first noticed in the third or fourth decade of life, mainly affecting the face, neck, and upper chest. Diagnosis of BHD is considered when at least five characteristic lesions are identified, with at least one confirmed histologically. The presence of typical skin lesions should lead to further BHD investigations, including renal and pulmonary screenings. In cases where differences are noted in lesion morphology, further evaluation with biopsy and genetic analysis is warranted.

B. Pulmonary Manifestations

The typical pulmonary manifestations of BHD syndrome is the presence of bilateral pulmonary cysts (seen in over 80% of patients). The mechanisms underlying cyst formation believed to involve dysregulated signaling pathways and cell-cell adhesion issues. These cysts, which vary in size, are bilateral and diffuse in distribution, significantly increasing the risk of spontaneous pneumothorax, a condition experienced by up to 24% of BHD patients with pulmonary cysts, and often presenting as the initial symptom. Notably, this risk is exacerbated by activities such as diving and air travel.

Despite the extensive involvement of lung parenchyma, patients typically maintain normal lung function, highlighting the unique pathology of BHD where structural changes in the lungs do not consistently correspond to functional impairment.

C. Renal Manifestations

In BHD syndrome, around 30% of patients have renal involvement, predominantly as FLCN-associated renal cell carcinomas (RCCs), which differ from sporadic RCCs. There is a significantly elevated risk of renal cancer in BHD patients, often diagnosed around age 50, though it can appear earlier. The tumours are usually multifocal and/or bilateral. The most common histological types in BHD are chromophobe RCC and mixed chromophobe RCC-oncocytoma, known for their lower malignant potential. In contrast, the clear cell RCC subtype, frequently seen in sporadic cases, is less common in BHD. While angiomyolipomas are uncommon in BHD, the presence of renal cysts is noted, with their significance in the disease yet to be fully understood.

The diagnosis of RCC in BHD typically is by symptom presentation or by incidental discoveries during imaging, or through familial screening. Metastatic disease in BHD, although observed, tends to progress in a relatively indolent manner. This highlights the need for early detection and management in BHD, considering the distinct nature of its renal involvement.

Table 21.1: Diagnostic criteria for BHD syndrome proposed by Menko et al	
Category	***Criteria***
Major criteria	1. At least five fibrofolliculomas or trichodiscomas, with at least one histologically confirmed, and of adult onset. 2. Pathogenic FLCN germline mutation.
Minor criteria	1. Multiple lung cysts: Bilateral, basally located lung cysts with no other apparent cause, with or without spontaneous primary pneumothorax. 2. Renal cancer: Early onset (<50 years) or multifocal/bilateral renal cancer, or renal cancer of mixed chromophobe and oncocytic histology. 3. A first-degree relative with BHD.

Note: For a BHD diagnosis, patients should fulfill either one major or two minor criteria.
Adapted from "Menko FH, et al. European BHD Consortium. Birt-Hogg-Dubé syndrome: diagnosis and management. Lancet Oncol. 2009 Dec;10(12):1199–206."

Confirmation of BHD diagnosis is based on the combination of clinical features and/or identification of a germline mutation of FLCN gene. Two diagnostic criteria have been proposed (Tables 21.1 and 21.2), but both of these criteria still await formal validation in larger patient cohorts.

Table 21.2: Diagnostic criteria for BHD syndrome proposed by Gupta et al	
Diagnostic category	***Criteria***
Definite pulmonary BHD	Characteristic[#] or compatible[¶] lung high-resolution CT (HRCT) chest findings and any one of the following: • Skin biopsy positive for fibrofolliculoma or trichodiscoma • Confirmed family history of BHD in a first- or second-degree family member • Tissue confirmation of renal chromophobe adenoma or oncocytoma • Genetic testing positive for BHD
Probable pulmonary BHD	• Characteristic HRCT, exclusion of tuberous sclerosis complex (TSC) and lymphangioleiomyomatosis (LAM), and personal or family history of pneumothorax. • Compatible HRCT, exclusion of TSC and LAM, and any of the following: – Family or personal history of renal tumours – Skin angiofibroma – Renal angiomyolipoma
Possible pulmonary BHD	Compatible or characteristic HRCT without other organ involvement

Note: [#]Multiple thin-walled round, elliptical or lentiform, well-defined air-filled cysts, without internal structure, in a basilar, medial and subpleural predominant distribution, with preserved or increased lung volume, and no other significant pulmonary involvement (specifically no interstitial lung disease)
[¶]Thin-walled cysts without the more typical elliptical shape or subpleural distribution
HRCT: High-resolution computed tomography; *TSC:* Tuberous sclerosis complex; *LAM:* Lymphangioleiomyomatosis.
Adapted from "Gupta N, Seyama K, McCormack FX. Pulmonary manifestations of Birt-Hogg-Dubé syndrome. Fam Cancer. 2013 Sep;12(3):387–96."

FURTHER READING

1. Raoof S, Bondalapati P, Vydyula R, Ryu JH, Gupta N, Raoof S, Galvin J, Rosen MJ, Lynch D, Travis W, Mehta S, Lazzaro R, Naidich D. Cystic Lung Diseases: Algorithmic Approach. Chest. 2016 Oct;150(4):945–965.

2. Rare diseases.org/ Birt-Hogg-Dubé syndrome.

3. Daccord C, Good JM, Morren MA, Bonny O, Hohl D, Lazor R. Birt-Hogg-Dubé syndrome. Eur Respir Rev. 2020 Sep 17;29(157):200042.

4. Gupta N, et al. Diffuse Cystic Lung Disease. Part II. *Am J Respir Crit Care Med.* 2015 Jul 1;192(1):17–29.

5. Gupta N, Seyama K, McCormack FX. Pulmonary manifestations of Birt-Hogg-Dubé syndrome. Fam Cancer. 2013 Sep;12(3):387–96.

Chapter 22

Approach to a Case of ILD: Non-Specific Interstitial Pneumonia

• *Anand Vijay* • *V Nagarjuna Maturu*

LEARNING POINTS

1. Nonspecific interstitial pneumonia (NSIP) is one of the radiologic and histologic types of interstitial lung disease.
2. NSIP can be idiopathic or associated with connective tissue disease (CTD), certain drugs, human immunodeficiency virus infection, and hypersensitivity pneumonitis.
3. Typical high-resolution computed tomography (HRCT) findings include ground-glass and reticular opacities, predominantly in the lower lung zones. Traction bronchiectasis and lobar volume loss may be present.
4. Identifying the underlying cause of NSIP in interstitial lung disease (ILD) is critical for initiating appropriate therapy and to prognosticate.

INTRODUCTION

Interstitial lung disease (ILD) is a common condition encountered in clinical practice, with various known etiologies. Its clinical presentation can vary based on the underlying cause, often initially manifesting with pulmonary symptoms without extrapulmonary involvement. The identification of clinical, radiological, and immunological features is key to determining the etiology, which is essential for targeted management and improved treatment outcomes. This report discusses the case of a middle-aged woman diagnosed with myositis-related ILD (CTD-ILD) and pneumomediastinum.

CASE VIGNETTE

A middle-aged woman, a teacher in her early fifties, visited our institution with a complaint of cough and breathlessness that had been ongoing for the past year. The cough, which began insidiously, was dry and showed no diurnal or postural variation. However, it had progressively worsened over the past two weeks. Her breathlessness, which had gradually intensified over the last month, had evolved from difficulty in climbing stairs to difficulty in walking on level ground. There was no postural or diurnal variation in her symptoms. She also reported experiencing pain and stiffness in the small joints of both hands for the last year, accompanied by fatigue and an unintentional weight loss of eight kilograms. She denied any history of fever, hemoptysis, wheezing, chest tightness, fever, skin rashes, hair loss, skin thickening, dysphagia, raynauds phenomenon, red eyes and dryness of the mouth or eyes. She had never smoked and had no exposure to pets, molds, or organic dust.

Her past medical history revealed no prior respiratory conditions. Despite use of oral cough suppressants, her symptoms persisted and continued to worsen without any relief.

Upon presentation, her vitals were as follows: pulse rate of 90 beats per minute, blood pressure at 110/80 mmHg, respiratory rate of 24 breaths per minute, temperature at 98.6°F, and oxygen saturation of 92% on room air. General examination revealed grade one clubbing and mechanic's hands (Fig. 22.1A). Auscultation of the chest indicated fine inspiratory crackles bilaterally in the infrascapular, infra-axillary, and interscapular regions. Other systemic examinations were normal.

Initial laboratory workup results (complete blood picture, renal and liver function tests) were within normal limits. An echocardiogram showed normal left ventricular function with no valvular abnormalities. A chest radiograph revealed bilateral lower zone reticular opacities (Fig. 22.1B). High-resolution computed tomography (HRCT) of the thorax showed multiple diffuse, ill-defined patchy ground-glass opacities predominantly in subpleural locations of all lobes bilaterally with basal predominance. This was associated with interlobular septal thickening and pneumomediastinum, extending along the paratracheal region and mediastinal vasculature into bilateral fissures (Fig. 22.1C to E).

The HRCT findings were indicative of a lower lobe predominant non-specific interstitial pneumonia pattern (NSIP). Rheumatology and immunology workups were conducted. Rheumatoid factor and anti-cyclic citrullinated peptide levels were negative

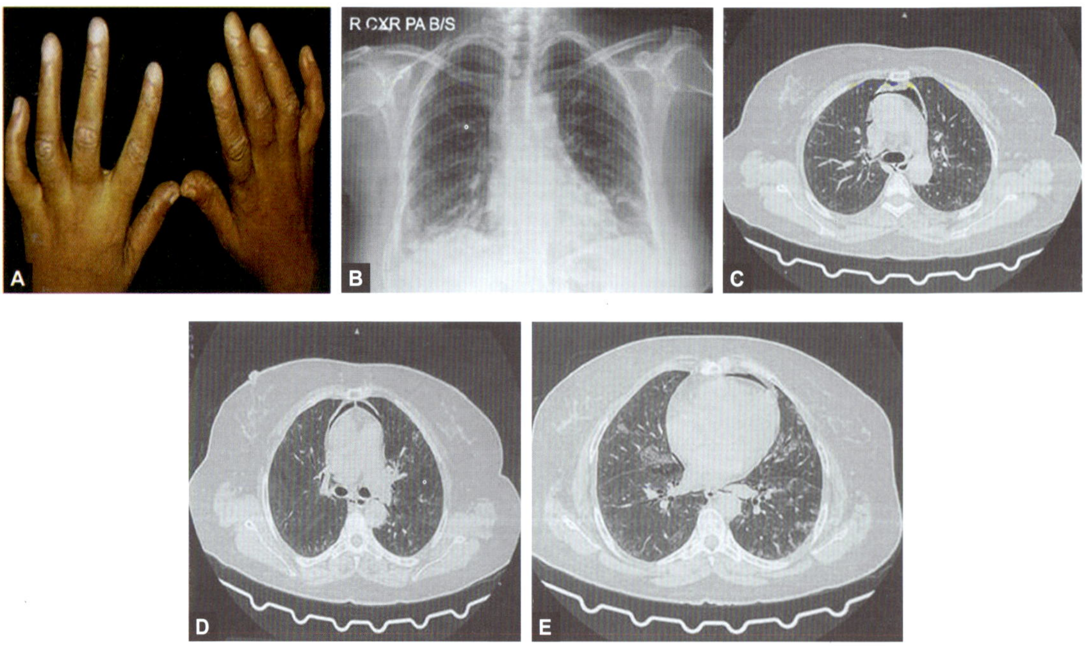

Fig. 22.1: (A) Image showing mechanic's hands in the index case; (B) Chest radiograph showing bilateral lower zone infiltrates; (C) HRCT chest axial view showing pneumomediastinum; (D) HRCT chest axial view, lung window showing ground glassing in bilateral middle lobes; (E) HRCT chest axial view, lung window showing ground glassing in bilateral lower lobes.

(11 IU/ml and <0.5 U/ml, respectively). The autoimmune workup showed strong positivity for Ro52 and PL-7 antibodies, establishing myositis-related ILD as the etiology. She however did not exhibit any features of clinically significant muscle involvement.

A diagnosis of PL-7 associated anti-synthetase syndrome associated with NSIP pattern ILD was made. The patient was initiated on induction immunosuppression with intravenous pulse corticosteroids therapy and rituximab. She exhibited significant improvement in her cough and breathing discomfort. Subsequently, she was transitioned to oral prednisone and was also enrolled in a pulmonary rehabilitation program. She received supportive treatments, including calcium supplementation, oral bisphosphonates and *Pneumocystis jirovecii* prophylaxis.

One-month post-treatment, the patient showed significant improvement in breathlessness and cough. Her resting saturation level was 96%. During a six-minute walk test, she covered a distance of 290 metres, experiencing only mild breathing discomfort without desaturation. Presently, the patient is on a tapering dose of oral steroids and remains under close observation.

DISCUSSION

Non-specific interstitial pneumonia (NSIP) is characterized as a chronic interstitial lung disease, marked by homogeneous expansion of the alveolar walls with varying degrees of interstitial inflammation and fibrosis. It was labelled as 'non-specific' due to the absence of the specific histopathological features found in other IIP subtypes like usual interstitial pneumonia (UIP), desquamative interstitial pneumonia (DIP) and lymphocytic interstitial pneumonia (LIP). Unlike UIP pattern ILD which is seen predominantly in elderly men and smokers, NSIP pattern ILD more often presents at younger age, and more often seen in women and non-smokers. NSIP usually affects both lungs and often involves the lower lobes. NSIP pattern is further classified as being cellular NSIP (inflammation predominant) or fibrotic NSIP (inflammation with associated fibrosis or predominantly fibrotic). The prognosis for NSIP is significantly better than that for UIP, with fibrotic NSIP thought to have a worse prognosis than the inflammatory, cellular NSIP.

Diagnosis of NSIP Pattern ILD

Diagnosis of NSIP pattern is by assessment of HRCT and/or histopathology (HPE) findings. HRCT of the thorax is the initial investigation of choice in all cases of ILD, as it helps in assessing the pattern of ILD and may provide clues to the probable etiology. The typical HRCT findings in NSIP include ground-glass opacities, irregular linear (reticular) opacities, and traction bronchiectasis, predominantly in the lower lung zones (Table 22.1). Ground-

Table 22.1: HRCT features of NSIP pattern interstitial lung disease

HRCT feature	*Characteristic*
Ground glass opacities (GGO)	• Present throughout (no zonal predilection) or basal predominant • Can be diffuse of patchy in distribution
Findings of fibrosis	• Traction bronchiectasis and bronchiolectasis • Intralobular interstitial thickening (reticulations) • Irregular interlobular septal thickening
Honeycombing	• Uncommon and typically mild if present, usually seen in end-stage fibrotic NSIP
Distribution of abnormalities	• Lower lung predominance of ground glassing and reticulations • Basal and peripheral predominance of ground glassing
Subpleural areas	• Relative sparing

glass opacities, present in 76 to 100% of patients, are mainly seen in the cellular NSIP pattern. Reticular opacities and septal thickening are mainly observed in the fibrotic NSIP pattern. Honeycombing, a feature typical of UIP pattern can sometimes be seen in fibrotic NSIP. It is important to recognize that even when honeycombing is present, it is often an associated but not predominant HRCT finding.

NSIP typically spares the immediate subpleural lung (*subpleural sparing*) in the lower lobes, a feature that helps distinguish fibrotic NSIP from UIP, which is most severe in the subpleural regions. This subpleural sparing is however seen in only 20–40% of the cases (less sensitive but a specific HRCT finding of NSIP pattern).

Identification of associated esophageal dilation is important and this points towards scleroderma as the cause of NSIP pattern. Similarly, presence of multi-compartment involvement (associated pleuropericardial effusions, ILD with a disproportionate pulmonary dilation) point towards CTD as the probable cause of ILD. Presence of certain HRCT findings (anterior upper lobe sign, four corner sign, straight edge sign) also point towards an autoimmune cause for the NSIP pattern. When the ground glass or reticular opacities are associated with small airway disease (air trapping, centrilobular nodules) a possibility of hypersensitivity pneumonitis needs to be considered.

Surgical biopsy via video-assisted thoracoscopic surgery (VATS) or thoracotomy is considered the gold standard for diagnosing diffuse interstitial lung disease. Transbronchial cryobiopsy is now fastly replacing VATS as the initial investigation of choice, offering a diagnostic yield similar to surgical lung biopsy. Biopsies when performed should be obtained from more than one lobe. NSIP histopathology is characterized by temporally homogeneous inflammatory and fibrosing interstitial processes. Fibroblastic foci and peripheral accentuation are typically absent, differentiating it from UIP. NSIP on histopathology is divided into three groups:

1. Predominantly interstitial inflammation.
2. A combination of inflammation and fibrosis.
3. Predominantly fibrosis.

Not all cases with NSIP pattern ILD on HRCT chest will need a biopsy. Biopsy will need to performed only when the pattern is indeterminate (difficulty in differentiating UIP from NSIP) or when the cause for NSIP pattern remains obscure after non-invasive investigations.

Causes and Etiologic Evaluation of NSIP Pattern ILD

The etiology of NSIP is varied. It can be idiopathic or secondary to several causes. Secondary causes of NSIP include connective tissue disorders (CTD), drug-induced ILDs, organic exposures, infectious pathologies, among others (Table 22.2). It is increasingly recognized that most NSIP pattern ILDs are due to secondary causes and are less often idiopathic. Hence, in the latest classification of idiopathic interstitial pneumonias, idiopathic NSIP has been reclassified into a less common ILD. Whenever a NSIP pattern is diagnosed in histopathology or radiology, it is imperative to extensively evaluate for the presence of associated diseases/ exposures which can cause this pattern. Several infections (viral pneumonias and atypical pneumonias) can also have a NSIP like pattern on imaging and have to be differentiated from the non-infectious ILDs by history and necessary investigations. A stepwise approach (Fig. 22.2) and a diagnostic algorithm (Fig. 22.3) for the assessment of ILD characterized by an NSIP pattern are proposed.

Idiopathic NSIP is classified under idiopathic interstitial pneumonia (IIP). Other IIPs include usual interstitial pneumonia (UIP), desquamative interstitial pneumonia (DIP),

Table 22.2: Causes of NSIP pattern interstitial lung disease on a HRCT chest		
Category	***Specific etiologies***	
1. Connective tissue diseases/ autoimmune cause of associated ILD	• Systemic sclerosis • Polymyositis/dermatomyositis • Rheumatoid arthritis	• Sjögren's syndrome • ANCA associated vasculitis • Systemic lupus erythematosus
2. Interstitial pneumonia with autoimmune features	No well-defined CTD identified, but features of an autoimmune disease are identified	
3. Drug-induced ILD	• Amiodarone • Methotrexate • Nitrofurantoin	• Chemotherapeutic agents • Statins
4. Exposure-related ILD	Hypersensitivity pneumonitis	
5. HIV infection		
6. Others	• IgG4-related systemic disease • Graft-versus-host disease • Familial interstitial pneumonia	• Radiation pneumonitis • Sarcoidosis
7. Idiopathic NSIP		

NSIP pattern on HRCT (predominant ground-glass opacities) can also be seen in several acute viral and atypical infections of the lung. These have to be differentiated from non-infectious ILDs by history and appropriate testing.

History
Common symptoms—cough, shortness of breath, fever, weight loss
CTD symptoms
Past history, exposure history, drug history

Clinical examination
Fine inspiratory crackles
Clubbing
CTD-related features like joint deformity, skin rashes, etc.

Blood investigation
Complete blood count, renal and liver functions
Serology—ANA (IF), ANA profile, RA factor, anti-CCP and myositis profile

Imaging
HRCT thorax—investigation of choice
Chest X-ray

Pulmonary function test
Spirometry, DLCO, blood plethysmography
6 minute walk test helps to monitor the progression of disease as well as response to the treatment

Lung biopsy
Surgical/VATS lung biopsy is gold standard
Cryo lung biopsy is more safer and has a similar diagnostic yield

Fig. 22.2: A stepwise approach to a case with presumed NSIP pattern interstitial lung disease.

ANA: Antinuclear antibody; *CTD:* Connective tissue disease; *CCP:* Cyclic citrullinated peptide; *DLCO:* Diffusion capacity of lung for carbon monoxide; *HRCT:* High resolution computed tomography; *RA:* Rheumatoid arthritis; *VATS:* Video-assisted thoracoscopic surgery.

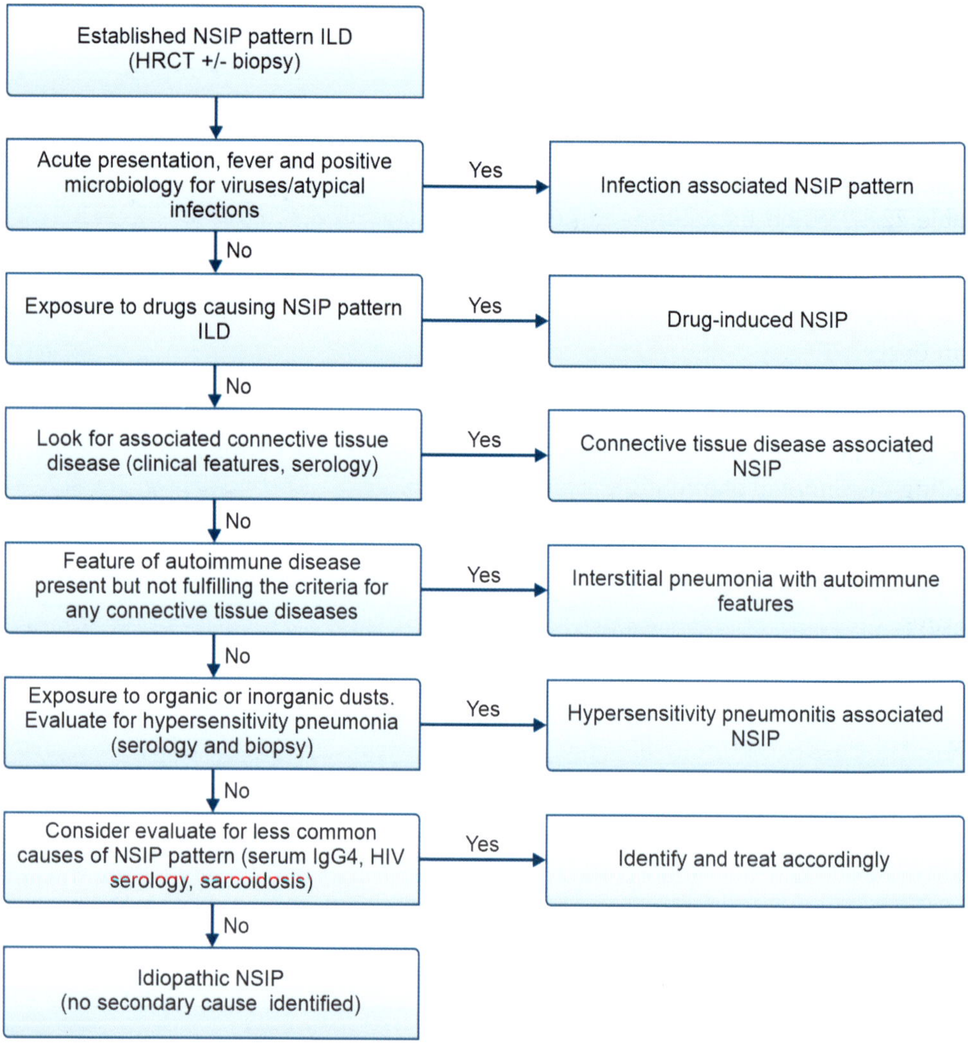

Fig. 22.3: Flowchart shows diagnostic algorithm for evaluation of a case with NSIP pattern.

respiratory bronchiolitis-associated interstitial lung disease (RB-ILD), acute interstitial pneumonia (AIP), lymphocytic interstitial pneumonia (LIP), and cryptogenic organising pneumonia (COP). Idiopathic NSIP is more commonly observed in middle-aged women, particularly those who have never smoked.

CTD-related NSIP is one of the commonest causes of secondary NSIP pattern. NSIP is the predominant pattern in patients with systemic sclerosis and myositis, whereas usual UIP is more common in patients with rheumatoid arthritis. Myositis-related ILD typically has NSIP with organizing pneumonia overlap (NSIP-OP) pattern. Some patients with idiopathic interstitial pneumonia, such as NSIP or UIP, exhibit features of autoimmune disease. However, these findings are insufficient for a definitive diagnosis of a specific CTD. This group is categorised as having interstitial pneumonia with autoimmune features (IPAFs).

Drug-induced ILD is also an important consideration as early identification and removal of offending drug helps in changing the course of disease. Some of the drugs which are implicated include nitrofurantoin, methotrexate, amiodarone, cyclophosphamide and other chemotherapeutic agents, and rituximab. A temporal correlation between the drug intake and onset of ILD is often the diagnostic clue.

Management of NSIP Pattern ILD

The management strategy for NSIP varies based on the etiology and disease severity (detailed in Table 22.3). When the NSIP is mild in severity and non-progressive, a wait and watch strategy may be considered. Most symptomatic NSIP patients, however benefit from a trial of immunosuppressants. The intensity of immunosuppression depends on the severity of disease at presentation and the underlying etiology. When the disease progresses and fibrosis sets in despite therapy, antifibrotics (nintedanib or pirfenidone) need to be added. Lung transplantation remains the only option when medical therapies fail to halt the progression of disease.

For secondary causes of NSIP, addressing the underlying cause is the primary treatment, including the removal of offending drugs in drug-induced ILD or treating CTDs. In the case presented, antisynthetase syndrome-related NSIP was diagnosed and treated with rituximab, systemic steroids, and other supportive treatments. Prophylaxis against *Pneumocystis jirovecii* pneumonia is mandatory for all patients receiving immunosuppression. General supportive measures, such as pneumococcal and influenza vaccinations and pulmonary rehabilitation, are also important. Treating associated comorbidities like obstructive airway disease, obstructive sleep apnea, and obesity is also crucial.

Antisynthetase Syndrome (ASS)

ASS is an autoimmune condition characterized by antibodies against an aminoacyl-transfer RNA synthetase, accompanied by clinical features such as ILD, non-erosive arthritis, myositis, Raynaud's phenomenon, unexplained fever, or mechanic's hands. ASS, an idiopathic

Table 22.3: An overview of the treatment of NSIP stratified as per severity of disease and response to therapy

Severity of NSIP	*Treatment strategy*
Initial therapy	
Mild disease and nonprogressive	• Close follow-up
Moderate to severe disease	• Systemic steroids (prednisolone 1mg/kg per day, max 60 mg daily)
Severe disease	• Pulse steroid therapy (1 g per day for 3 days) followed by oral corticosteroids
Very severe disease	• Cyclophosphamide, rituximab, or calcineurin inhibitors
Maintenance therapy	
Good response to initial OCS therapy	• Gradually taper dosage of OCS
Steroid-dependent disease	• Consider steroid-sparing agents (azathioprine, mycophenolate mofetil, methotrexate)*
Progressively fibrotic lung disease	• Antifibrotics (pirefenidone or nintedanib)
Severe refractory disease	• Lung transplantation

OCS: Oral corticosteroids.

*May be initiated from the beginning in diseases which are expected to require longer/more intense immunosuppression (autoimmune diseases).

inflammatory myopathy (IIM), has a higher prevalence of ILD compared to dermatomyositis (DM) and polymyositis. The ILD in ASS patients is often severe and rapidly progressive, contributing significantly to the increased morbidity and mortality associated with ASS compared to other IIMs. Connor's and Solomon's criteria are used for diagnosing ASS. The case described fulfils both criteria. Specific antibodies related to ASS include anti-Jo1, which is the most common associated antibody, and anti-PL7 and anti-PL12, which are antibodies associated with more severe ILD.

FURTHER READING

1. Belloli EA, Beckford R, Hadley R, Flaherty KR. Idiopathic non-specific interstitial pneumonia. Respirology. 2016 Feb;21(2):259–68.
2. Teoh AKY, Corte TJ. Non-specific Interstitial Pneumonia. Semin Respir Crit Care Med. 2020 Apr;41(2):184–201.
3. Leslie KO. My approach to interstitial lung disease using clinical, radiological and histopathological patterns. *Journal of Clinical Pathology*. 2009 May 1;62(5):387–401.
4. Tomassetti S, Ryu JH, Piciucchi S, Chilosi M, Poletti V. Non-specific Interstitial Pneumonia: What is the Optimal Approach to Management? Semin Respir Crit Care Med. 2016 Jun;37(3):378–94.
5. Solomon J, Swigris JJ, Brown KK. Myositis-related interstitial lung disease and antisynthetase syndrome. *Journal of Brasileiro de pneumologia*. 2011;37:100–109.

Chapter 23

Approach to a Patient with Pulmonary Calcification

• *Hari Prasad Kalpakam* • *M Punita* • *Srikant Kashinath Malegaonkar*

LEARNING POINTS

1. Pulmonary calcification identified on a chest CT scan is not uncommon and can be because of varying causes (metastatic calcification, dystrophic calcification or pulmonary alveolar microlithiasis).
2. Metastatic pulmonary calcification (MPC) is a rare condition occurring in the setting of hypercalcemia, and frequently involves the upper lung zones.
3. Presence of abnormal serum calcium homeostasis and CT scans showing parenchymal and vascular calcifications can provide a conclusive diagnosis of MPC, potentially eliminating the need for a biopsy.
4. In cases with MPC, timely correction of hypercalcemia is crucial for favorable patient outcomes.
5. Pulmonary alveolar microlithiasis is a rare genetic condition which leads to pulmonary calcification. The diagnosis can be established by characteristic radiology, genetic testing or a lung biopsy.

INTRODUCTION

Abnormal calcification of the lung parenchyma is an often seen clinical condition and can be caused by several disease processes. It is broadly classified as being metastatic or dystrophic. Calcification occurring in a normal lung parenchyma due to an abnormal calcium homeostasis is metastatic pulmonary calcification (MPC). Calcification occurring in a diseased lung tissue in the presence of a normal calcium homeostasis is dystrophic pulmonary calcification. Another uncommon genetic cause of pulmonary calcification is pulmonary alveolar microlithiasis. The cases below illustrate two distinct clinical presentations of diseases with pulmonary calcification. Prompt identification of the disease and etiology is crucial because timely intervention can be life-saving.

CASE VIGNETTE 1

A 53-year-old male salesman with a history of end-stage renal disease (ESRD) presented with a three-week cough, accompanied by scanty mucoid expectoration and exertional dyspnea.

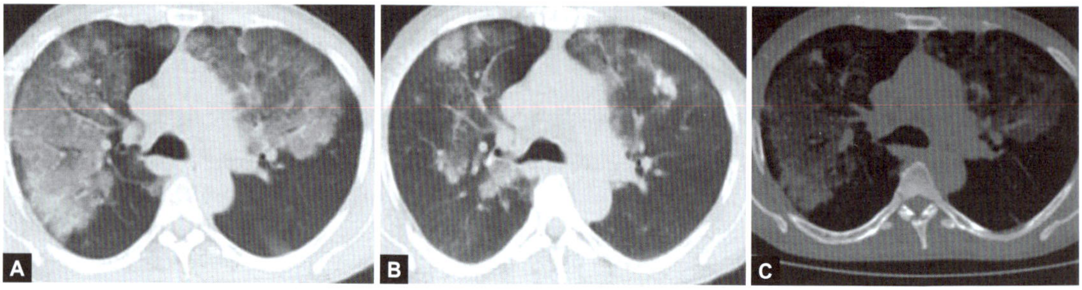

Fig. 23.1: (A) High resolution computed tomography scans (HRCT) lung parenchymal window showing ground-glass opacities with septal thickening involving bilateral upper lobe at presentation; (B) HRCT showing interval resolution of opacities post-treatment; (C) HRCT mediastinal window showing parenchymal calcification seen in metastatic pulmonary calcification.

He had no fever, weight loss, appetite loss, or hemoptysis. Although hemodynamically stable, he required 2 liters of oxygen to maintain a saturation of 93%. Apart from bilateral pitting pedal edema and bibasilar fine inspiratory crepitations on chest auscultation, his examination was unremarkable. A chest X-ray, performed to evaluate these findings, showed bilateral patchy inhomogeneous opacities. Further, a thorax computed tomography (CT) scan revealed extensive bilateral ground-glass opacities with septal thickening and calcification, predominantly in the upper lobes and right lower lobe (Fig. 23.1A). The mediastinal window of the CT chest revealed calcifications in right upper lobe (Fig. 23.1C).

Due to respiratory failure, the patient was hospitalized for management. Laboratory tests and sputum analysis were conducted, and intravenous third-generation cephalosporin was administered along with supportive treatment. Laboratory results showed elevated serum calcium (11.3 mg/dl) and phosphorus levels (5.4 mg/dl), with a high serum parathyroid hormone level (119 pg/ml). The sputum workup was negative for infectious agents. Hemodialysis was initiated as conservative medical treatment for hypercalcemia proved ineffective. Post-dialysis, respiratory failure improved, and serum calcium levels normalised. Lung infiltrates also showed improvement following hemodialysis and calcium level correction (Fig. 23.1B).

The patient was diagnosed with MPC secondary to chronic kidney disease, as no underlying lung injury was present previously, ruling out dystrophic calcification. He recovered without complications and was discharged. At a two-year follow-up, he remains asymptomatic, continuing maintenance hemodialysis.

CASE VIGNETTE 2

An 18-year-old girl presented to our outpatient department with symptoms of nonprogressive breathlessness on climbing stairs for two years. She had no other pulmonary or constitutional symptoms. At presentation, she was thin built and was comfortable at rest. General physical examination and respiratory system examination were normal. Chest radiograph was performed which showed fine reticular opacities in the lower lung fields (Fig. 23.2A). A HRCT thorax was then performed which showed the presence of lower lobe predominant micronodules and interlobular septal thickening (Fig. 23.2B).

A possibility of interstitial lung diseases/granulomatous lung disease was considered and she then underwent a bronchoscopic transbronchial lung cryobiopsy which revealed the presence of intra-alveolar lamellar microliths (Fig. 23.2C). A diagnosis of pulmonary alveolar microlithiasis was established. This was further confirmed by genetic testing which revealed a

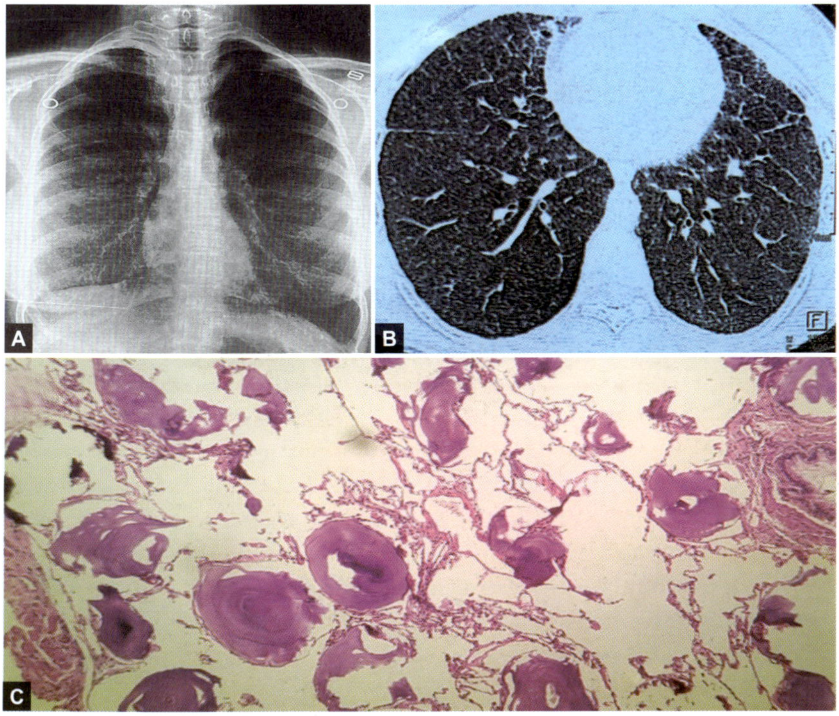

Fig. 23.2: (A) Chest radiograph showing fine reticular opacities in basal lung fields; (B) HRCT chest showing diffusely distributed micronodules in the lung parenchyma and associated smooth interlobular septal thickening in the anterior aspect; (C) Histopathology image (H&E stain; 40X) of the cryobiopsy showing lamellated intra-alveolar microliths.

homozygous mutation in SCL34A2 gene. Spirometry showed the presence of mild restrictive ventilatory defect. She has been initiated on a low phosphate diet and is under follow-up since the last two years and continues to remain only mildly symptomatic and stable.

DISCUSSION

Pulmonary calcification is defined as the deposition of calcium salt in the lung parenchyma and is identified on HRCT thorax as areas of high attenuating lung parenchymal lesions with HU of >200 units. There are several causes for pulmonary calcification and they can broadly be classified into three groups: (a) Metastatic pulmonary calcification, (b) dystrophic pulmonary calcification, (c) pulmonary alveolar microlithiasis. In addition, pulmonary calcification also needs to be differentiated from pulmonary ossification which is defined as the formation of bone tissue (with or without marrow elements) in the lung parenchyma. A brief description of the various causes of pulmonary calcification is provided below.

A. Metastatic Pulmonary Calcification

Metastatic pulmonary calcification (MPC) is defined as deposition of calcium salts in normal lung tissue. This condition arises from abnormalities in calcium and phosphate metabolism, alkaline phosphatase activity, and changes in local physiochemical conditions like pH variation. Various disease states can lead to MPC, with ESRD being the most prevalent risk factor, as outlined in Table 23.1.

Table 23.1: Benign and malignant causes of metastatic pulmonary calcification

Benign	*Malignant*
Renal failure	Parathyroid adenoma
Hyperparathyroidism	Multiple myeloma
Resorption of bone tissue	Lymphoma/leukaemia
Disorders of vitamin D	Synovial sarcoma
Aluminium intoxication	Breast carcinoma
Orthotopic liver transplantation	Choriocarcinoma

Pulmonary infiltrates in ESRD are often due to infections, volume overload, or diffuse alveolar hemorrhage. These conditions can often be excluded based on clinical assessments and laboratory findings, such as positive sputum microbiology tests and a decrease in hemoglobin levels. However, when these common causes are ruled out, it is necessary to consider rarer etiologies, such as pulmonary calcification. In ESRD, acidosis and hyperparathyroidism can elevate blood calcium and phosphate levels. Additionally, intermittent alkalosis during dialysis may cause these minerals to precipitate in tissues. The upper pulmonary lobes, having higher ventilation–perfusion ratios and alkalotic environments are common sites for calcium deposition.

Patients with MPC often exhibit symptoms like cough and progressive breathlessness or may be diagnosed incidentally through radiographic findings. MPC can manifest as septal thickening, nodular opacities, or ground-glass opacities, with pulmonary and vascular calcifications being characteristic signs. Diagnostic tools like bone scintigraphy using Tc-99m methylene diphosphonate (MDP), which reveals uptake of the radioactive tracer in lung parenchyma, or high-resolution computed tomography (HRCT) chest with mediastinal windows, can confidently identify MPC, often making further evaluations unnecessary.

Bronchoscopy might show nodular and linear lesions on the surface of the trachea and main bronchi, and calcifications can be identified in endobronchial biopsies using routine hematoxylin and eosin stains or specific stains like Von Kossa and Alizarin red.

Treatment typically involves correcting the underlying abnormal calcium metabolism through medical management, hemodialysis, or transplantation. In the presented case, clinical and radiological improvement was observed following the initiation of hemodialysis (Fig. 23.1A and B).

B. Dystrophic Pulmonary Calcification

Dystrophic pulmonary calcification (DPC) is defined as calcification that occurs in areas of previously diseased/abnormal tissue. Prior tissue injury can be due to infections, non-infectious granulomatous processes (sarcoidosis, silicosis) or fibrotic interstitial lung diseases. Infections which lead to dystrophic calcification include granulomatous infections like *Histoplasma capsulatum*, *Coccidioides immitis*, and *Mycobacterium tuberculosis*, viral infections (e.g. Varicella), parasitic infections (e.g. *Paragonimus westermani*) and *Pneumocystis jirovecii* pneumonia.

In cases with DPC, serum calcium levels are normal. There is excess local tissue production of 1,25 vitamin D by macrophages, and this leads to excess calcium and phosphate absorption into the tissue even in the absence of serum hypercalcemia. Dystrophic calcification is often identified as an incidental abnormality on the HRCT chest. It is evident as calcification within areas of nodules, masses, fibrotic lung or consolidation. There may be associated calcification of mediastinal nodes and the pleura. Treatment is usually of the disease which causes the lung infiltrates and no specific therapy is necessary for the calcification which is irreversible. The co-occurrence of hypercalcemia and presence of vascular calcification in MPC can aid in distinguishing MPC from these other causes.

C. Pulmonary Alveolar Microlithiasis

Pulmonary alveolar microlithiasis (PAM) is a rare, autosomal recessive interstitial lung disease characterized by deposition of calcium phosphate microliths diffusely in the lungs. Mutations in the gene SCL34A2, which encodes a sodium dependent phosphate transporter is the cause for PAM. Functional defects of this phosphate transporter in type 2 pneumocytes make them unable to transport phosphate from degraded surfactant phospholipids in alveolar spaces. This leads to the formation of intra-alveolar microliths.

Most patients are diagnosed under the age of 50 years. Many patients with PAM have typical clinico-radiologic dissociation—paucity of clinical symptoms and signs despite the presence of extensive radiographic calcification. The disease may be identified as an incidentally picked radiographic abnormality. Symptoms develop late in the course of disease, and include dry cough and dyspnea. HRCT thorax is often diagnostic and patients have characteristic radiographic findings (sand storm appearance, black pleura sign) (Fig. 23.3). When in doubt, genetic tests for identifying the SCL34A2 mutation or a lung biopsy (showing intra-alveolar lamellar microliths) will help in confirming the diagnosis. In the index case 2, the HRCT was performed in the pre-calcific initial phase and showed only lung micronodules. Lung biopsy and genetic testing confirmed the diagnosis of PAM in the index case.

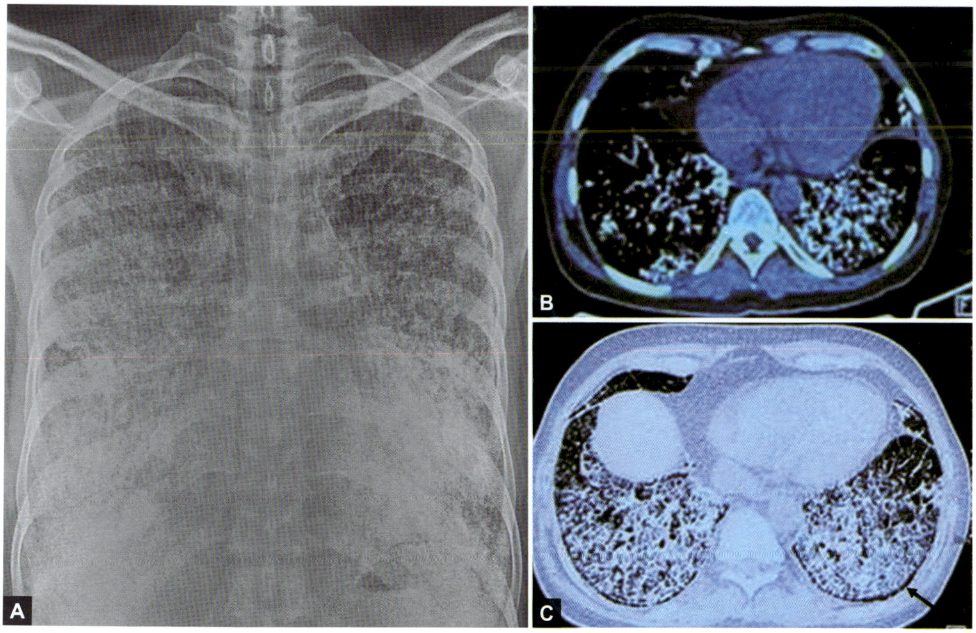

Fig. 23.3: Characteristic radiographic appearances in another proven case of pulmonary alveolar microlithiasis. (A) Chest X-ray showing "sand storm appearance"—find sand-like micronodules; (B) HRCT chest mediastinal window showing the presence of lower lobe predominant dense calcified lesions in the parenchyma; (C) HRCT chest lung parenchymal window showing the characteristic "black pleura sign"—a linear zone of radiolucency between the ribs and calcific lung parenchyma (black arrow).

There is no established therapy for PAM. Several centers initiate patients with PAM on a low phosphate diet.

Differentiating between the above three causes of parenchymal calcification is important. Associated clinical diseases, pattern of lesions on a HRCT chest, distribution of the calcification, and serum levels of calcium and phosphorus help in identifying the correct etiology. Table 23.2 highlights the differences between the three causes of pulmonary calcifications.

Table 23.2: Clinical, laboratory and radiologic features of the various types of pulmonary calcification

	Radiologic pattern	*Distribution of lesions*	*Associated calcifications*	*Abnormal calcium homeostasis*	*Clinical presentation*
Metastatic pulmonary calcification	Ground-glass opacities with calcifications within (most common presentation). Can also present as calcified nodules or a high attenuation consolidation	Upper lobe predominant	Calcification of mediastinal vessels, chest wall vessels and myocardium may be seen	Always present. Elevated serum calcium, phosphorus levels, and elevated serum parathormone or vitamin D levels	Symptoms can be of varying severity and depend on the underlying disease
Dystrophic pulmonary calcification (DPC)	Calcific nodules or masses (>5 mm in size) Calcification within the areas of underlying lung disease	Depends on the underlying disease which leads to DPC	Calcification of mediastinal nodes/pleura may be present	Normal serum calcium and phosphorus levels	Asymptomatic and incidentally identified on radiology Symptoms when present are due to the underlying disease process
Pulmonary alveolar microlithiasis	Calcified micronodules (0.01–1 mm) diffusely distributed. Stage 1: Pre-calcific stage (Tc-99 MDP scan can identify abnormality in this stage) Stage 2: Sand storm appearance Stage 3: Increasing opacities Stage 4: White our lungs with sub-pleural sparing (black pleura sign)	Lower lobe predominant	Up to 1/3rd can have extra pulmonary calcifications—kidneys, ovaries/testes, prostate, intestine and pancreas	Normal serum calcium and phosphorus levels	Asymptomatic or mildly symptomatic at diagnosis Clinico-radiologic dissociation is usually present Slowly progressive and symptoms worsen in the 4th to 5th decade of life

FURTHER READING

1. Chan ED, Morales DV, Welsh CH, McDermott MT, Schwarz MI. Calcium deposition with or without bone formation in the lung. *Am J Respir Crit Care Med.* 2002;165(12):1654–69.

2. Hartman T, Müller N, Primack S, Johkoh T, Takeuchi N, Ikezoe J, et al. Metastatic pulmonary calcification in patients with hypercalcemia: findings on chest radiographs and CT scans. *AJR Am J Roentgenol.* 1994;162(4):799–802.

3. Hochhegger B, Marchiori E, Soares Souza Jr A, Soares Souza L, Palermo L. MRI and CT findings of metastatic pulmonary calcification. *Br J Radiol.* 2012;85(1011):e69–72.

4. Kosciuk P, Meyer C, Wikenheiser-Brokamp KA, McCormack FX. Pulmonary alveolar microlithiasis. Eur Respir Rev. 2020 Nov 27;29(158):200024.

5. Saito A, McCormack FX. Pulmonary Alveolar Microlithiasis. Clin Chest Med. 2016 Sep;37(3):441-8. doi: 10.1016/j.ccm.2016.04.007.

SECTION VI

Sleep Disorders

Chapter 24

Approach to a Case of Insomnia

• *Prakhar Agarwal* • *Ravi Gupta* • *Abhishek Goyal*

LEARNING POINTS

1. Insomnia is a prevalent sleep disorder and poses a significant risk to health if untreated.
2. Multiple etiologies are associated with insomnia, which need to be identified and treated accordingly.
3. Comorbid insomnia and sleep apnea (COMISA) is a common treatable cause of insomnia, and if suspected, should be evaluated by polysomnography.
4. Pharmacotherapy for insomnia encompasses various drugs and should be initiated only after identifying the cause of insomnia.
5. Cognitive behavioural therapy for insomnia (CBTi) is an emerging treatment option for patients with insomnia, and specialist consults should be sought wherever needed.

INTRODUCTION

Insomnia is a common disorder characterized by difficulty in initiating or maintaining sleep (waking up during sleep with difficulty in returning to sleep, or having a final awakening too early or well before the desired rising time) which is often accompanied by symptoms such as irritability, headache, low mood, poor concentration, memory deficits or fatigue during wakefulness.

CASE VIGNETTE

A 54-year-old female, housewife, was referred to our sleep clinic for the evaluation of insomnia. From the last seven months, she had complaints of inability to fall asleep and recurrent and often prolonged arousals from sleep. Her husband did not observe any snoring and she denied any complaints of excessive daytime sleepiness. Her Epworth Sleepiness Score (ESS) was 6 out of 24. She however, reported feeling tired throughout the day, and confirmed the presence of nocturia (at least two episodes per night). During each voiding, volume of the urine was adequate without any other urinary complaints. She suffered from hypothyroidism and hypertension, both of which were well controlled with her regular medications. Her body mass index (BMI) was 26 kg/m^2, there was no retrognathia or micrognathia and her modified mallampatti was grade 2. Her Insomnia Severity Index (ISI) score was 24 out of 28, which was suggestive of severe insomnia.

Patient was advised to maintain a sleep diary for a period of two weeks. It showed that her time to go to bed was around 10 pm and time to wake up was 6 AM. After going to bed it took her around 30 minutes to one hour to fall sleep and she generally woke up at around 2 AM and then again fell asleep at around 3:30 AM to 4 AM. She consumed tea only once a day in the morning and had a sedentary lifestyle.

Her overnight polysomnography comprised of 420.4 minutes of recording time of which she slept only for 211 minutes (sleep efficiency 50.19%). Her sleep latency was 31.5 minutes and apnea–hypopnea index (AHI) was 23.8/hour. Mean SpO_2 was 94%, and nadir SpO_2 was 87%. She was diagnosed to have positional OSA as her supine AHI was 44.3/hour and lateral AHI was 16/hour.

Subsequently, she underwent a full night manual positive airway pressure (PAP) titration. Adequate titration was achieved at continuous positive airway pressure (CPAP) of 7 cm of H_2O with a nasal mask. After one month of usage of CPAP, she had remarkable improvements in her symptoms. Her insomnia resolved, and her ISI score decreased to 8 (mild insomnia). There were no complaints of nocturia, and her daytime fatigue improved. Her subjective duration to sleep onset decreased to 10 minutes.

DISCUSSION

Insomnia is one of the major sleep disorders with a huge impact on public health. The prevalence of chronic insomnia in Indian population is found to be between 15 and 33% with increased incidence found with increasing age, diabetes and comorbid chronic physical illness. Prevalence of insomnia is found to be more in women as compared to men. Insomnia is a risk factor for psychiatric disorders and is associated with poor short-term as well as long-term outcomes of depression and alcohol dependence. Risk of other medical disorders, viz. hypertension, coronary heart disease and metabolic syndrome is increased by untreated insomnia. Untreated insomnia can lead to impaired function, poor academic performance, increase risk of motor accidents, decrease productivity of work and irritability.

Classification of Insomnia

The International Classification of Sleep Disorders-third edition (ICSD-3) classification categorises insomnia into three major categories—chronic, short-term, and other insomnia disorders.

A. Chronic Insomnia

Chronic insomnia disorder includes night-time complaints of at least one of the three problems—difficulty initiating sleep (DIS), difficulty maintaining the sleep (DMS) and early morning awakening (EMA) for at least three times a week for at least three months. However, many patients present with combination of any of the three or all of the night-time symptoms, which may be present in the same night or keep changing in successive nights during the period of illness. Night-time symptoms must be associated with daytime impairment, e.g. *mood changes*—low mood or irritability, *cognitive changes*—attention and memory lapses and *somatic symptoms*, viz. fatigue, mild headache. Lastly, the symptoms must be present despite the patient having adequate opportunity to sleep (e.g. dark and safe room with adequate duration to sleep). In absence of daytime symptoms and adequate opportunity for the sleep, diagnosis of insomnia cannot be made.

B. Short-term Insomnia

Short-term insomnia disorder encompasses sleep/wake challenges that do not meet the minimal duration criteria required for the diagnosis of chronic insomnia disorder. However, requirement of all the three components—night time symptoms, daytime symptoms as well as adequate opportunity for sleep must be met.

C. Other Insomnia Disorders

A diagnosis of other insomnia disorders includes rare cases that fail to meet criteria for either chronic or short-term insomnia disorder but yet have symptoms of insomnia. Largely, this category shall include individuals with night-time symptoms with absence of daytime symptoms. In some of the literature this condition has been termed "insomnia symptoms".

It is important to note that presence of other medical, psychiatric or use of addictive substance or medications along with insomnia do not preclude the diagnosis of insomnia, unless one is sure that present of these factors are solely responsible for insomnia. In clinical practice, it is extremely difficult to decide if the insomnia can be attributed solely to any of these factors. Similarly, individuals who are taking any hypnotics and are not able to sleep without them should be diagnosed as having chronic insomnia disorder.

Insomnia symptoms often accompany comorbid medical illnesses, psychiatric disorders, and other sleep disorders such as circadian rhythm sleep-wake disorders (CRSWD), restless leg syndrome (RLS), periodic leg movement disorder (PLMS), and obstructive sleep apnea (OSA) (Fig. 24.1).

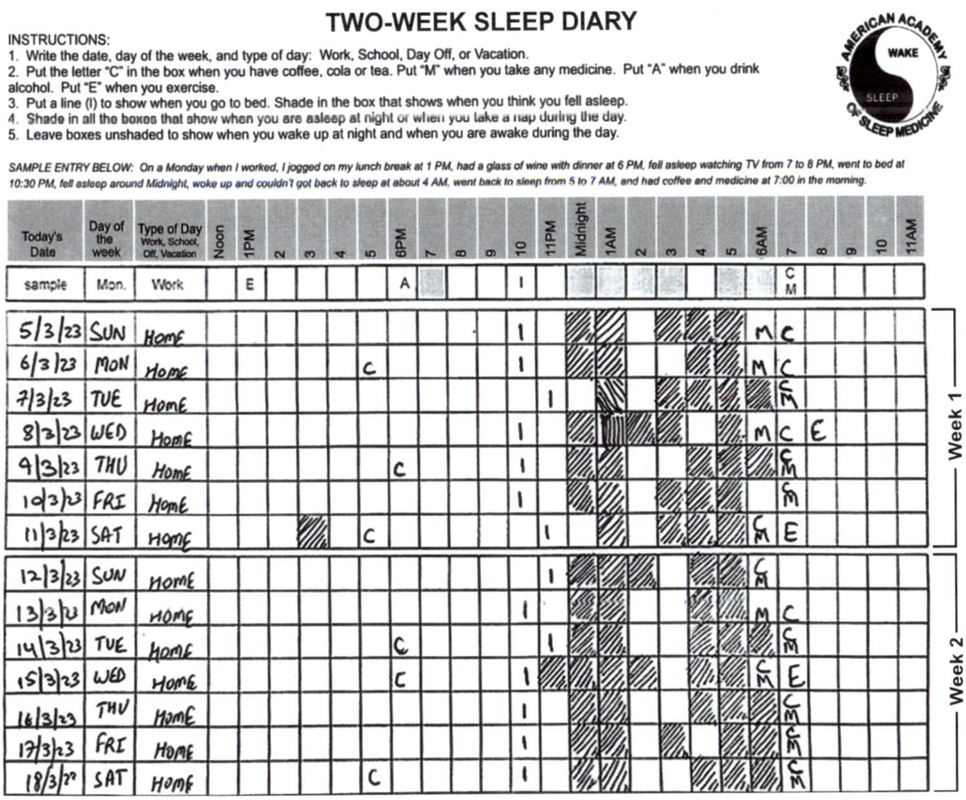

Fig. 24.1: A two-week sleep diary for evaluation of Insomnia.

OSA and insomnia often coexist together and terminology called COMISA (co-morbid insomnia and sleep apnea) is used for the same. Patients with COMISA usually have worse outcome than either insomnia or OSA individually, and have higher management costs. Around 39% of patients with OSA have comorbid insomnia and around 10.7% of patients with insomnia has concomitant OSA. Increased sympathetic tone in OSA is associated with physiologic arousal and contributes to insomnia. Moreover, in patients of OSA, multiple respiratory events are present throughout the night which may be associated with either recurrent micro-arousals or complete arousals leading to chronic insomnia.

Evaluation of a Case of Insomnia

It is important to acknowledge that insomnia is a subjective clinical diagnosis. A thorough sleep history is crucial for confirming the diagnosis and devising optimal treatment for individuals experiencing insomnia. This includes sleep/wake schedule, bedtime routine, nocturnal behaviour, and daytime dysfunction of memory, fatigue, mood, and success at work or school. Duration and frequency of symptoms need to be recorded for classification of insomnia into various subtypes. Any history suggestive of psychiatric disorder needs to be asked for specially pertaining to anxiety disorder, depression and substance use disorder. History of snoring, nocturia, witnessed apnea episodes and excessive daytime sleepiness along with insomnia are suggestive of COMISA (Fig. 24.2).

Insomnia symptoms can also arise with the use, abuse, or exposure to certain substances. Medications history needs to be reviewed as various medications can influence sleep.

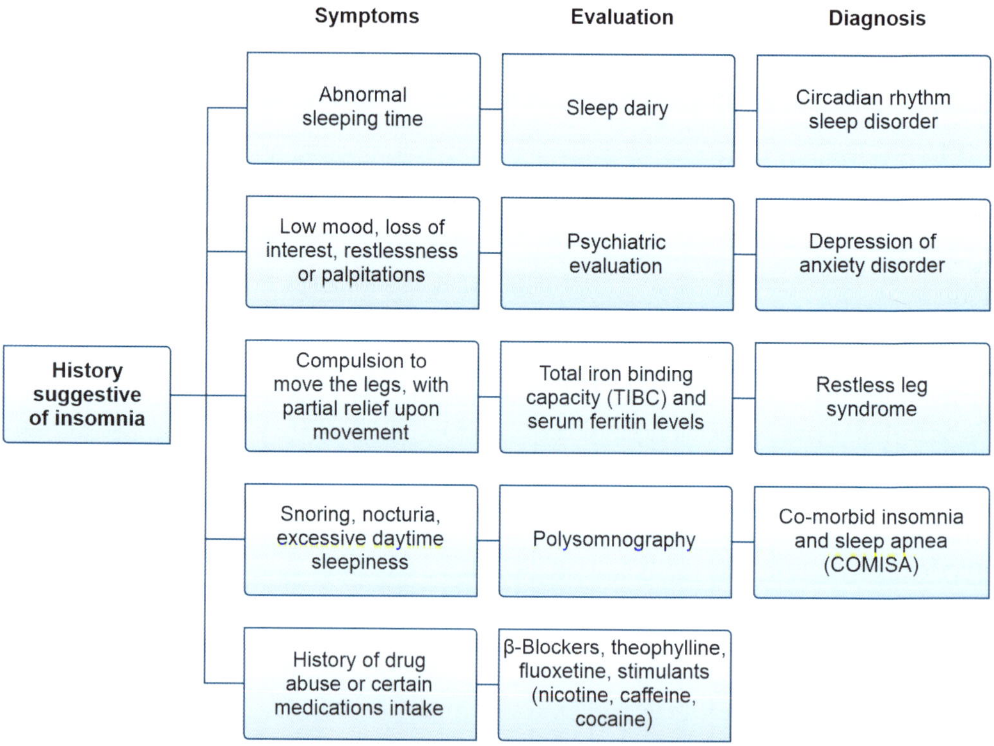

Fig. 24.2: Proposed diagnostic approach to patient of insomnia.

Table 24.1: Medicines and substances that can contribute to insomnia	
Antidepressants	Selective serotonin reuptake inhibitors (SSRIs), serotonin norepinephrine reuptake inhibitors (SNRIs), and monoamine oxidase inhibitors (MAOIs)
Respiratory medicines	Salbutamol, theophylline
Decongestants	Pseudoephedrine, phenylephrine (available over-the-counter)
Stimulants	Caffeine, nicotine, amphetamines, cocaine, and methylphenidate
Substance withdrawal	Alcohol, benzodiazepines, or opioid withdrawal
Antihypertensives	Blockers, α-blockers, and diuretics

It is important to gather a comprehensive list of medications, encompassing both prescription and non-prescription drugs, as well as substances that might be misused (Table 24.1). The quantity and timing of caffeine, usage of nicotine, and alcohol should be asked in history.

Various assessment tools aid in the diagnostic evaluation of insomnia. These include a sleep diary which helps to identify the total sleep time, disruptions in sleep, and factors influencing sleep quality. Insomnia Severity Index is a questionnaire used to assess the severity of the insomnia disorder (score 8–14: mild insomnia, and 15–21: moderate insomnia; 22–28: severe insomnia), impact on daily life and treatment response. Pittsburgh Sleep Quality Index (PSQI) questionnaire can be used for assessing sleep quality over a 1 month period. However, it does not diagnose insomnia.

Polysomnography is a very useful tool for diagnosing patients of COMISA. However, the consideration of a referral to a sleep laboratory for polysomnographic diagnosis should be limited to cases where there is suspicion of another primary sleep disorder, like OSA or periodic limb movement disorder.

Treatment of Insomnia

Treatment of insomnia involves treating the associated conditions, if any. In case of any suspicion of psychiatric illness, an individual should be referred for formal psychiatric evaluation. Associated circadian rhythm sleep disorders are treated with changing of daily sleep routine, melatonin, bright light therapy, and cognitive behaviour therapy for insomnia (CBTi). Individuals with associated restless leg syndrome require iron supplements (when there is associated iron deficiency) and drugs (dopamine agonists, opioids). Treatment of COMISA involves primarily weight reduction in obese patients and overnight PAP therapy. After ruling out above causes if insomnia persists, then it should be managed with CBTi along with pharmacotherapy. CBTi is a multicomponent therapy that involves stimulus control therapy, sleep restriction, relaxation therapies, cognitive therapy, paradoxical intention, sleep hygiene education and behavioural intervention.

Pharmacotherapy for insomnia includes various drugs such as benzodiazepines, selective H1 antagonists, dual orexin/hypocretin receptor antagonists, anti-depressants, anti-psychotics, non-selective antihistamines, etc. Pharmacotherapy for insomnia and CBTi is a specialized field and must be dealt with a specialist. It is important not to start patients on sedatives for insomnia without ruling out and treating common causes.

FURTHER READING

1. American Academy of Sleep Medicine. The International Classification of Sleep Disorders-Third Edition (ICSD-3) Darien, IL: American Academy of Sleep Medicine; 2014.
2. Ohayon MM. Epidemiology of insomnia: What we know and what we still need to learn. Sleep Med Rev. 2002 Apr;6(2):97–111.
3. Roth T. Insomnia: Definition, Prevalence, Etiology, and Consequences. *J Clin Sleep Med.* 2007 Aug 15;3(5 Suppl):S7–10.
4. Riemann D, Spiegelhalder K, Feige B, Voderholzer U, Berger M, Perlis M, et al. The hyperarousal model of insomnia: a review of the concept and its evidence. Sleep Med Rev. 2010 Feb;14(1):19–31.
5. Krakow B, Melendrez D, Ferreira E, Clark J, Warner TD, Sisley B, et al. Prevalence of insomnia symptoms in patients with sleep-disordered breathing. Chest. 2001 Dec;120(6):1923–9.
6. Smith S, Sullivan K, Hopkins W, Douglas J. Frequency of insomnia report in patients with obstructive sleep apnoea-hypopnea syndrome (OSAHS). Sleep Med. 2004 Sep;5(5):449–56.

Chapter

25

Approach to a Case with Hypersomnia/Hypersomnolence

• Kirti Kadian • Abhishek Goyal

LEARNING POINTS

1. Hypersomnolence/excessive daytime sleepiness is a common problem that leads to a serious impact on an individual's health, safety, functioning, and quality of life.
2. Obstructive sleep apnea is one of the most common causes of hypersomnolence.
3. An accurate and a definite diagnosis of the underlying cause by a proper algorithmic approach (proposed) will help in proper medical management of the disorder.

INTRODUCTION

Hypersomnolence is defined as the inability to sustain wakefulness or alertness during the major waking periods of the day. It differs from fatigue, which relates to a subjective lack of physical or mental energy. The prevalence of hypersomnolence in the general population ranges from 10 to 15%. Common causes of hypersomnolence are obstructive sleep apnea (OSA), insufficient sleep, depression, medications, and comorbid medical and psychiatric disorders. Less common causes are hypersomnia's of central origin (narcolepsy, idiopathic hypersomnia), and malingering. However, physicians must recognize that there is substantial overlap between individuals who are pathologically sleepy and those who are considered "normal" (often sleep-deprived) individuals.

CASE VIGNETTE

A female in her mid-40s, with a body mass index (BMI) of 35 kg/m^2, presented to the emergency room with shortness of breath and altered sensorium for one day. Her arterial blood gas analysis (ABG) showed type II respiratory failure (pH:7.120; pCO_2: 101 mm of Hg; HCO_3: 35 mmol/L; pO_2: 55 mm of Hg). She was intubated and put on invasive mechanical ventilation. Gradually her parameters improved and she was weaned off invasive ventilation in the next 2 days. Her daytime sleepiness persisted after being weaned from the ventilator.

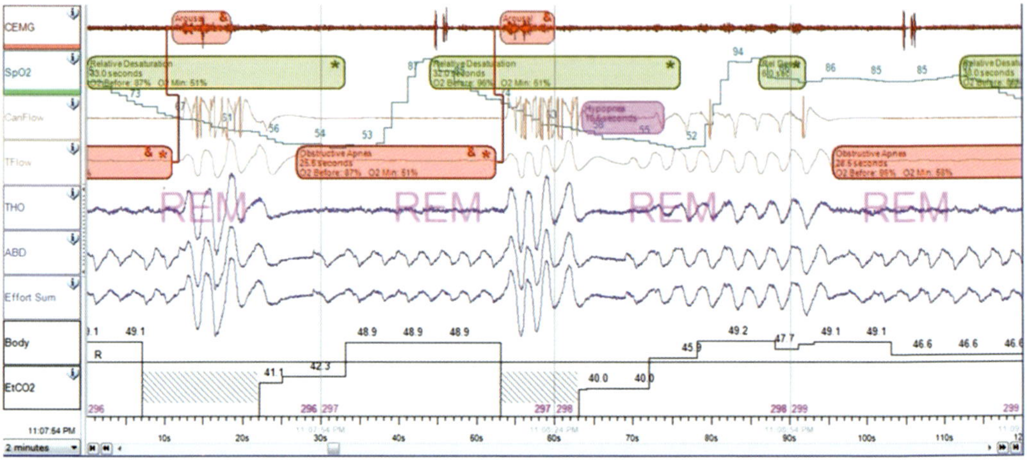

Fig. 25.1: A PSG epoch from the level 1 PSG, showing obstructive apnea, hypopnea, relative desaturation and arousal during REM sleep.

The patient had no addictions or history of biomass fuel exposure. She was a known diabetic for which she regularly took medications. She had a history of loud snoring for 2 years and complained of excessive daytime sleepiness (EDS) from the last 5 months. Her Epworth Sleepiness Score (ESS) was 21 (normal ≤0). Her husband had witnessed episodes of apnea and she had experienced choking during her sleep. She gave a history of leg discomfort which was worse in the evenings. She had an urge to move her legs when at rest and the discomfort improved on movement. She had nocturia for which she had to wake up 4–5 times during the night. In her normal routine she usually slept around 10 pm and would awaken around 6 am. She did not have any history of cataplexy, sleep attacks, hypnagogic hallucinations, or sleep paralysis.

She gave history of depressed mood, loss of interest in daily activities, low energy, poor concentration, thoughts of worthlessness or guilt, and recurrent thoughts of death or suicide. On examination, she had macroglossia and her modified mallampati was grade IV. There was no evidence of micrognathia or retrognathia.

She underwent chest radiograph, electrocardiography, spirometry, and 2D echocardiography, which revealed no abnormality. To evaluate further an overnight level I polysomnography (PSG) was performed in which her apnea–hypopnea index (AHI) was found to be 121/hour (Fig. 25.1). Thus, she was diagnosed as a case of severe OSA with restless leg syndrome (RLS). Subsequently, a manual positive airway pressure (PAP) titration was done. As she continued to have apneas even at a PAP of 18 cm H_2O, she was shifted to bi-level PAP (BiPAP) during titration. Iron profile was done to investigate for RLS which was normal.

The patient was advised BiPAP therapy with inspiratory PAP 25 cm H_2O and expiratory PAP 14 cm H_2O with a full face mask throughout her sleep. She was advised a diet plan (1200 kcal/day) and exercise sessions under observation 2 times a week. She was also prescribed ropinirole for her RLS. After 2 months, her compliance data was checked and it was found to be adequate. Her symptoms of snoring and nocturia resolved. She lost 8 kg and her ESS improved to 4 (Fig. 25.2). Symptoms of RLS and depression also improved.

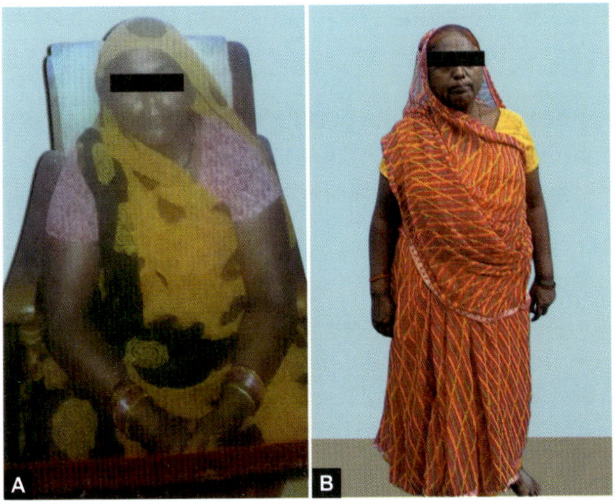

Fig. 25.2: (A) Before and (B) after treatment photographs of the patient demonstrating reduction in her BMI.

DISCUSSION

Hypersomnolence and excessive daytime sleepiness (EDS) are often used interchangeably and represent daily episodes of an irrepressible need to sleep or daytime lapses into sleep. Population-based surveys by National Sleep Foundation found that about 30% of the respondents suffer from enough EDS to interfere with their quality of life. The causes of hypersomnolence are numerous and broadly divided into the following four categories.

A. **Sleep-related breathing disorders** (OSA, central sleep apnea (CSA), sleep related hypoventilation disorders, and sleep related hypoxemia disorders.

B. **Circadian rhythm sleep-wake disorders** (Jet lag disorder, delayed sleep-wake phase disorder, advanced sleep-wake phase disorder, irregular sleep-wake rhythm disorder, non-24-hr sleep-wake rhythm disorder, shift work disorder, circadian rhythm sleep-wake disorders not otherwise specified).

C. **Sleep-related movement disorders** (Restless legs syndrome, periodic limb movement disorder).

D. **Central disorders of hypersomnolence:**
   - Narcolepsy type I, narcolepsy type II, idiopathic hypersomnolence, Kleine-Levin syndrome
   - Hypersomnia due to a medical disorder (encephalitis, multiple sclerosis, Parkinson's disease, and other genetic disorders).
   - Hypersomnia associated with a psychiatric disorder (depression).
   - Hypersomnia due to medication or substance abuse/overuse
   - Insufficient sleep syndrome

Mechanisms of Hypersomnolence

Several neuronal mechanisms located in various regions of the brain such as the brainstem, thalamus, hypothalamus, and basal forebrain control wakefulness and sleep. The action of different neurotransmitters like noradrenaline, serotonin, histamine, and orexin (hypocretin) promote wakefulness. On the other hand, neurotransmitters acetylcholine and GABA are involved in initiating and maintaining sleep. Decreased activity of wake-promoting systems results in increased activity of sleep-promoting systems thus causing hypersomnia.

a. **Obstructive sleep apnea:** In the general population, the prevalence of OSA is approximately 35% in adult men and 24% in adult women in Indian population (unpublished study). Only approximately 15% of OSA patients have hypersomnia (ESS ≥11). Although anatomically compromised airway accounts for the major predisposition to OSA, a patient's arousal threshold and factors related to the central control of breathing are also important.

   During an episode of obstructive apnea, airway obstruction and apnea/hypopnea leads to a reduction in the oxygen levels in the blood. This is detected by peripheral chemoreceptors in carotid bodies, which send signals to the brainstem, including reticular activating system (RAS). This leads to an arousal which is accompanied by increased muscle tone, including the muscles of the upper airway, which helps to reopen the obstructed airway. After the arousal, once normal breathing and oxygenation are restored, the individual may resume sleep. However, these cycles of apneas followed by arousals repeat numerous times throughout the night in individuals with OSA, leading to a poor sleep quality.

   The frequent awakenings prevent individuals from achieving the deeper stages of sleep, particularly rapid eye movement (REM) sleep and slow-wave sleep, which is essential for restorative and cognitive functions. Long-term intermittent hypoxia is associated with oxidative injury which in turn produces wake impairments.

b. **Insufficient sleep syndromes:** Insufficient sleep means not getting enough sleep specifically for that age. As per the American Academy of sleep medicine (AASM), adults need at least 7 hours of sleep. Lack of sleep leads to sleep debt, causing daytime sleepiness, obesity, impaired immune function, diabetes, hypertension, heart disease, depression, and a greater risk of accidents.

c. **Narcolepsy:** Narcolepsy is a neurological disorder characterized by EDS, often leading to sudden, uncontrollable episodes of sleep. Hypersomnia in narcolepsy stems from a complex interplay of factors including hypocretin deficiency, autoimmune destruction of hypocretin-producing neurons, neurotransmitter imbalances, sleep fragmentation, genetic predisposition, neural network abnormalities, and potential environmental triggers. These factors collectively disrupt the normal regulation of sleep-wake cycles and contribute to the excessive daytime sleepiness characteristic of narcolepsy.

d. **EDS due to drugs/comorbid diseases:** Sleepiness caused by medication use or withdrawal as well as in other medical conditions, is linked to an increase in sleep-inducing neurotransmitters or a decrease in alertness-inducing neurotransmitters.

e. **Cyclical hypersomnolence:** Kleine-Levin syndrome presents with episodic profound sleepiness frequently triggered by infection or alcohol consumption. Sometimes, a similar syndrome occurs in connection with the menstrual cycle in girls.

Approach to the Evaluation of a Patient with Hypersomnolence

An algorithmic approach to a patient with hypersomnolence is proposed in Fig. 25.3.

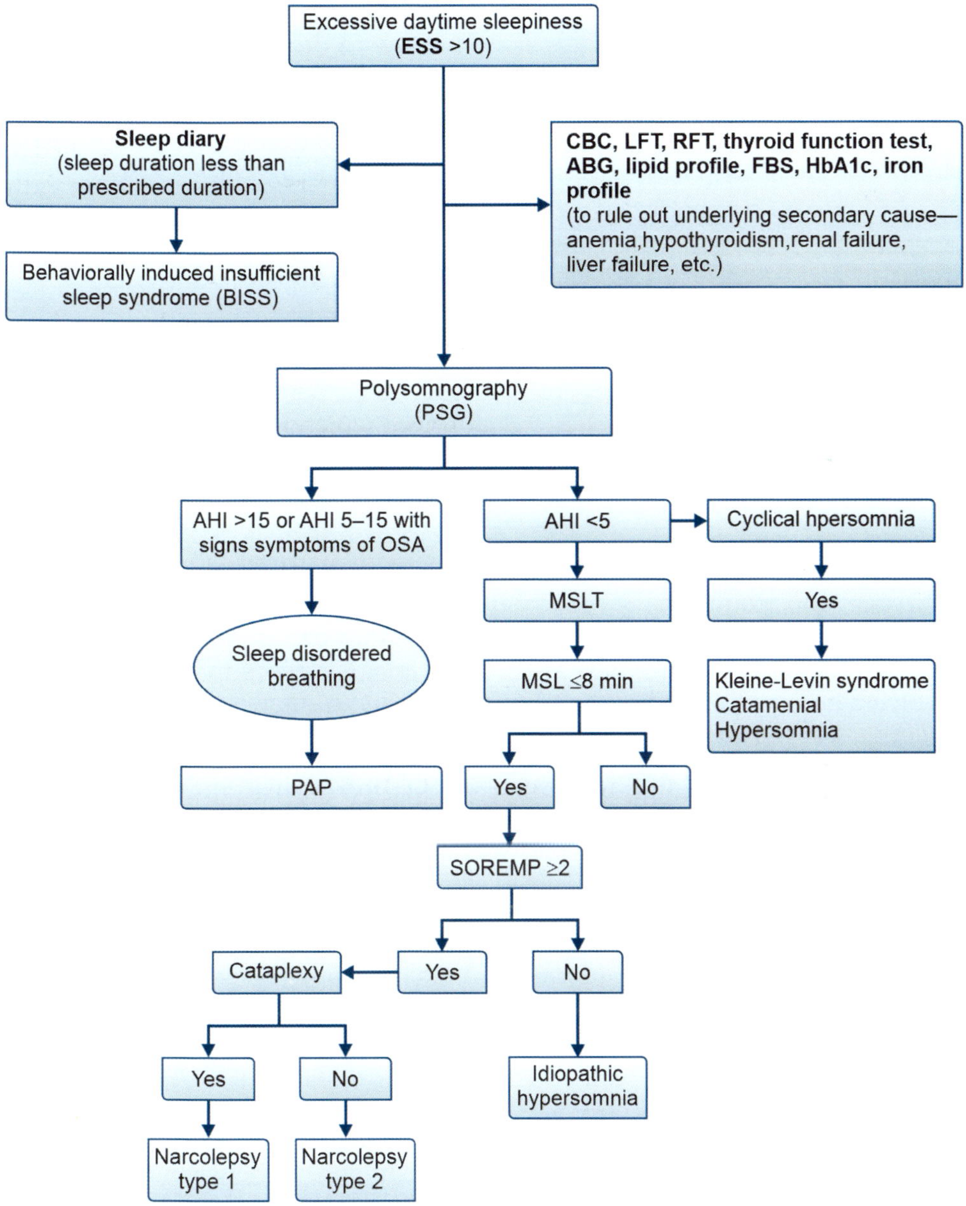

Fig. 25.3: Approach to patient with excessive daytime sleepiness.

ESS: Epworth sleepiness score; *CBC:* Complete blood cell count; *LFT:* Liver function test; *RFT:* Renal function test; *ABG:* Arterial blood gas analysis; *FBS:* Fasting blood sugar; *AHI:* Apnea–hypopnea index; *MSLT:* Multisleep latency test; *MSL:* Mean sleep latency; *SOREMP:* Sleep onset REM periods.

Step 1: History taking and examination: The initial step involves identifying EDS and other symptoms suggestive of specific disorders through history taking, examination, blood investigations, and subjective and objective assessment of sleep (Table 25.1).

Table 25.1: Specific disorders causing excessive daytime sleepiness and their symptoms	
Disorder	*Symptoms*
Sleep apnea	Habitual snoring, witnessed apneas, EDS, tiredness, obesity, nocturia
Restless leg syndrome	Urge to move legs at rest increases in the evening and improves with movement
Narcolepsy	Sleep attacks, hypnagogic or hypnopompic hallucination, cataplexy
Kleine-Levin syndrome	Episodic symptoms of cognitive dysfunction, derealization, major apathy, disinhibited behavior
Depression	Loss of interest, poor concentration, low energy, depressed mood
Medication use	Antidepressants, anxiolytics, antiepileptics, analgesics, antihistamines
Substance abuse	Alcohol
Comorbidities	Diabetes mellitus, hypothyroidism, anemia, renal failure
CNS disorders	Infections, head injury, parkinsonism, dementia
Genetic	Myotonic dystrophies

A detailed examination should include measuring waist circumference, BMI, neck circumference, and examining for micrognathia, retrognathia, macroglossia, tonsillar enlargement and mallampati Score. Blood investigations are to be conducted to rule out metabolic disorders (if clinically indicated). Brain imaging needs to be performed only if CNS involvement is suspected.

Subjective assessment of sleepiness: Epworth sleepiness score.

Objective Assessment of sleepiness: Sleep log/diaries for sleep wake routines, autography.

Step 2: Polysomnography: As per AASM scoring, a frequency of obstructive respiratory events ≥15 AHI or 5–15 AHI with associated signs/symptoms of sleep apnea confirms the diagnosis of OSA. For central sleep apnea, the total number of central apneas plus central hypopneas must be >50% of the total number of apneas and hypopneas. In our patient, OSA diagnosis was established on PSG (Fig. 25.1).

Step 3: Multisleep latency test (MSLT): Patient with sleepiness and AHI <5 or persistence of symptoms despite CPAP treatment require further evaluation with MSLT. Presence of a mean sleep latency of ≤8 minutes and two or more sleep-onset REM periods (SOREMPs) on an MSLT performed according to standard techniques, suggests narcolepsy. The presence of cataplexy and low CSF hypocretins (≤110 pg/ml) distinguishes between narcolepsy type 1 and type 2. Presence of a mean sleep latency of 8 minutes and absence of SOREMPs on MSLT suggest idiopathic hypersomnia.

Treatment options for hypersomnolence include:
1. Weight reduction for obese patients
2. Counseling about sleep hygiene
3. PAP therapy for sleep apnea
4. Medication for restless legs syndrome
5. Stimulants for central disorders of hypersomnolence
6. Avoidance of medications causing hypersomnia

FURTHER READING

1. Sateia MJ. International Classification of Sleep Disorders-Third Edition. Chest. 2014;146:1387–94.

2. Young TB. Epidemiology of Daytime Sleepiness: Definitions, Symptomatology, and Prevalence. *J Clin Psychiatry*. 2004; 65:12–6.

3. Johns MW. A new method for measuring daytime sleepiness: the Epworth sleepiness scale. Sleep. 1991;14:540–5.

4. Watson NF, Badr MS, Belenky G, Bliwise DL, Buxton OM, Buysse D, et al. Recommended Amount of Sleep for a Healthy Adult: A Joint Consensus Statement of the American Academy of Sleep Medicine and Sleep Research Society. Sleep. 2015;38:843–4.

5. Trotti LM, Arnulf I. Idiopathic Hypersomnia and Other Hypersomnia Syndromes. Neurotherapeutics. 2021 Jan;18(1):20-31.

6. Pérez-Carbonell L, Mignot E, Leschziner G, Dauvilliers Y. Understanding and approaching excessive daytime sleepiness. Lancet. 2022 Sep 24;400(10357):1033–1046.

Chapter 26

Approach to a Case with Parasomnia

• *Khushboo Saxena* • *Avishek Kar* • *Abhishek Goyal*

LEARNING POINTS

1. Video polysomnography is considered the gold standard investigation when sleep related abnormal movements are associated.
2. Multiple sleep related disorders may co-exist.
3. Obstructive sleep apnea can present with parasomnia, and should be considered while evaluating a case of parasomnia.

INTRODUCTION

Parasomnias are undesirable physical experiences or events that occur during sleep or transition of sleep stages. Identifying cause of such movements or behavior is often challenging due to mimics and overlapping of symptoms with other sleep-related movement disorders and sleep-related epilepsy. A detailed history and examination including neurological examination plays a very important role. Indications of polysomnography are limited but should include extended EEG electrodes, EMG and synchronized audio and video recording whenever indicated. Indications for polysomnography include injurious or disruptive behavior, or if it is accompanied with excessive daytime sleepiness, or when associated with abnormal medical, psychiatric or neurological findings.

CASE VIGNETTE

A man in his mid-twenties presented to sleep clinic along with his mother for complaints of abnormal involuntary movements during sleep, excessive daytime sleepiness, and choking spells when asleep for three-month duration. He also had loud snoring for the past 10 years. He has no known comorbidities and works in a software company. He was not married, and patient prefers to sleep alone. As per his mother he was snoring loud enough to be heard in other rooms but it used to subside on lateral positioning.

Patients mother had also noticed excessive and abnormal body movements during his sleep. She describes his movements during sleep as trying to lift his head and moving both upper limbs in air (right more than left) along with continuous lower limb movements.

He also rubs his chest often with his right-hand during sleep. She has also heard some incomprehensible sounds that he makes during sleep. He is normal while awake and denies memory of any of above-mentioned events and tells that he is not aware of all these events. No history suggestive of focal neurological deficit or epilepsy was present. Patient denies any complaints of headache or aura or foreboding of any such events.

She also observed that he is excessively sleepy throughout the day and he would sleep and snore even while talking or watching mobile phone or while sitting alone. His Epworth sleepiness score (ESS) was 24. He has even fell down twice in past two months and injured his knee. She was now more worried about frequent choking spells observed during sleep for past four months which were absent previously.

There is no history of similar episodes in childhood. He achieved all milestones at due age. His academic performance was satisfactory. There was no history of sudden fall or loss of muscle tone with laughter or anger, no history suggestive of sleep walking or night terrors. Significant family history includes chronic depression in father with suicidal tendencies.

On examination, he was well oriented to time, place and person. His Glasgow Coma Scale was 15. He was hemodynamically stable with SpO_2 98% with ambient air. He was 158 cm tall and weighed 88.9 kg (body mass index of 35.6 kg/m^2). He had macroglossia, mallampati grade 4 along with retrognathia. His neck circumference was 46 cm, abdominal circumference was 112 cm, and waist circumference was 120 cm. Other systemic examination including neurological examination was normal. His mother also shared videos of him while asleep which confirmed the history provided by her.

As per the history provided by patient and his mother, the following differential diagnoses were considered:

- Severe obstructive sleep apnea
- Narcolepsy
- REM behavior disorder
- Nocturnal frontal lobe epilepsy

He underwent diagnostic level 1 video polysomnography using ALICE 6 LDxS®™ system. As soon as the study started, video monitoring revealed continuous stereotypic, repetitive body movements like rhythmic banging type up and down movements of neck into the pillow, rubbing of chest using left hand and upward thrust of torso (Fig. 26.1). EEG was

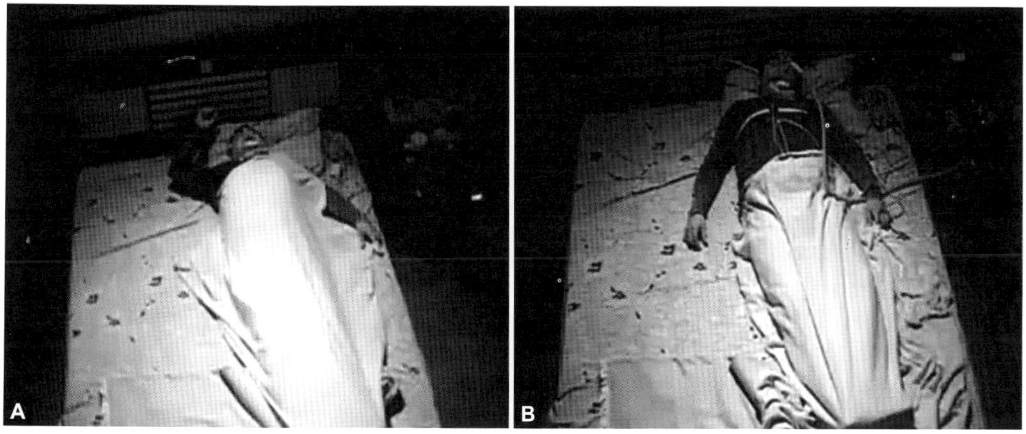

Fig. 26.1: (A) Picture of video monitoring showing stereotypical right upper limb movement; (B) Representative image showing resolution of autonomous movements during CPAP titration.

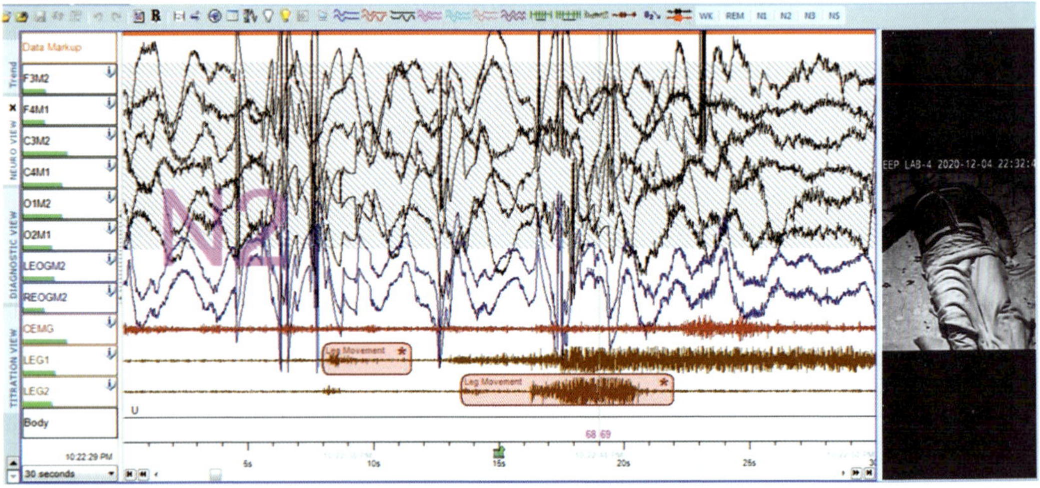

Fig. 26.2: EEG during diagnostic study showing unreadable waveforms due to motion artifacts.

incomprehensible due to obscuration of signals by muscular artefacts (Fig. 26.2). However, respiratory channels showed frequent respiratory events with apneas lasting as long as 30 seconds and lowest SpO_2 recorded was 68% associated with events (Fig. 26.3).

Average apnea–hypopnea index (AHI) for two hours was more than 40 events per hour, and patient was initiated on manual titration using continuous positive airway pressure therapy. Patient's EEG stabilized and he had rebound REM sleep for >60 minutes. Optimal titration was achieved at a pressure of 16 cm of water using nasal mask.

Neurology consultation was sought and his neurological examination and relevant investigations including imaging was normal. Psychiatry consultation and counseling was done for depression.

Final diagnosis: A final diagnosis of severe OSA with sleep-related rhythmic movement disorder was made, and he was advised to use nocturnal CPAP therapy at 16 cm water with nasal mask for entire sleep duration. He was also advised for calorie restriction and weight reduction, along with sleep hygiene and lifestyle modifications.

He was followed up after four weeks. He was following advise meticulously and was using CPAP for more than six hours daily. His daytime sleepiness resolved (ESS <10). Abnormal movements during sleep subsided completely. Patient symptomatically improved and realized that he is now fresher and more efficient during daytime. Work efficiency also improved.

DISCUSSION

The term parasomnia is derived from two words—*para* and *somnus*. Para is a Greek word meaning "alongside of", and *somnus* is a Latin word meaning "sleep". It is a undesirable motor, verbal or experiential phenomenon which occurs while in sleep or during transition from sleep to wakefulness or from wakefulness to sleep.

Diagnosing parasomnia is often challenging due to wide overlapping of symptoms and history with sleep related rhythmic disorders and sleep related epilepsy. A detailed and meticulous history which should include nature of movements, age at onset, time of these episodes and a detailed systemic and neurological examination is the key to reach towards diagnosis.

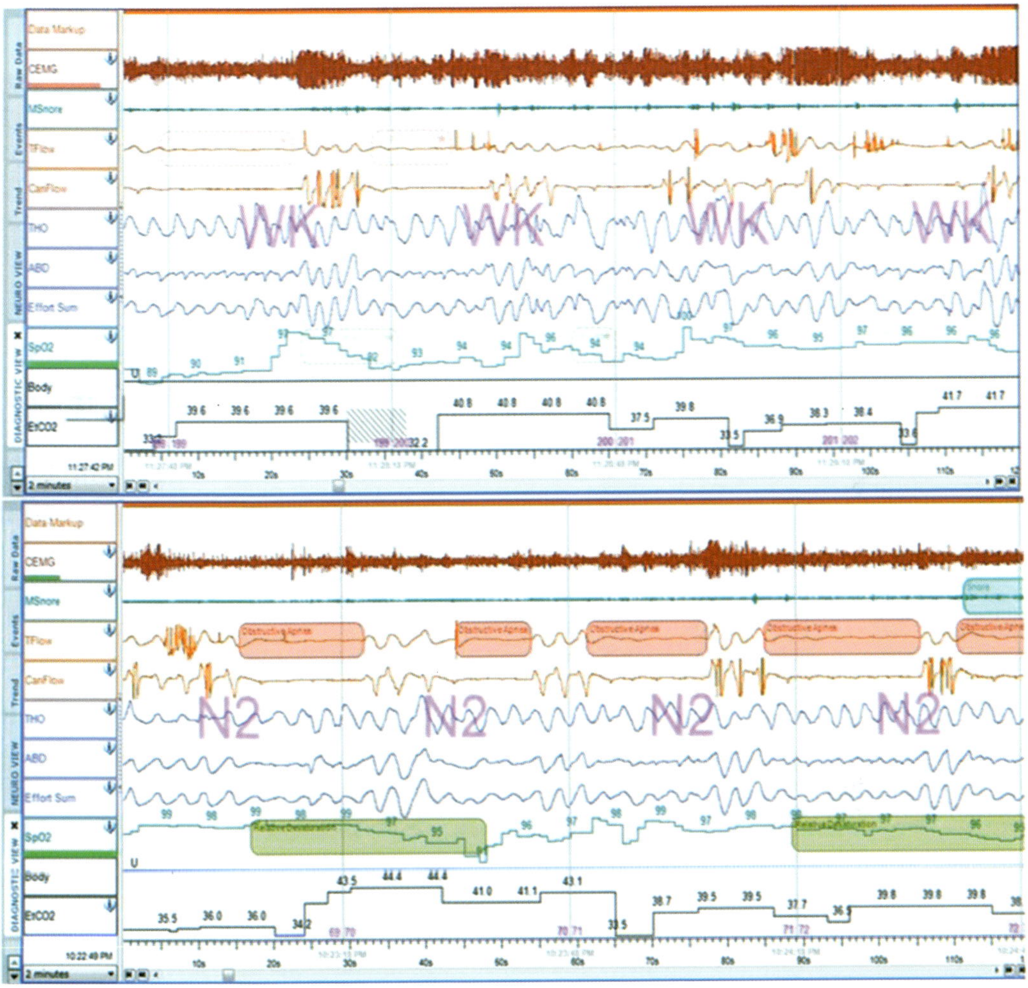

Fig. 26.3: Respiratory events (apneas) observed during diagnostic sleep study.

Polysomnography is not indicated for all parasomnias but is recommended when it is associated with potentially violent or injurious behavior, when the behaviour becomes disruptive to family members, when it results in excessive daytime sleepiness, and when it is associated with other medical, psychiatric or neurological symptoms.

A. Sleep-related Rhythmic Disorders

These comprises stereotyped, repetitive and rhythmic motor movements involving large muscle groups. These movements interfere with normal sleep resulting in significant impairment in daytime function. These may cause injuries if preventive measures are not used. Epilepsy should be ruled out in such conditions. These are usually seen in but are not limited to children and infants. The various movement types include rocking of the body, banging the head, rolling the head or combined movements. Rhythmic humming and inarticulate sounds may also be present associated with events.

These movements can also be associated with restless leg syndrome, narcolepsy, obstructive sleep apnea, or parasomnias like REM behaviour disorder. Sleep apneas can trigger these rhythmic motor events via a respiratory-related arousal mechanism in subjects who are genetically predisposed. Video polysomnography is useful in diagnosis.

B. Parasomnia

Parasomnias are undesirable physical events which occur during entry into sleep, during sleep, or while arousal from sleep. Parasomnias have significant impact on quality-of-life, have prognostic and also forensic implications for patients as well as their bed-partners. Commonly seen in children, they may persist into adulthood, or may present in adulthood also. Parasomnias can be seen in NREM as well as REM stages of sleep. Sleep-related hypermotor epilepsy should be ruled out as an important differential of parasomnias (Table 26.1).

Parasomnias encompass abnormal sleep-related movements, behaviors, emotions, perceptions, dreams, and autonomic nervous system activity. NREM parasomnias occur during slow wave, or stage N3 sleep. NREM parasomnias include disorders of arousal such as confusional arousals, sleepwalking and sleep terrors. REM behavior disorder (RBD) is the representative of REM parasomnia. REM parasomnias also include recurrent isolated sleep paralysis and nightmare disorder. NREM and REM parasomnias may co-exist, and sometimes confounded by other sleep associated diseases like obstructive sleep apnea.

RBD usually manifests as complex, injurious, and violent sleep or dream-related behaviors in adults. In general, RBD is manifested as an attempted enactment of unpleasant, aggressive dreams. These usually occur a few hours after sleep onset and result in a rapid awakening from an episode. In contrast, sleepwalking and sleep terror episodes often occur in the first two hours after sleep onset, are not associated with awakening, and are rarely associated with dreaming.

C. Sleep-related Epilepsy

Sleep-related epilepsy presents with repetitive, stereotypical behaviors. A seizure is a paroxysmal event resulting from a sudden excessive discharge of the cerebral cortex neurons. Epilepsy is a condition of recurrent un-provoked seizures. Sleep facilitates both epileptic activity and seizures.

The different types of nocturnal frontal lobe epilepsy (NFLE) can cause sleep disruption, resulting in poor sleep quality, daytime fatigue, and excessive daytime sleepiness. The

Table 26.1: International Classification of Sleep Disorder for parasomnias (3rd edition)

NREM parasomnias	1. Confusional arousals 2. Sleepwalking 3. Sleep terrors and sleep-related eating disorder
REM parasomnias	1. REM sleep behavior disorder 2. Recurrent isolated sleep paralysis 3. Nightmare disorder
Other parasomnias	1. Exploding head syndrome 2. Sleep-related hallucinations 3. Sleep enuresis 4. Parasomnia due to a medical disorder 5. Parasomnia due to a medication/substance 6. Parasomnia, unspecified
Isolated symptoms and normal variants	Sleep talking

movements also may be severe enough to lead to physical injuries. Up to one-third to one-half of patients with NFLE can also have occasional seizure episodes during the day, although these daytime events may not necessarily be of the same type as those occurring during night.

NFLE can Present in Three Ways

1. Nocturnal paroxysmal arousal
2. Nocturnal paroxysmal dystonia, or
3. Episodic nocturnal wanderings.

The seizures in NFLE can often be confused with non-epileptic parasomnias.

In the case described above, video polysomnography played a crucial role in diagnosis. Usage of titration therapy resolved the movements as well as obstructive events in patient suggestive of overlap of multiple sleep disorders.

An approach to abnormal movements during sleep is illustrated in Fig 26.4.

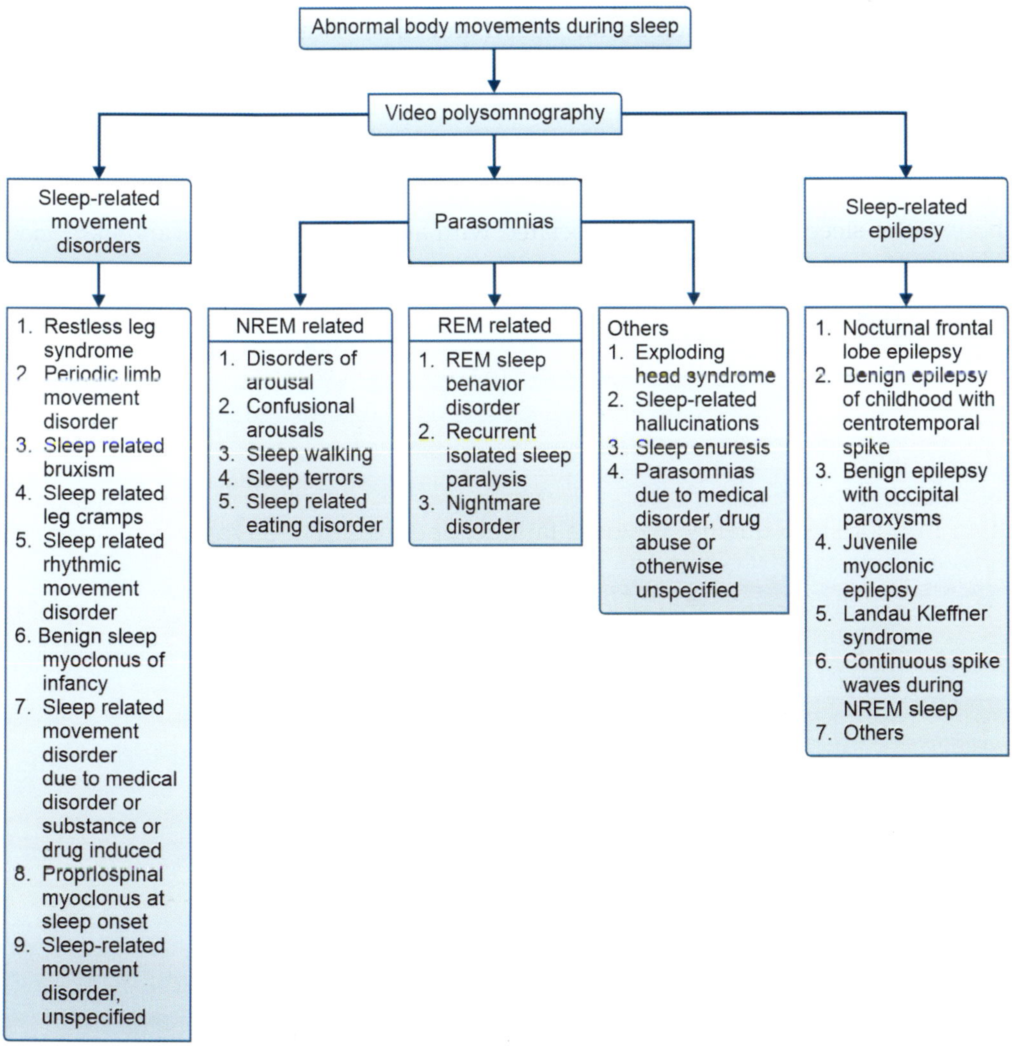

Fig. 26.4: Differential diagnosis for abnormal sleep movements during sleep.

FURTHER READING

1. American academy of sleep medicine. International classification of sleep disorders. 3rd ed. Darien, il : american academy of sleep medicine; 2014.
2. Chiaro G, Maestri M, Riccardi S, Haba-rubio J, Miano S, Bassetti CL, Heinzer RC, Manconi M. Sleep-related rhythmic movement disorder and obstructive sleep apnea in five adult patients. *J Clin Sleep Med* 2017;13:1213–1217.
3. Fleetham JA, Fleming JA. Parasomnias. CMAJ. 2014 May 13;186(8):E273–80.

SECTION VII

Miscellaneous

Chapter

27

Approach to a Case of Granulomatous Mediastinal Lymphadenopathy

• BR Rinoosha • V Nagarjuna Maturu

LEARNING POINTS

1. Granulomatous mediastinal lymphadenopathy is a common clinical presentation and the causes are myriad, tuberculosis and sarcoidosis being the most common.
2. EBUS sampling of the nodes (aspirate or biopsy) is the preferred technique for sample acquisition in cases of undifferentiated mediastinal lymphadenopathy. It is important to triage the sample appropriately for pathologic and microbiologic studies.
3. Necrotizing GML can be secondary to many infections other than tuberculosis and hence, these need to be considered while evaluating a case of necrotizing GML, where the microbiologic workup for tuberculosis is negative.

INTRODUCTION

Granulomatous inflammation is an immune response characterized by the formation of granulomas, which are organized collections of epithelioid macrophages. When there is enlargement of lymph nodes due to a granulomatous inflammation it is labelled as granulomatous mediastinal lymphadenopathy. This can arise from various causes, both benign and malignant. The etiology often varies based on demographic factors, with tuberculosis and sarcoidosis being the most common causes in the Indian context. Thoracic imaging plays a crucial role in detecting mediastinal lymph nodes. We present a case of an elderly male with uncontrolled diabetes who presented with mediastinal lymphadenopathy, and ultimately diagnosed as necrotizing granulomatous lymphadenitis due to melioidosis.

CASE VIGNETTE

A farmer in his sixties, with a medical history of diabetes and chronic kidney disease, presented to our centre with a two-month history of high-grade, intermittent fever accompanied by chills and rigor, relieved by antipyretics, and a progressively worsening dry cough. He had also experienced a loss of appetite and a weight loss of 5 kg in two months.

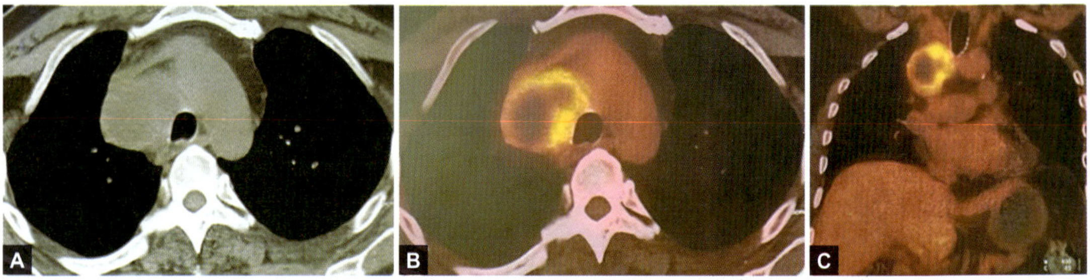

Fig. 27.1: (A) CT chest axial view showing presence of enlarged lymph node at station 4R; (B and C) Axial and coronal sections of PET-CT scan showing a large necrotic FDG avid node (37 × 47 × 42 mm) in the right paratracheal region with heterogeneously increased FDG uptake (SUV_{max} of 8.9).

Upon examination, he had a fever of 101.1°F, a pulse rate of 108 beats per minute, oxygen saturation of 97% on room air, blood pressure of 120/80 mmHg, and a respiratory rate of 16 breaths per minute. General examination showed no pallor, cyanosis, clubbing, icterus, or peripheral lymphadenopathy, and his respiratory system examination was normal. His blood reports indicated leukocytosis (16,000 cells/cu mm), elevated C reactive protein (120 mg/L), uncontrolled blood sugars (HbA1c 9.5%), mildly elevated creatinine (1.4 mg/dl), while other investigations were within normal limits. A chest X-ray revealed widening of the right paratracheal stripe, likely indicating lymph node enlargement. Computed tomograph (CT) and PET-CT scans confirmed the presence of necrotic right paratracheal lymph nodes. (Fig. 27.1A to C).

Endobronchial ultrasonography (EBUS) revealed a large, heterogeneous lymph node with signs of coagulation necrosis. Pus aspirated from the lymph node was sent for microbiological evaluation, including acid fast bacillus (AFB) smear, Xpert MTB/Rif, AFB culture, bacterial culture, and fungal smear. EBUS aspirate cytology identified numerous necrotizing granulomas (Fig. 27.2), but workup for tuberculosis was negative. However, the bacterial culture grew *Burkholderia pseudomallei*, thus confirming a diagnosis of mediastinal melioidosis. He was commenced on triple antibiotic therapy with trimethoprim-sulfamethoxazole, levofloxacin, and a cephalosporin with which his symptoms resolved.

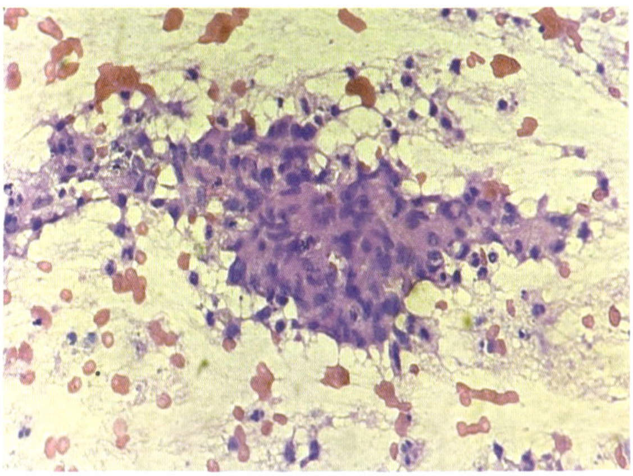

Fig. 27.2: Microscopic view of cytology slide showing presence of granuloma with central necrosis.

DISCUSSION

Granulomatous involvement of mediastinal lymph nodes is a common clinical presentation. The various causes of granulomatous mediastinal lymphadenopathy (GML) are detailed in Table 27.1. The two common causes of GML in a tuberculous endemic country like India are tuberculosis and sarcoidosis. Tuberculosis is a chronic granulomatous infection caused by *Mycobacterium tuberculosis* complex. Sarcoidosis is a multi-systemic granulomatous disease

Table 27.1: Causes of granulomatous mediastinal lymphadenopathy	
Infectious	***Non-Infectious***
Tuberculosis	Sarcoidosis
Histoplasmosis	Lymphomas
Melioidosis	Sarcoid-like reactions
Fungal infections	Berylliosis
Toxoplasmosis	Common variable immunodeficiency
Nontuberculous mycobacteria	Kikuchi's disease
Nocardiosis	Silicosis

which predominantly affects the lungs and the mediastinal nodes. Differentiating tuberculosis and sarcoidosis is extremely important as the treatment approach is different.

Non-necrotic granulomas resembling sarcoidosis can be seen in a regional lymph node(s) when there is an underlying disease such as a solid organ malignancy. This is termed sarcoid-like reaction (SLR), and has to be differentiated from systemic sarcoidosis by clinical presentation. Though malignancy is the commonest cause of a SLR in mediastinal nodes, SLR can happen secondary to a local immune response to infections, chemicals, tumor or a foreign body. When a GML is diagnosed, it is important to accurately determine the cause for it. A stepwise approach to diagnosing the cause of GML is described below.

A. Clinical History

A comprehensive patient history is the initial step in evaluation of patients presenting with mediastinal lymphadenopathy. Symptoms such as fever, night sweats, and weight loss in the context of mediastinal lymph nodes raise suspicion for infectious causes or lymphomas. Tuberculosis is the commonest cause of GML in tuberculosis endemic countries like India. It is however important to realize that many chronic infections other than tuberculosis can cause a similar clinical presentation and granulomatous reaction in the lymph nodes. Some of them include non-tuberculous mycobacterial (NTM) disease, brucellosis, melioidosis, nocardiosis and other endemic fungal infections. It is important to look at the immune status of the patient while considering the possible differentials. People who are immunosuppressed (HIV infection, uncontrolled diabetes, immunosuppressive drugs) are more likely to develop GML due to opportunistic pathogens.

It is also important to look at the patient's travel history, particularly time spent in areas endemic for certain diseases. Occupational exposure to silica and other inorganic dusts is important to consider the diagnosis of silicosis or berylliosis, both of which can cause GML. A past or present history of malignancies is to be taken, as sarcoid-like reactions can be a cause of GML in individuals with solid organ malignancies or lymphomas.

During physical examination, a thorough assessment for peripheral lymphadenopathy is essential, as these nodes are more easily accessible for biopsy.

B. Radiologic Evaluation

Often the initial radiologic sign for the presence of mediastinal lymphadenopathy is either a widened right paratracheal stripe (>4 mm in diameter) or presence of hilar prominence on a chest radiograph. Multi-detector chest CT scans are considered the gold standard for assessing lymph node characteristics (size, texture, presence of calcification, relationship with surrounding structures), and any associated changes in lung parenchyma. Sometimes, what appears to be lymphadenopathy in a chest radiograph might be identified as large pulmonary arteries or a distinct mass on CT imaging. The scan also aids in determining the most suitable approach for potential biopsy.

Presence of asymmetric nodes, necrotic nodes and associated centrilobular nodules or lung cavity points toward tuberculosis as the possible cause. Presence of bilateral symmetric nodes, non-necrotic nodes and associated peribronchovascular thickening and nodules point towards sarcoidosis as the possible cause.

C. Pathologic/Cytologic Evaluation

EBUS bronchoscopy is a minimally invasive, safe procedure that facilitates adequate sample collection for microbiological and histopathological analysis. Cytologic or histologic examination is the gold standard for confirming a granuloma. On pathology, granulomas are classified into two types: necrotizing and non-necrotizing (Table 27.2). Microscopically, necrotizing granulomas have a central necrosis with a palisaded lymphohistiocytic reaction, and a cuff of chronic inflammation. Non-necrotizing granulomas are characterized by the collection of epithelioid histiocytes and giant cells with minimal peripheral chronic inflammation. While cytology is sufficient to diagnose granulomas in majority, in cases where cytology is inconclusive, obtaining a biopsy from lymph node (EBUS-guided biopsy or mediastinoscopic biopsy) can identify granulomas.

Necrotizing granulomatous lymphadenopathy primarily occurs in chronic infectious conditions such as tuberculosis, NTM disease, histoplasmosis, nocardiosis, endemic fungal infections and acute bacterial infections like melioidosis. Non-infectious causes of necrotizing granulomas include treated or untreated lymphoma, necrotizing sarcoid granulomatosis, and Kikuchi's disease. It is important to realize that necrotizing granulomas is not always tuberculosis and many diseases, both infectious and non-infectious, can lead to necrotizing granulomas.

Conversely, non-necrotizing granulomas are commonly found in non-infectious conditions such as sarcoidosis, berylliosis, sarcoid-like reactions, CVID associated granulomatous lymphadenitis and lymphomas. Sarcoid-like reactions histologically resemble sarcoidosis, except for the presence of a population of B cells, which is not observed in sarcoidosis. Non-necrotic granulomas can also be found in infectious conditions like tuberculosis and toxoplasmosis (Table 27.2). It is again important to realize that non-necrotic granulomas does not always mean a non-infectious cause. Diseases like tuberculosis can have non-necrotic granulomas as their clinical presentation.

Table 27.2: Etiologies of necrotizing and non-necrotizing granulomatous inflammation

Necrotizing granulomas	*Non-Necrotizing granulomas*
Tuberculosis	Sarcoidosis
Histoplasmosis	Sarcoid-like reactions
Melioidosis	Berylliosis
Fungal infections	GPA
Hodgkin's lymphoma	Lymphomas
Necrotizing sarcoid granulomatosis	Tuberculosis
Kikuchi's disease	

D. Microbiologic Evaluation

Microbiologic positivity remains the gold standard for confirming tuberculosis and other infectious diseases. A positive AFB smear, Xpert MTB/Rif or a positive MTB culture confirms the diagnosis of mediastinal tuberculosis. However, being extra-pulmonary and paucibacillary in nature, not all patients with mediastinal tuberculosis will have a positive microbiological result. In tuberculosis endemic countries like India, presence of granulomatous lymphadenitis (necrotizing or non-necrotizing), absence of alternate etiology, and a positive tuberculin skin test can be considered as probable tuberculosis and started on a trial of anti-tuberculous therapy. When culture and histological results are combined with a high clinical suspicion, endobronchial ultrasound-guided transbronchial needle aspiration (EBUS-TBNA) demonstrates excellent diagnostic accuracy and negative predictive value (NPV) for the diagnosis of mediastinal TB lymphadenitis. We suggest that in immune-compromised hosts and in instances when frank pus is aspirated from the lymph node, further microbiological workup for bacterial culture and fungal smear be undertaken.

An algorithmic approach to a patient with granulomatous mediastinal lymphadenopathy is illustrated in Fig. 27.3.

Melioidosis, often dubbed the 'great mimicker' due to its varied clinical presentations, can be challenging to diagnose. Its presentation as isolated mediastinal lymphadenopathy is rare and can be easily confused with tuberculosis or malignancy. For patients with uncontrolled

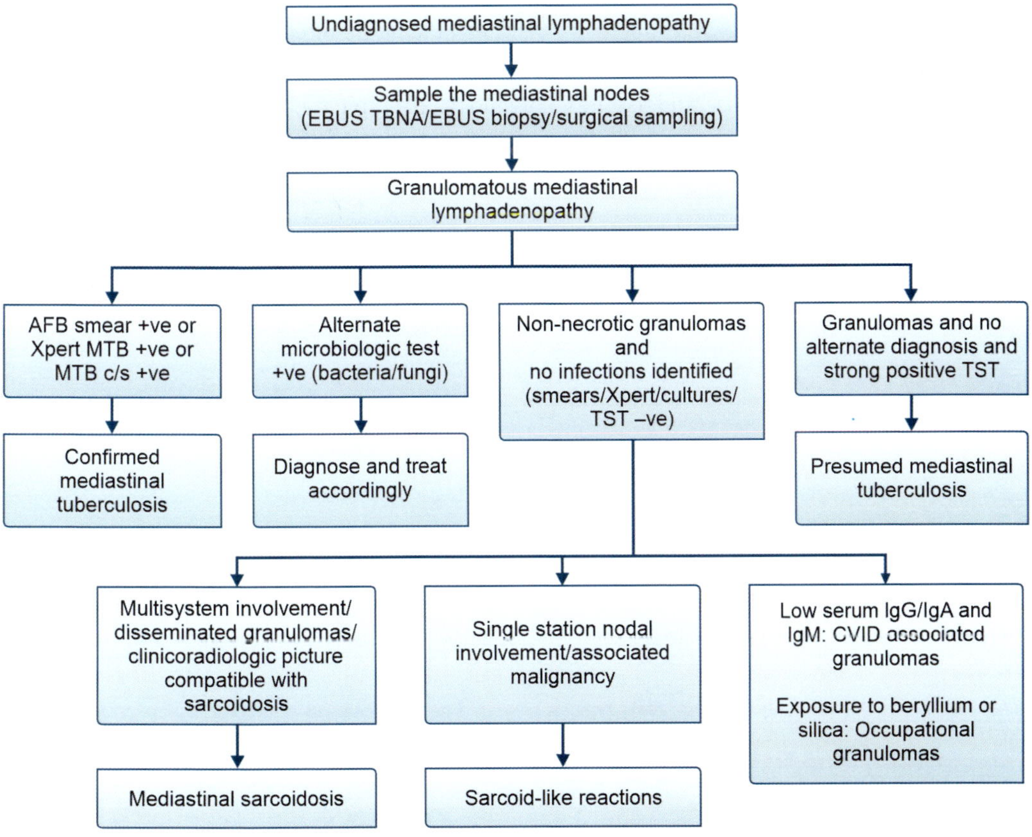

Fig. 27.3: An algorithmic approach to a patient with granulomatous mediastinal lymphadenopathy.

diabetes and other comorbidities, while tuberculosis is a common initial differential diagnosis, other less common etiologies should also be considered. This case underscores the importance of considering diverse etiologies, including less common infections, in granulomatous lymphadenopathies, particularly in patients with comorbidities.

FURTHER READING

1. Nyanti LE, Lee SSY, Shanmugam V, Muien MZBA, Othman AA, Chia YL, Huan NC, Ramarmuty HY, Kannan KKS. Clinical-radiological features and diagnostic modalities for mediastinal melioidosis. *Int J Tuberc Lung Dis*. 2023 Oct 1;27(10):724–728.
2. Tchernev G, Tana C, Schiavone C, Cardoso JC, Ananiev J, Wollina U. Sarcoidosis vs. Sarcoid-like reactions: The Two Sides of the same Coin? Wien Med Wochenschr. 2014 Jul;164(13-14):247–59.
3. Kaur H, Ahuja J, Singh P, Dhillon NK, Samagh N, Tiwari P. Necrotic mediastinal lymphadenopathy: Tuberculosis or Sarcoidosis, a diagnostic conundrum: A case report and review of the literature. *Journal of Family Medicine and Primary Care*. 2022 Nov;11(11):7425.
4. Geake J, Hammerschlag G, Nguyen P, Wallbridge P, Jenkin GA, Korman TM, Jennings B, Johnson DF, Irving LB, Farmer M, Steinfort DP. Utility of EBUS-TBNA for diagnosis of mediastinal tuberculous lymphadenitis: a multicentre Australian experience. *J Thorac Dis*. 2015 Mar;7(3):439–48.
5. Smith-Rohrberg D, Sharma SK. Tuberculin skin test among pulmonary sarcoidosis patients with and without tuberculosis: its utility for the screening of the two conditions in tuberculosis-endemic regions. Sarcoidosis Vasc Diffuse Lung Dis. 2006 Jun;23(2):130–4.

Chapter

28

Approach to a Patient with Unexplained Pulmonary Hypertension

• *Lakshmi Narasimhan R*

LEARNING POINTS

1. Pulmonary hypertension (PH) is a heterogeneous disease encountered commonly, and can present with non-specific symptoms.
2. Evaluating a case of pulmonary hypertension requires a systematic approach, attention to detail, and expertise from various medical disciplines. It is essential to get an early and accurate diagnosis so as to provide appropriate management and to improve patient outcomes.
3. Chronic thromboembolic PH (CTEPH) is often missed and requires a high index of suspicion; V/Q scan remains the initial screening test of choice, but CTPA is widely available and can also be used if V/Q scan is unavailable.
4. The treatment of choice for CTEPH is pulmonary endarterectomy (PEA), along with lifelong anticoagulation. For those unfit for PEA, other options include riociguat and balloon pulmonary angioplasty.

INTRODUCTION

Pulmonary hypertension (PH), a disease characterized by elevated pressures of the pulmonary vasculature usually presents with shortness of breath, fatigue, palpitation, angina, syncope and may lead to progressive right heart failure. The diagnosis is often delayed as the symptoms are nonspecific. Here we present a patient who was symptomatic for one year with progressive unexplained PH before he was diagnosed and treated successfully.

CASE VIGNETTE

An advocate in his early forties presented with history of progressive breathlessness and fatigue for one year duration. The symptoms were insidious in onset and slowly progressive, and by the time he presented to us, he was breathless on performing daily activities (mMRC grades 3 to 4). He also reported on-and-off episodes of mild exacerbations in symptoms characterized by increased breathlessness along with wheeze. Of late he also had noticed swelling in legs.

He was a reformed smoker who had quit smoking 5 years ago, and had no other comorbidities. He had also recovered 2 years ago from a moderate COVID-19 pneumonia requiring admission, but no oxygen or ICU care. Over the last one year he had consulted various physicians, cardiologists and pulmonologists and had been labelled and treated for "long COVID", "asthma", "COPD", "cor pulmonale" and "heart failure". He claimed marginal benefit with inhaled bronchodilators and diuretics but his symptoms continued to relentlessly progress.

On examination, he was thin built and well nourished. He was comfortable at rest but short of breath on walking: with SpO_2 of 93% at rest, dropping to 83% after a short walk. There was bilateral pitting pedal edema with mild varicose veins and elevated JVP with a loud P2 on auscultation. Respiratory system examination revealed occasional wheeze and a few scattered fine crackles.

Clinically, a diagnosis of pulmonary hypertension (PH) with right heart failure was made based on above findings. A 2D echocardiography was performed which revealed moderate pulmonary arterial hypertension (PAH), with a right ventricular systolic pressure (RVSP) of 55 mmHg. Plain computed tomography (CT) scan of the chest done earlier revealed a few small non-specific fibrotic bands bilaterally, which could not explain his breathlessness or PH.

It was decided to do a detailed workup to evaluate for the cause of PH. Differential diagnoses for PH considered in the index case were:
1. COPD/small airways disease
2. Diffuse parenchymal lung disease (interstitial lung disease/ILD)
3. Connective tissue disease-related PH
4. Obstructive sleep apnea (OSA)
5. Congenital heart disease with delayed presentation in adult
6. Chronic thromboembolic pulmonary hypertension (CTEPH)
7. Idiopathic PAH (a diagnosis of exclusion after all above causes are ruled out).

The relevant investigations to rule out the above causes were done. Pulmonary function test was normal—hence ruling out significant COPD or ILD. His Epworth Sleepiness Scale score was only 3, and STOP-BANG questionnaire score was 2, and he did not have any characteristic OSA symptoms. He did not have any symptoms of connective tissue disease and his antinuclear antibody (ANA) and rheumatoid arthritis (RA) factor were negative. His HIV serology by ELISA was also negative. A detailed 2D echo was repeated which revealed severe PAH with severe tricuspid regurgitation and an RVSP of 76 mmHg. Also, there was no congenital or valvular or left heart disease. Six-minute walk distance was 420 meters with a 10% drop in SpO_2.

With all other common causes of PH ruled out and a past history of moderate COVID-19 pneumonia—it was decided to do a CT pulmonary angiogram (CTPA) to rule out CTEPH. The CTPA revealed hypodense filling defects in right lower lobe pulmonary artery extending to segmental and subsegmental level, along with near complete nonvisualization of left upper and left lobar branches with multifocal areas of mosaic perfusion, hence confirming the diagnosis of CTEPH (Fig. 28.1). Procoagulant (thrombophilia) workup including antiphospholipid antibody (APLA) workup was negative.

A multidisciplinary team meeting was held with a pulmonologist, cardiologist, cardiothoracic surgeon, and the patient was started on optimal medical treatment including

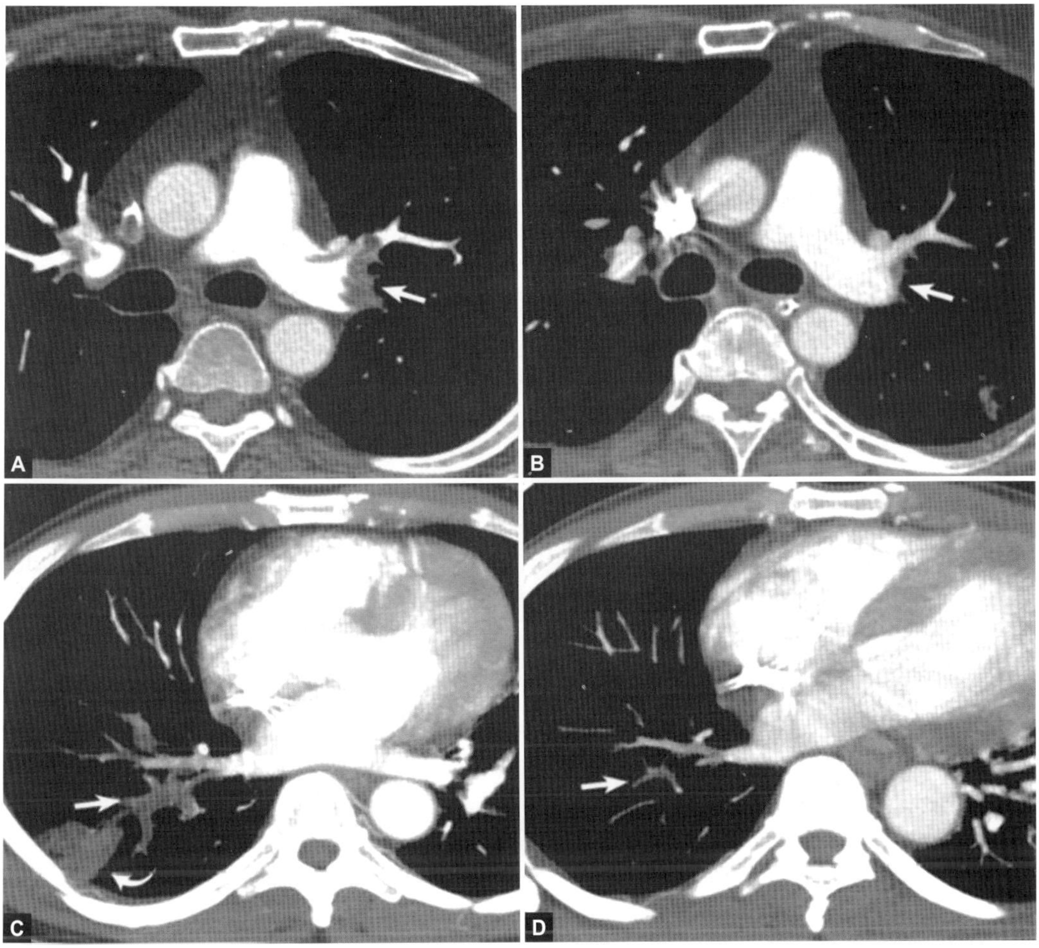

Fig. 28.1: CT pulmonary angiogram. (A) Filling defect in distal left main pulmonary artery; (B) Filling defect in left upper lobar pulmonary artery; (C) Filling defect in right lower lobar pulmonary artery; (D) Filling defect in right lower lobar segmental and subsegmental artery.

warfarin, riociguat, diuretic and domiciliary oxygen support. Ventilation–perfusion scan (V/Q scan) revealed absent perfusion in entire left lung and also the superior, lateral basal and posterior basal segments of right lower lobe (Fig. 28.2).

Right heart catheterization was performed which revealed mean pulmonary artery pressure (PAP) of 60 mmHg, with pulmonary capillary wedge pressure (PCWP) of 16 mmHg, and a pulmonary vascular resistance (PVR) of 7 Wood units confirming severe precapillary PH.

He was counselled for pulmonary endarterectomy (PEA) and after necessary pre-anesthetic workup, he underwent PEA. During the surgery both right pulmonary artery (RPA) and left pulmonary artery (LPA) were opened and clots were removed to the maximum possible extent. He had significant postoperative improvement in PA hemodynamics on repeat right heart catheterization. He had an uneventful postoperative recovery and within 2 weeks' postoperative he was weaned completely off O_2 and currently

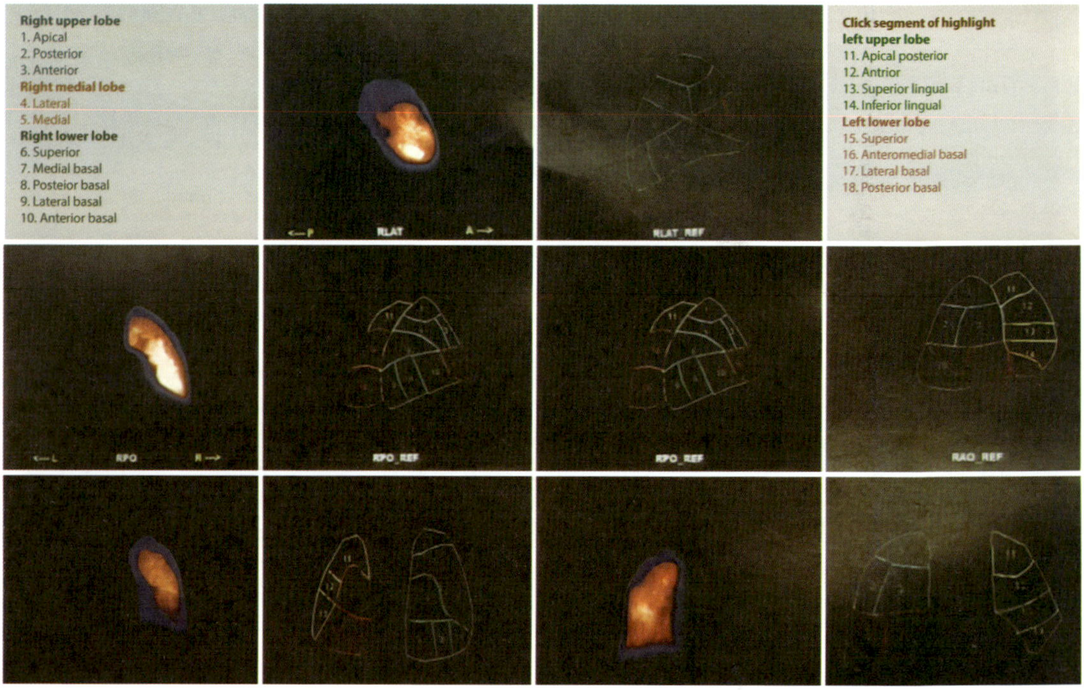

Fig. 28.2: Ventilation–perfusion scan showing absent perfusion in entire left lung and some segments of right lower lobe.

is on regular follow-up with SpO_2 >95% at room air and warfarin dose adjusted as per weekly INR readings.

DISCUSSION

A. Diagnosing Pulmonary Hypertension

Patients with pulmonary hypertension present with non-specific symptoms, such as shortness of breath, fatigue, chest pain, palpitation and syncope. Uncommon symptoms include cough, hemoptysis (pulmonary infarction), hoarseness of voice (dilated left pulmonary artery pressing on the recurrent laryngeal nerve) and wheeze. Release of serotonin—a potent bronchoconstrictor—from platelets in the clots is one of the mechanisms of wheeze in PH associated with thromboembolism. This causes many CTEPH patients to be incorrectly treated as asthma or COPD for months/years.

A diagnosis of PH is often delayed because the presenting symptoms and clinical signs are not specific to the diagnosis. Also many patients (40–50%) with CTEPH do not give a definite history of DVT or acute PE. Box 28.1 lists the common clinical scenarios when a clinician should suspect pulmonary hypertension.

Early diagnosis and management is of paramount importance to improve patient outcomes. It is estimated that more than 20% of patients with PH remain undiagnosed for up to two years after onset of symptoms. This often leads to significant morbidity and mortality.

Pulmonary hypertension (PH) is currently defined by presence of elevated mean pulmonary artery pressure, specifically greater than 20 mm Hg at rest, when measured

Box 28.1: Clinical scenarios when a clinician should suspect pulmonary hypertension.

- Unexplained dyspnea or unexplained effort intolerance.
- Dyspnea which is disproportionate to the existing pulmonary/cardiac disease.
- Dyspnea with associated pedal edema.
- Dyspnea/hypoxemia with a normal lung parenchyma on chest radiograph/CT scan.
- Presence of loud P2 on auscultation.
- Presence of hilar prominence/prominent right descending pulmonary artery on chest radiograph.
- ECG showing p-pulmonale.

by right heart catheterization (RHC). Hemodynamic definitions of pre-capillary and post-capillary pulmonary hypertension are elucidated in Table 28.1. Given the impracticality of performing RHC on all individuals, echocardiographic criteria are frequently employed for PH identification. An elevated right ventricular systolic pressure (RVSP), as determined by 2D echocardiography, is commonly used for diagnosing PH. However, RVSP measurements obtained via 2D echocardiography are operator-dependent and may be inaccurate in patients with sub-optimal acoustic windows, such as those with obesity or emphysema. Additionally, in the absence of a tricuspid regurgitant (TR) jet, RVSP cannot be calculated, yet the patient may still have significant PH.

Echocardiographic assessment for PH, particularly in symptomatic patients, primarily involves measuring the peak tricuspid regurgitation velocity (TRV) alongside other diagnostic indicators. This approach facilitates the stratification of PH probability into three categories.

1. **Low probability:** This is characterized by a peak TRV of ≤2.8 m/s and absence of other 2D echo features indicative of PH.
2. **Intermediate probability:** Defined by a peak TRV ranging from 2.9 to 3.4 m/s, regardless of the presence of additional signs, or a peak TRV of ≤2.8 m/s when accompanied by other indicators of PH.

Table 28.1: Hemodynamic definitions of pre-capillary and post-capillary pulmonary hypertension

Definitions	*Hemodynamic characteristics*
PH	• mPAP >20 mmHg
Pre-capillary PH	• mPAP >20 mmHg • PAWP ≤15 mmHg • PVR >2 WU
Isolated post-capillary PH (IpcPH)	• mPAP >20 mmHg • PAWP >15 mmHg • PVR ≤2 WU
Combined pre- and post-capillary PH (CpcPH)	• mPAP >20 mmHg • PAWP >15 mmHg • PVR >2 WU
Exercise PH	• mPAP/CO slope between rest and exercise >3 mmHg/L/min

PH: Pulmonary hypertension; *mPAP:* Mean pulmonary arterial pressure; *PAWP:* Pulmonary arterial wedge pressure; *PVR:* Pulmonary vascular resistance; *WU:* Wood units; *CO:* Cardiac output

Adapted from: 2022 ESC/ERS Guidelines for the diagnosis and treatment of pulmonary hypertension. Eur Heart J. 2022 Oct 11;43(38):3618–3731.

Table 28.2: Additional echocardiographic signs suggestive of PH

*The ventricles**	*Pulmonary artery**	*IVC and RA**
RV/LV basal diameter/area ratio >1.0	RVOT AT <105 m/s and/or mid-systolic notching	IVC diameter >21 mm with decreased inspiratory collapse (<50% with a sniff or <20% with quiet inspiration)
Flattening of the interventricular septum (LVEI >1.1 in systole and/or diastole)	Early diastolic pulmonary regurgitation velocity >2.2 m/s	RA area (end-systole) >18 cm^2
TAPSE/sPAP ratio <0.55 mm/mmHg	PA diameter >AR diameter PA diameter >25 mm	

PH: Pulmonary hypertension; *PA:* Pulmonary artery; *IVC:* Inferior vena cava; *RA:* Right atrium; *RV:* Right ventricle; *LV:* Left ventricle; *RVOT AT:* Right ventricular outflow tract acceleration time; *LVEI:* Left ventricle eccentricity index; *TAPSE:* Tricuspid annular plane systolic excursion; *sPAP:* systolic pulmonary arterial pressure; *AR:* Aortic root.

*Echocardiographic signs from at least 2 categories (A/B/C) must be present to alter the level of echocardiographic probability of PH.

Adapted from: European Society of Cardiology & European Respiratory Society 2023: European Respiratory Journal 61(1) 2200879; DOI: 10.1183/13993003.00879-2022. Published 6 January 2023.

3. **High probability:** Indicated by a peak TRV of ≥3.4 m/s, or a peak TRV within the 2.9 to 3.4 m/s range combined with other signs suggesting PH, such as evidence of right ventricular dysfunction or dilation.

Other echocardiographic signs contributing to the diagnosis of pulmonary hypertension are elucidated in Table 28.2. While echocardiography serves as an effective screening tool for PH, it does not provide a definitive diagnosis. A conclusive diagnosis of PH requires right heart catheterization.

B. Diagnosing the Cause of Pulmonary Hypertension

The causes of PH are myriad, and it is important to ascertain the cause of PH, as the treatment options differ, and the prognosis is varied. The latest European Society of cardiology (ESC)/ European Respiratory Society (ERS) 2022 clinical classification of pulmonary hypertension classifies patients into five groups (Table 28.3). Not all cases of PH have clear underlying causes, leading to the term "unexplained" or "idiopathic" pulmonary hypertension.

Evaluating a case of PH requires a comprehensive stepwise approach that involves a combination of clinical assessments, diagnostic tests, and collaboration among various medical specialists.

Step 1: Obtain Comprehensive Medical History

Gather detailed information about the patient's symptoms, including the onset, duration, and progression of symptoms such as shortness of breath, fatigue, chest pain, and syncope. Ask about any underlying medical conditions, past medical history, surgical history, and family history of cardiovascular diseases or thrombophilia.

Inquire about risk factors for pulmonary hypertension and thromboembolism, such as a history of thrombotic events, connective tissue disorders, sarcoidosis, interstitial lung disease (ILD), obstructive sleep apnea (OSA), chronic obstructive pulmonary disease (COPD), prolonged immobility, major surgery, recurrent abortions (APLA) or exposure to drugs (oral contraceptives, anorectics) and toxins/fumes.

Table 28.3: Clinical classification of pulmonary hypertension (ESC/ERS 2022)

Group	Category	Subcategories and notes
1.	Pulmonary arterial hypertension (PAH)	1.1 Idiopathic 1.2 Heritable 1.3 Associated with drugs and toxins 1.4 Associated with: 1.4.1 Connective tissue disease 1.4.2 HIV infection 1.4.3 Portal hypertension 1.4.4 Congenital heart disease 1.4.5 Schistosomiasis 1.5 PAH with features of venous/capillary involvement (PVOD/PCH) 1.6 Persistent PH of the newborn
2.	PH associated with left heart disease	2.1 Heart failure with preserved or reduced ejection fraction 2.2 Valvular heart disease 2.3 Congenital/acquired cardiovascular conditions leading to post-capillary PH
3.	PH associated with lung diseases and/or hypoxia	3.1 Obstructive lung disease or emphysema 3.2 Restrictive lung disease 3.3 Lung disease with mixed restrictive/obstructive pattern 3.4 Hypoventilation syndromes 3.5 Hypoxia without lung disease (e.g. high altitude) 3.6 Developmental lung disorders
4.	PH associated with pulmonary artery obstructions	4.1 Chronic thromboembolic PH 4.2 Other causes of pulmonary artery obstructions
5.	PH with unclear and/or multifactorial mechanisms	5.1 Hematological disorders 5.2 Systemic disorders 5.3 Metabolic disorders 5.4 Chronic renal failure with or without hemodialysis 5.5 Pulmonary tumour thrombotic microangiopathy 5.6 Fibrosing mediastinitis

Adapted from *2022 ESC/ERS Guidelines for the diagnosis and treatment of pulmonary hypertension. Eur Heart J. 2022 Oct 11;43(38):3618-3731.*

Step 2: Perform Detailed and Focused Physical Examination

It is essential to assess the patient's heart rate, blood pressure, and oxygen saturation. Look for cyanosis (hypoxia, congenital heart disease, Raynaud's phenomenon in systemic sclerosis), clubbing (congenital heart disease, bronchiectasis, ILD), lymphadenopathy (HIV, sarcoidosis) and pedal edema (right heart failure, DVT, post-phlebitis syndrome). Also look for markers of connective tissue disease (sclerodactyly, skin changes, alopecia).

Examine the chest for signs of right ventricular hypertrophy (enlargement), such as a prominent precordial impulse or a left parasternal heave. Listen for abnormal heart sounds, including an accentuated pulmonary component of the second heart sound (P2) and a tricuspid regurgitation murmur.

Presence of pulmonary bruits (high-pitched blowing sounds) over the lung fields which gets accentuated on inspiration or a breath hold are characteristic for CTEPH and can be seen in up to 30% of patients with CTEPH. They arise due to blood followed through narrowed and partially thrombosed pulmonary arteries. It is important to carefully auscultate for the presence of bruits in a case with unexplained PH.

Step 3: Perform Investigations to Diagnose, Etiotypes and Prognosticate Pulmonary Hypertension

Once a patient is diagnosed with PH, it is important to ascertain the cause for PH, stratify into groups, assess severity of disease and prognosticate. Investigations which need to be performed are listed in Tables 28.4 and 28.5.

Table 28.4: Diagnostic tests and their utility in patients with pulmonary hypertension

Test	Utility
2D echo cardiography (Transthoracic/transesophageal)	Simple, non-invasive technique can provide valuable information about heart chamber sizes, valve function, rule out congenital cardiac lesions and estimate pulmonary artery pressures.
Electrocardiograph	Look for signs of right ventricular hypertrophy and strain, identify S1Q3T3 pattern, rule out arrhythmias like atrial fibrillation and atrial tachycardia.
Chest X-ray	Identify signs of enlarged pulmonary arteries (diameter of right descending pulmonary artery >16 mm in females and >18 mm in males) and to identify associated lung parenchymal and pleural diseases.
Pulmonary function test (PFT)—spirometry	Assess lung function and identify any underlying restrictive and obstructive lung diseases. PH *per se* can lead to a mild restrictive defect on spirometry.
Six minute walk distance	To assess patient's baseline functional status, and to monitor the response to therapy.
Ventilation–perfusion (V/Q) scan	Screening test of choice for CTEPH (>95% sensitivity). Detect perfusion defects or mismatch, which might indicate CTEPH. However, use is limited by lack of wide availability.
CT pulmonary angiography	Widely available and almost as good as V/Q scan. Provides information on the pulmonary artery clot burden and the size and extent of obstruction. Also provides information on the lung parenchyma simultaneously. It may, however, miss smaller peripheral clots and a few chronic lesions.
Right heart cardiac catheterization	Gold standard for measuring pulmonary artery pressures, diagnosing pulmonary hypertension, and evaluating the level and severity of PH. Vasoreactivity testing can also be done which predicts response to calcium channel blocker (CCB) therapy.
Polysomnography (PSG)	Overnight level 1 PSG should be done when obstructive sleep apnea as a cause of PH is suspected.
Brain natriuretic peptide (BNP) or N-terminal pro-BNP level	Assessment of severity of PH and to prognosticate the disease.
Autoimmune screen	Tests such as ANA (IF), ANA profile, RA factor, ANCA (ELISA) may be performed to identify underlying autoimmune disease as the cause of pulmonary hypertension.

Table 28.5: Investigations which may be performed in patients with pulmonary hypertension		
Investigations for confirming pulmonary hypertension	***Investigations for identifying etiology of pulmonary hypertension***	***Investigations to assess severity of pulmonary hypertension***
2D echocardiogram (RVSP)	2D echocardiogram (TTE/TEE): To look for left heart pathology, right to left shunts	2D echocardiogram
Right heart catheterization (mPAP, PAWP, PVR)	V/Q scan (when available)	Six-minute walk distance
Contrast enhanced CT chest (pulmonary artery diameter)	• CT pulmonary angiogram • Diagnostic sleep study • HIV serology • Autoimmune screen (ANA by immunofluorescence, ANA profile) • HRCT chest and spirometry (to look for associated pulmonary pathology) • Thyroid function test	• Serum BNP/NT pro BNP levels • Cardiopulmonary exercise testing • Spirometry/DLCO assessment

ANA: Anti-nuclear antibody; *BNP:* Brain natriuretic peptide; *CT:* Computed tomography; *DLCO:* Diffusion capacity of lung for carbon monoxide; *HRCT:* High resolution CT; *HIV:* Human immunodeficiency virus; *mPAP:* mean pulmonary artery pressure; *PAWP:* Pulmonary arterial wedge pressure; *PVR:* Pulmonary vascular resistance; *RVSP:* Right ventricular systolic pressure; *TTE:* Transthoracic echocardiogram; *TEE:* Transesophageal echocardiogram; *NT pro BNP:* N terminal pro brain natriuretic peptide.

C. Treatment of Pulmonary Hypertension

Based on the clinical symptoms and investigation results, the severity of pulmonary hypertension is to be determined. A treatment strategy tailored to the patient's classification and severity is to be determined. In group 2 and group 3 PH, vasodilator therapies play little role and it is important to treat the underlying left heart/lung disease.

Vasodilators are the mainstay of treatment in group 1 PH: Endothelin receptor antagonists (Bosentan, Ambrisentan, Macitentan); Prostacyclin analogues (Selexipag—oral, Epoprostenol, Treprostenil—parenteral), PDE-5 inhibitors (Sildenafil, Tadalafil) are the currently available vasodilators. A stepwise approach where one vasodilator is started and later others are added is recommended in mild cases. Upfront combination approach is recommended in moderate-severe cases. Diuretics, oxygen therapy (if PaO_2 <55 mmHg), are equally important along with cardiopulmonary rehabilitation and treatment of comorbidities/associated conditions (e.g. OSA, COPD, IHD, etc.).

When CTEPH is identified as the cause of PH, the treatment of choice is pulmonary endarterecomy (PEA). With advancements in surgical techniques, more distal clots can also now be cleared. Lifelong anticoagulation is also mandatory for all patients with CTEPH. Balloon pulmonary angioplasty is an alternative option for those medically unfit for PEA. Riociguat is the oral drug approved for use in CTEPH. It can be used as a bridge to surgery or as definitive therapy if surgery is not feasible.

FURTHER READING

1. Yang J, Madani MM, Mahmud E, Kim NH. Evaluation and Management of Chronic Thromboembolic Pulmonary Hypertension. Chest. 2023 Aug;164(2):490–502.
2. Hambly N, Alawfi F, Mehta S. Pulmonary hypertension: diagnostic approach and optimal management. CMAJ. 2016 Aug 9;188(11):804–812.
3. Gupta T, Shariati F, Krim SR. A Simplified Diagnostic and Therapeutic Approach to Pulmonary Hypertension. Curr Probl Cardiol. 2022 Apr;47(4):100857.
4. Maron BA. Revised Definition of Pulmonary Hypertension and Approach to Management: A Clinical Primer. *J Am Heart Assoc*. 2023;12:e029024.
5. Humbert M, Kovacs G, Hoeper MM, Badagliacca R, Berger RM, Brida M, Carlsen J, Coats AJ, Escribano-Subias P, Ferrari P, Ferreira DS. 2022 ESC/ERS Guidelines for the diagnosis and treatment of pulmonary hypertension: Developed by the Task Force for the diagnosis and treatment of pulmonary hypertension of the European Society of Cardiology (ESC) and the European Respiratory Society (ERS). Endorsed by the International Society for Heart and Lung Transplantation (ISHLT) and the European Reference Network on rare respiratory diseases (ERN-LUNG). European heart Journal. 2022 Oct 7;43(38):3618–731.

Chapter 29

Approach to a Case with Non-resolving Pneumonia

• *Lakshimikant Baburao Yenge*

LEARNING POINTS

1. Non-resolving pneumonia is a common clinical entity, and an algorithmic approach helps to establish the correct cause.
2. Pneumonia does not mean it is always infective. To avoid this confusion, it may be better to approach it as syndrome—non-resolving pneumonia syndrome (NRPS).
3. Once we start looking beyond infective causes, we shall recognize many missed non-infective conditions.

INTRODUCTION

Non-resolving pneumonia (NRP) is a radiological term. Though we commonly use this term, there is no clear and accepted definition as the time to resolution of pneumonia has wide variability, and is affected by many factors like causative agent, severity of pneumonia, associated bacteraemia, comorbidities and most importantly age. Resolution of pneumonia may be as rapid as two weeks in young patients without comorbidities especially when caused by agents such as *Streptococcus pneumoniae*. Resolution may take as long as two to three months in elderly patients with structural lung disease and other comorbidities, and with infective pathogens like Legionella. Here we present two relatively uncommon, but commonly missed causes of NRP.

CASE VIGNETTE 1

A young female in her early thirties presented with right-sided pleuritic chest pain, generalized weakness, evening rise of temperature, anorexia and weight loss of three kilograms over the last three weeks. While she has no known comorbidities, her obstetric history was significant for medical termination (MTP) of her first pregnancy and a stillbirth, a year ago. She was diagnosed with right lower lobe (RLL) pneumonia based on the chest X-ray findings of a right lower lobe consolidation, and treated with broad spectrum antibiotics which resulted in transient improvement of her symptoms.

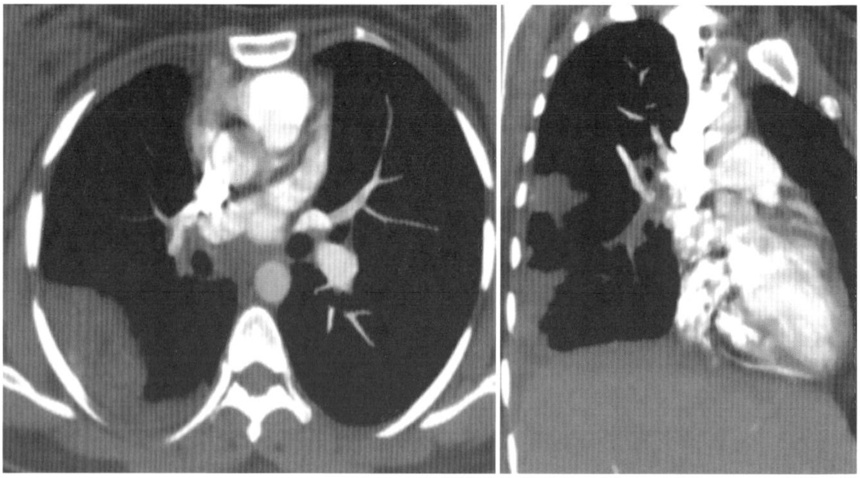

Fig. 29.1: CT pulmonary angiogram (CTPA) showing thrombus in distal right main pulmonary artery (MPA) extending to right descending pulmonary artery with wedge-shaped consolidation in right lower lobe.

She was further evaluated with a computed tomography (CT) chest which revealed the presence of persistent right lower lobe consolidation with minimal pleural effusion. Hematological workup revealed presence of normal leukocyte count of 10400 cells/mm^3, elevated erythrocyte sedimentation rate (ESR) of 115 mm, and an elevated C-reactive protein (CRP) of 71 mg/L. Her antinuclear antibody (ANA) by immunofluorescence (IF) was positive with end point dilution (EPD) of 1:1000. Patient had no clinical features suggestive of connective tissue disorder. Bronchoscopy and bronchoalveolar lavage (BAL) was performed. BAL was negative for tuberculosis and fungal pathogens. BAL culture revealed growth of Klebsiella and Chryseobacterium which were treated with appropriate antibiotics.

Despite adequate antibiotic therapy, she complained of persistent chest pain, low grade fever and generalized weakness. As she had a past history of a stillbirth and her ANA serology was positive, a non-infectious cause of NRP was considered. CT pulmonary angiography was performed and it revealed presence of thrombus in distal right pulmonary artery extending into the right descending pulmonary artery with associated consolidation in RLL and mild pleural effusion (Fig. 29.1). Subsequently, she was evaluated for antiphospholid syndrome (APS) and her antiphospholipid antibody (APLA) IgG (68 U/ml) and anti-β glycoprotein IgG antibody (35 U/ml) were found to be elevated and the corresponding IgM antibodies for both were negative. Echocardiography revealed mildly elevated right ventricular systolic pressure (RVSP) of 48 mm Hg.

She was treated with low molecular weight heparin (LMWH) and later switched to vitamin K antagonists (VKA) with international normalized ratio (INR) monitoring. At follow up after four months, the patient improved clinically, with improvement in her symptoms. There was complete resolution of the consolidation and decrease in the RVSP. She was continued on long-term anticoagulation with VKA, with a plan switch over to LMWH and aspirin when planning conception.

CASE VIGNETTE 2

A gentleman in his mid-fifties, presented with low-grade fever, myalgia, fatigue, anorexia and weight loss of four kilograms over the last five months. Patient is a well-controlled diabetic.

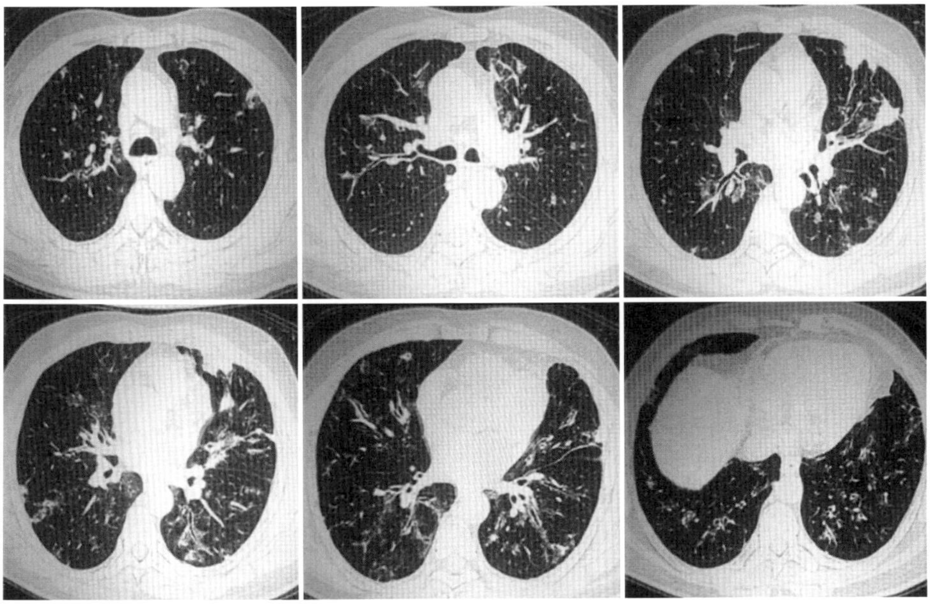

Fig. 29.2: Bilateral bronchial wall thickening with mild bronchiectasis and sub-segmental consolidations.

He was evaluated at a peripheral centre where X-ray chest revealed bilateral opacities. He was empirically started on anti-tubercular treatment (ATT). Patient completed nine months of ATT during which he improved symptomatically and gained two kilograms weight.

Six months after stopping ATT, the patient had recurrence of symptoms. CT chest was performed and it revealed presence of bilateral peribronchovascular and subpleural sub-segmental consolidations and bilateral bronchiectasis (Fig. 29.2). Spirometry revealed moderate obstruction with significant post-bronchodilator reversibility. Hematological workup revealed presence of normocytic normochromic anemia (Hb 10.9 gm/dl) with eosinophilia (5%).

Aspergillus specific IgM and IgG were negative and serum total IgE was only mildly elevated. Bronchoscopy revealed normal tracheobronchial tree with no evidence of mucus plugging. Bronchoalveolar lavage was performed from the lingula and sent for bacterial, fungal and tubercular cultures, all of which were sterile. BAL and serum galactomannan was also negative.

As diagnosis remained elusive, we revisited the history. Fatigue, generalized weakness, asthma and mild eosinophilia were positive findings noted. On further enquiry the patient complained of numbness in the 4th and 5th toes of left foot. The possibility of antineutrophil cytoplasmic antibody (ANCA) associated vasculitis (AAV) was considered. Antibodies directed against myeloperoxidase (anti-MPO) were found to be strongly positive. Nerve conduction study (NCS) revealed mononeuritis multiplex. Nerve biopsy was performed which showed features of vasculitic neuropathy. A final diagnosis of ACNA associated vasculitis—eosinophilic granulomatosis with polyangiitis (AAV- EGPA) was made (Table 29.1).

Patient had a five-factor score (FFS) of 2 and was started on prednisolone 1 mg/kg/day along with oral cyclophosphamide. He achieved remission with this regimen and was then continued on maintenance therapy with oral azathioprine and low dose prednisolone. After 2 years of remission, a treatment-free trial was given in view of pancytopenia, which

Table 29.1: Relevant investigations of Case 2 (non-resolving pneumonia)	
Investigation	***Result***
Spirometry	Moderate obstruction with significant bronchodilator reversibility.
CBC	10.9 gm/dl (NCNC)/11040 cells/cumm/377000 cells/cumm, AEC 530 (5%)
RFT/LFT	Mild hyperglobulinemia, rest normal.
ABPA work up	*Aspergillus fumigatus* specific IgE/IgG-negative, total IgE 208 (KIU/L)
Sputum	ZN stain X3, calcofluor stain-negative, culture—pan sensitive *E. coli*. Fungal culture—no growth.
Bronchoscopy	Normal tracheobronchial tree. No mucus plugs.
BAL	Negative for tuberculosis/fungal/bacterial pathogens
ESR/CRP	115 mm/75 mg/L.
Urine routine	Microscopic hematuria with proteinuria (5.4 gm/24 hr).
NCS	Axonal neuropathy bilateral lower limbs, left > right.
ANCA	Anti-PR3-negative, anti-MPO-125 (strong positive)
Nerve biopsy	Consistent with vasculitic neuropathy

ABPA: Allergic bronchopulmonary aspergillosis; *AEC:* Absolute eosinophil count; *ANCA:* Antineutrophil cytoplasmic antibody; *BAL:* Bronchoalveolar lavage; *CBC:* Complete blood count; *CRP:* C-reactive protein; *ESR:* Erythrocyte sedimentation rate; *IgE:* Immunoglobulin E; *IgG:* Immunoglobulin G; *LFT:* Liver function test; *MPO:* Myeloperoxidase; *NCS:* Nerve conduction studies; *PR-3:* Proteinase 3; *RFT:* Renal function test; *ZN:* Zeihl-Neelsen.

was likely due to azathioprine. However, he had a relapse with pulmonary and renal involvement within 9 months of treatment-free trial. At this time in view of relapse and uncontrolled diabetes he was initiated on rituximab plus prednisolone which was tapered rapidly. Presently he is in remission and is on rituximab maintenance therapy.

DISCUSSION

Non-resolving pneumonia (NRP) is a common clinical entity and accounts for approximately 15% of all pulmonology consultations, and 8% of bronchoscopies. However, it is not clearly defined and there are no validated criteria. Those who are not showing satisfactory clinical and radiological response (despite appropriate antibiotic use) at four to twelve weeks are considered to have NRP.

The first step in evaluating non-resolving pneumonia is to discriminate between expected versus actual rate of resolution of pneumonia. The rate of resolution can be looked at as a spectrum: from expected resolution, slow resolution to non-resolution and progressive pneumonia (Table 29.2). Normal resolution is combination of a good clinical response and at least 50% radiological resolution at 4 weeks. Slowly resolving pneumonia (SRP) is good clinical response but <50% radiographic resolution after 4 weeks. Progressive pneumonia (PP) is when there is clinical and radiological progression on appropriate treatment. While labelling a case as SRP, NRP or PP, it is important to take into account factors that affect the expected rate of resolution (Table 29.3). In SRP, it is prudent to wait for radiological infiltrates to resolve. However, in PP it may be disastrous to wait and we should perform early additional diagnostic tests to arrive at appropriate diagnosis.

It is also important to recognize that NRP is not always due to an infectious cause, and many cases of NRP are due to non-infectious causes (Table 29.4). So, it is better to consider it as non-resolving pneumonia syndrome (NRPS).

Table 29.2: Proposed definitions based on rate of resolution of pneumonia

Clinical syndrome	*Definition*
Expected resolution of pneumonia	Resolution of clinical symptoms by 2 weeks and resolution of radiologic infiltrates (>50% resolution from baseline) by 4 weeks
Slowly resolving pneumonia (SRP)	Satisfactory clinical response to therapy but lack of radiologic resolution (<50% resolution from baseline) at 4 weeks
Non-resolving pneumonia (NRP)	Lack of clinico-radiologic response to therapy at 4 weeks.
Progressive pneumonia (PP)	Progression of clinical symptoms and/or radiologic infiltrates at 2 weeks despite therapy

Table 29.3: Factors affecting rate of resolution of pneumonia

Sl. No.	*Factor*	*Slow resolution*
1.	Agent factors	• *Legionella pneumophila, Haemophilus influenzae* • Tuberculosis, other mycobacteria • Fungi, nocardia, actinomyces • Resistant pathogens
2.	Host factors	• Older age • Comorbid conditions: COPD, alcoholism, diabetes mellitus, neurological disorders, ischemic heart disease, malignancy and renal failure • Structural causes: Endobronchial obstruction • Hypogammaglobulinemia: Congenital and acquired. • HIV infection
3.	Treatment-related factors	• Inappropriate drug • Inappropriate dose • Inappropriate duration of therapy
4.	Complications	• Lung abscess • Empyema

COPD: Chronic obstructive pulmonary disease; *HIV:* Human immunodeficiency virus

Table 29.4: Non-infectious causes of non-resolving pneumonia syndrome

Sl. No.	*Group*	*Specific pathology*
1.	Neoplastic	Endobronchial obstruction—post-obstructive pneumonia Lepidic adenocarcinoma Lymphoma Metastatic malignancy
2.	Immunologic	Vasculitis Organizing pneumonia Eosinophilic pneumonia syndromes Acute interstitial pneumonia Pulmonary alveolar proteinosis Sarcoidosis

(Contd.)

Table 29.4: Non-infectious causes of non-resolving pneumonia syndrome (*Contd.*)

Sl. No.	*Group*	*Specific pathology*
3.	Drug induced	Bleomycin Amiodarone Nitrofurantoin Methotrexate
4.	Cardiovascular	Pulmonary embolism Pulmonary edema
5.	Miscellaneous	Lipoid pneumonia Pulmonary contusions

Approach to a Case with Non-resolving Pneumonia

After ascertaining that it is a case of NRPS, next step is to establish the causes of NRPS. We need to evaluate for infectious causes of pneumonia first as they are more common and once specific pathogen is identified, it obviates need for further extensive work up. Review of history and clinical course for any pointers towards non-bacterial infectious pathogens for NRPS like tuberculosis, fungal infections, nocardia, pneumocystis, etc. should be considered. Sputum evaluation with special stains for these pathogens is to be considered, if not done already.

If NRPS remains undiagnosed despite sputum evaluation, a high-resolution computed tomography (HRCT) chest is next investigation to be performed. Two specific CT studies to be considered are: (a) CT pulmonary angiography for suspected pulmonary embolism; and (b) CT aortogram for suspected sequestration. If these two pathologies are not under consideration, non-contrast HRCT scan followed by contrast enhanced CT chest is be performed. If HRCT is diagnostic, management follows disease-specific guidelines.

If the cause for NRPS remains unclear after a CT chest, next step is to consider tissue sampling. Bronchoscopic versus image guided sampling depends on location and pattern of pathology, clinical possibilities under consideration, availability and accessibility of these tests and preferences of clinician and patient. Bronchoscopic sampling (bronchoalveolar lavage and lung biopsy) is safe and yields adequate information to obviate further evaluation in more than 90% of NRPS. Image-guided sampling is preferred if pathology is subpleural and non-infectious or invasive mould infection is most likely diagnosis, as negative predictive value (NPV) of bronchoscopic sampling in these cases is low.

NRPS remaining undiagnosed with this usual work up deserves to be reviewed again with fresh perspective, and focus should shift towards non-infectious causes at this point. We would re-emphasize here that infectious causes cannot be completely ruled out with above evaluation alone. Two most common non-infectious pathologies to be considered are autoimmune/inflammatory diseases and neoplastic causes. Targeted laboratory work up and multispecialty inputs are to be considered at this point. Larger tissue acquisition, preferably via transbronchial lung cryobiopsy or a video-assisted thoracoscopic surgery (VATS) is usually the final step in diagnostic evaluation of NRPS. Cryolung biopsy is a bronchoscopic technique which can procure larger tissue samples and has a diagnostic yield similar to a VATS biopsy. Addition of radial endobronchial ultrasound to accurately identify the lesion before sampling will further improve the yield of a cryobiopsy. An algorithm for approach to a case with non-resolving pneumonia is provided in Fig. 29.3.

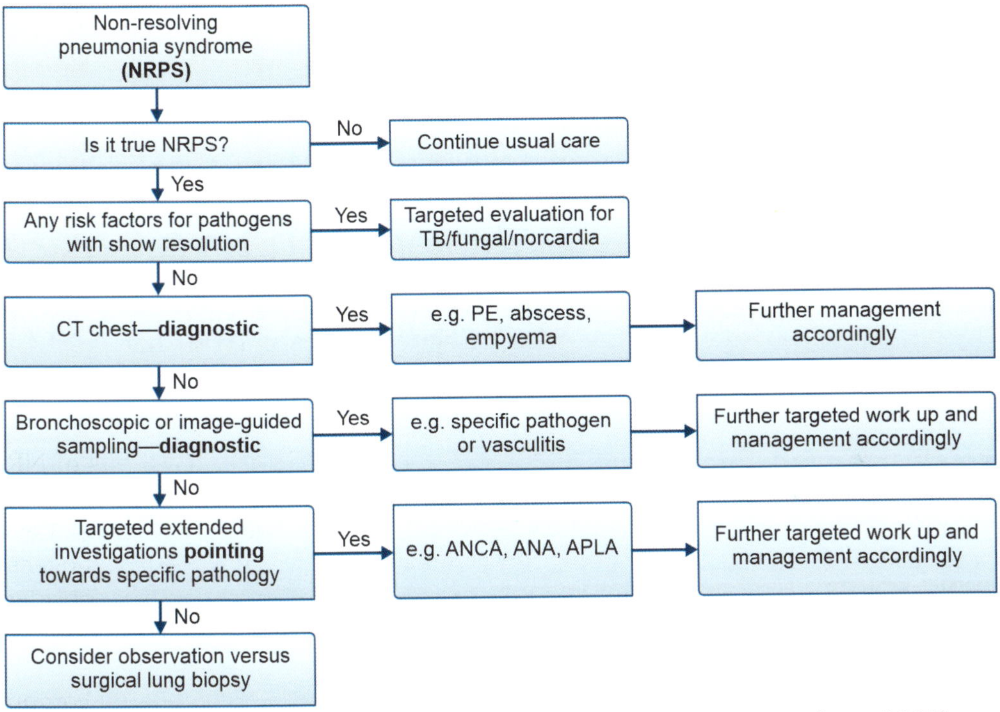

Fig. 29.3: Algorithmic approach to a case with non-resolving pneumonia syndrome (NRPS).

FURTHER READING

1. El Solh AA, Aquilina AT, Gunen H, Ramadan F. Radiographic resolution of community-acquired bacterial pneumonia in the elderly. *J Am Geriatr Soc*. 2004 Feb;52(2):224–9.
2. Palkar AV, Rapose A. 'Non-resolving' pneumonia. BMJ Case Rep. 2012 Sep 7;2012:bcr 2012006861.
3. Weyers CM, Leeper KV. Nonresolving pneumonia. Clin Chest Med 2005; 26:143–58.
4. Chaudhuri AD, Mukherjee S, Nandi S, Bhuniya S, Tapadar SR, Saha M. A study on non-resolving pneumonia with special reference to role of fiberoptic bronchoscopy. Lung India 2013;30:27–32.

Chapter

30

Approach to a Case of Unexplained Lung Cavity

• *Alekhya lakkam* • *V Nagarjuna Maturu*

LEARNING POINTS

1. The presence of a cavity in the lung does not always indicate pulmonary tuberculosis. It is essential to consider other possible diagnoses as well.
2. Radiological characteristics of a cavity are crucial in deciphering the underlying nature of the disease. Features such as size, location, wall characteristics, and associated imaging findings play a significant role in narrowing the differentials.
3. Confirmed diagnosis and therapy is always to be preferred over empiric therapy based on radiologic features alone.

INTRODUCTION

A pulmonary cavity, as defined by the Fleischner Society, is 'a gas-filled space within a zone of pulmonary consolidation or within a mass or nodule, with a wall thicker than four mm'. Cavities arise from liquefactive necrosis and the expulsion of debris from bronchial trees. A wide array of pathological conditions presents with cavities, including infectious and non-infectious causes such as malignancy, autoimmune diseases, and congenital abnormalities. The radiological characteristics of cavities help to narrow the differential diagnosis. In this case report, a middle-aged woman presented with unexplained weight loss and a lung cavity was initiated on empiric anti-tuberculous treatment (ATT), but her weight loss continued. Follow-up imaging revealed a persistent lung cavity, and evaluation confirmed non-tuberculous mycobacteria as the underlying cause.

CASE VIGNETTE

A female homemaker in her fifties presented to our outpatient department with a two-year history of progressive weight loss. She has no other cardinal symptoms or known comorbidities. She has no addictions and an unremarkable medical history.

Eighteen months' prior, a chest X-ray which was performed for evaluation for weight loss identified the right upper zone infiltrates. Despite receiving symptomatic treatment,

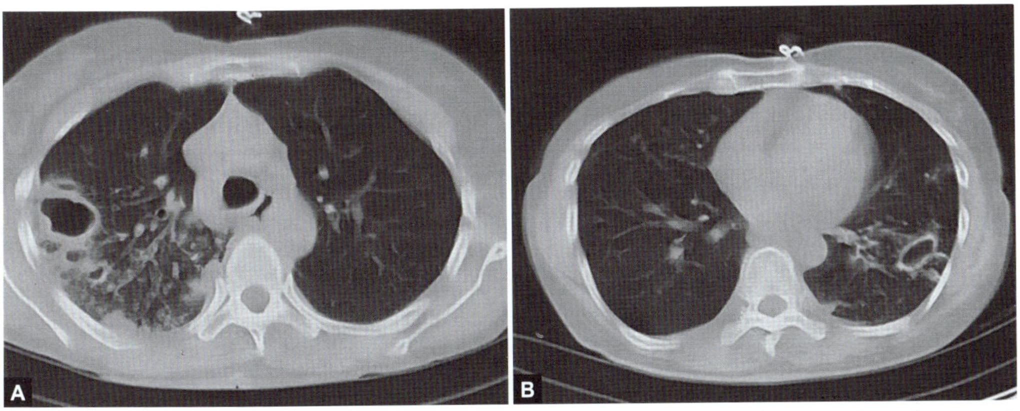

Fig. 30.1: HRCT chest showing (A) thick-walled cavity with pericavity consolidation in the right upper lobe and; (B) Cavity in the left lower lobe.

and empiric antibiotics her weight loss and weakness persisted. Six months later, a high-resolution computed tomography (HRCT) of the chest was performed which revealed cavities in the right upper lobe and left lower lobe, accompanied by surrounding consolidation (Fig. 30.1A and B). Bronchoalveolar lavage (BAL) was performed from the right upper lobe to evaluate the cause of lung cavity. However, all infective workup turned out to be negative. An autoimmune workup showed weak positivity for the Pm-Scl antibody. A CT-guided biopsy from the right upper lobe cavity wall was then performed which showed necrotizing granulomatous inflammation. Based on these findings, she was commenced on anti-tubercular therapy (ATT) for six months. However, she showed no radiological improvement and continued to experience weakness and weight loss.

At presentation to our hospital, her vital signs were as follows: pulse rate at 92 beats per minute, blood pressure at 100/60 mmHg, respiratory rate at 20 per minute, a temperature of 98°F, and oxygen saturation at 96% on room air. She was underweight, looked weak and her general examination was normal. A repeat HRCT chest revealed bilateral cavitary lesions with inhomogeneous opacities (Fig. 30.2A and B). A repeat bronchoscopy was performed, and the BAL analysis showed a positive AFB smear but negative Xpert MTB/RIF. BAL DNA PCR for MTB/MOTT and MTB culture detected *Mycobacterium intracellulare*. A diagnosis

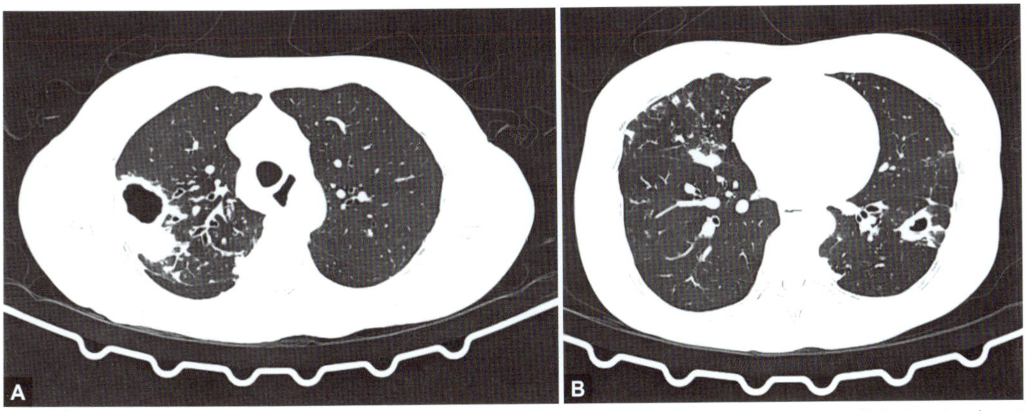

Fig. 30.2: HRCT chest showing (A) persistent thick-walled cavity with pericavity consolidation in the right upper lobe; (B) Persistent cavity with pericavity consolidation in the left lower lobe.

of non-tuberculous mycobacterial disease was thus confirmed. The patient has since been started on rifampicin, clarithromycin and ethambutol and is currently under follow-up.

DISCUSSION

This case features a patient with cavitary lung lesions evident on radiography and necrotizing granulomatous inflammation on histopathology, who did not respond to anti-tuberculosis therapy (ATT). Subsequent evaluation revealed non-tuberculous mycobacteria (NTM), necessitating a change in therapy. This highlights the fact that cavitary lung lesions can result from various causes, and also to the fact that a correct diagnosis of the cause of cavity is important to initiate appropriate therapy. A four step approach to a patient with pulmonary cavity is presented here.

Step 1: Differentiate Cavity From Cavity Mimics

It is crucial to distinguish true cavities from mimics like cysts, emphysema, infected bullae, and cystic bronchiectasis (Table 30.1). The thickness of the wall is the important radiologic feature which differentiates emphysema (no wall), bulla (<1 mm thick wall), cyst (<3 mm thick wall) and cavity ($\geq$4 mm thick wall). Presence of associated bronchiectasis is a clue to the possibility of cystic bronchiectasis presenting as multiple cavities.

Step 2: Assess History and Clinical Presentation

A clinical assessment is very important which trying to ascertain the cause for the pulmonary cavity.

1. Duration of symptoms: Acute or subacute cavities are defined as those less than 6 weeks old, while chronic cavities persist for more than 6 weeks. When the clinical presentation is acute or subacute, the possibility of infections is higher. Malignancies, inflammatory diseases and other causes usually have a more chronic clinical presentation.
2. Presence of fever and other constitutional symptoms point towards infectious or noninfectious inflammatory diseases (vasculitis) as the cause of cavities.
3. Immune status of the individual is also an important clinical consideration. Presence of cavities in an immunocompromised host should raise the suspicion of invasive fungal and other opportunistic infections (nocardia, melioidosis, etc.) in addition to the usual causes of an infectious cavity.
4. Associated systemic diseases also need to be looked into. History suggestive of connective tissue disease or vasculitis is to be taken. Presence of extrapulmonary malignancy should raise the suspicion of possible cavitary metastases.

Table 30.1: Various cavity mimics and their definitions

Cavity mimic	*Description*	*Characteristics*
Cysts	Round circumscribed spaces surrounded by an epithelial or fibrous wall.	Wall thickness is usually less than 3 mm.
Emphysema	Permanently enlarged air spaces with alveolar wall destruction.	Can be focal or diffuse, usually without a visible wall.
Bulla	Sharply demarcated, rounded, low attenuated areas.	Features an imperceptible wall (<1 mm)
Cystic bronchiectasis	Irreversible bronchial dilatation.	No bronchial tapering on CT, size larger than adjacent artery.

5. Other risk factors for primary lung malignancy need to be assessed. Tobacco smoke exposure, elderly age, asbestos exposure when present in a patient presenting with a thick walled cavity raise the clinical probability of bronchogenic carcinoma presenting as lung cavity.

Step 3: Assess Radiologic Characteristics of Cavity

This is a very important step in assessing a case of a pulmonary cavity. Several radiologic features need to be assessed on a HRCT chest.

1. **Number of cavities:** Cavities can be solitary or multiple. Solitary cavities typically occur in active pulmonary tuberculosis, sequelae of tuberculosis, aspergilloma, lung abscess, or primary lung carcinoma. Multiple cavitary lesions are more common in conditions such as granulomatosis with polyangiitis (GPA), septic emboli, active pulmonary tuberculosis and its sequelae, or invasive fungal infections (Table 30.2).
2. **Cavity wall characteristics:** The thickness of cavity wall is an important diagnostic factor. Cavities with a thinner wall are more likely to be benign and those with a thicker wall are more likely malignant. Thickness of the wall alone is however not a very reliable feature in distinguishing benign from malignant cavities. Invasive fungal infections and vasculitis also can present as thick walled cavities. Irregular/nodular walls of the cavity point towards infectious or a neoplastic process, whereas smooth walls are seen in diseases such as vasculitis, rheumatoid arthritis, septic emboli, etc.
3. **Location of cavity:** The cavity's location also provides diagnostic insights. Typically, post-primary tuberculosis affects the upper lobe's posterior segments and the lower lobe's superior segments. Lung abscesses, commonly a result of aspiration pneumonia, are found in the lower lobe's superior segment. Upper lobes frequently show old tubercular cavities and aspergillomas, while lung carcinomas usually appear in the upper lobe's anterior segment. Septic emboli, stemming from hematogenous spread, initially manifests in the lower lobes before progressing to the upper lobes.
4. **Intracavitary contents:** Presence of intra-cavitary contents also needs to be assessed. An air fluid level indicates a lung abscess or a cavity with superadded bacterial infection.

Table 30.2: Causes of cavitating pulmonary diseases

Cause	*Solitary/Few*	*Multiple*
Infectious cause	• Tuberculosis/non-tuberculous mycobacterial disease • Lung abscess/necrotizing pneumonia • Fungal infections (Aspergillus/Mucormycosis) • Nocardiosis	• Septic pulmonary emboli • Tuberculosis
Malignancy	• Bronchogenic carcinoma	• Cavitating metastases • Cavitating papillomas • Lymphomas
Inflammatory (non-infectious)		• Granulomatosis with polyangiitis • Rheumatoid nodules
Congenital causes	• Pulmonary sequestration • Congenital cystic adenomatoid malformation	
Miscellaneous	• Pulmonary infarct • Post-RF ablation of lung mass • Pulmonary laceration	• Pulmonary Langerhans cell histiocytosis • Pulmonary amyloidosis

Presence of an air crescent sign is suggestive of invasive aspergillosis. Other causes of intra-cavitary contents include aspergilloma, intracavitary clot or a Rasmussen's aneurysm.

5. **Surrounding lung parenchyma/structures:** Assessing lung parenchyma surrounding the cavity is also important. Presence of centrilobular nodules or pericavitary consolidation is common in infectious causes of a lung cavity. Cavity which invades the adjacent pericavitary structures is suggestive of invasive malignancy or an invasive infection (zygomycetes, actinomycetes).
6. **Presence of a feeding vessel or a feeding bronchus:** Presence of a feeding vessel into the cavity indicates a hematogenous spread of disease and is seen in septic emboli, vasculitis and invasive fungal infections. Presence of bronchus going into the cavity does not narrow the differential, but point to the fact that bronchoscopic approach is likely feasible in reaching to the cavity.

Step 4: Acquire Samples for Microbiologic/Histologic Diagnosis

Though a HRCT chest helps in narrowing the differentials, it cannot help in confirming the etiology. Sputum examination (when feasible) for bacteria, tuberculosis and fungal infections needs to be performed. When sputum is not produced or is non-contributory, a broncho-alveolar lavage is the best test for diagnosing infectious causes of a cavity. Serologic tests in

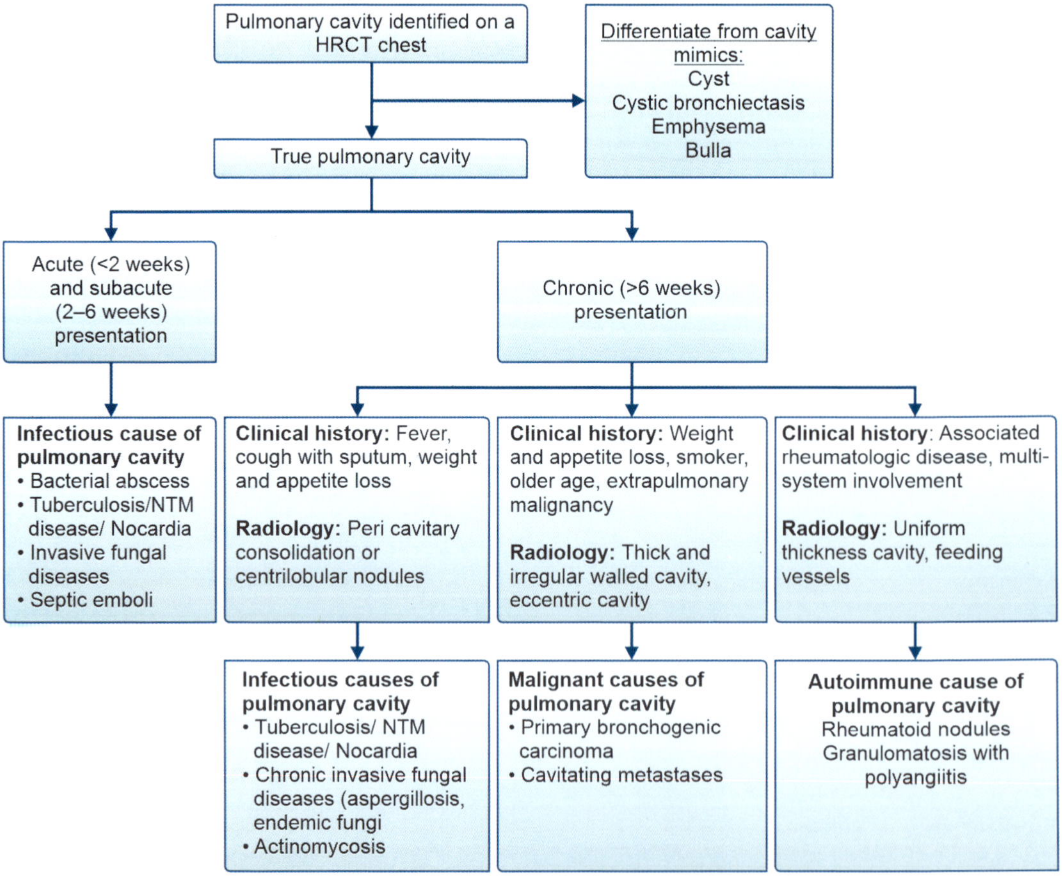

Fig. 30.3: Approach to cavitary lung disease (a radiologic algorithm).

the correct clinical context help in diagnosing inflammatory conditions like vasculitis and rheumatoid arthritis.

A biopsy is essential for confirming the diagnosis of malignancy. A biopsy can be performed from the wall of the cavity via a transthoracic approach (CT or USG-guided) or a bronchoscopic approach (using a radial EBUS). A biopsy also helps in diagnosing granulomatous infections and other invasive fungal infections.

Diagnosing the etiology for a cavitary lung disease is complex due to various differential diagnoses and presentations. An algorithmic approach is crucial for effective evaluation and management (Fig. 30.3).

FURTHER READING

1. Duong TB, Ceglar S, Reaume M, Lee C. Imaging Approach to Cavitary Lung Disease. Annals of the American Thoracic Society. 2020 Mar;17(3):367–71.
2. Gafoor K, Patel S, Girvin F, Gupta N, Naidich D, Machnicki S, Brown KK, Mehta A, Husta B, Ryu JH, Sarosi GA. Cavitary lung diseases: a clinical-radiologic algorithmic approach. Chest. 2018 Jun 1;153(6):1443–65.
3. Canan A, Batra K, Saboo SS, Landay M, Kandathil A. Radiological approach to cavitary lung lesions. *Postgraduate Medical Journal*. 2021 Aug;97(1150):521–31.

Chapter

31

Approach to a Case with Reversed Halo Sign on CT Chest

• *Narendra Kumar Narahari* • *Rakesh Kodati*

LEARNING POINTS

1. In patients presenting with a reversed halo sign (RHS) on a HRCT chest, which can be seen in both infectious and noninfectious diseases, obtaining a microbiologic or a histopathologic diagnosis is essential.
2. Assessment of clinical presentation, immune status, and radiologic findings is crucial for accurate differential diagnosis in RHS cases.
3. In immunocompromised patients with RHS, immediate initiation of antifungal therapy for suspected mucormycosis is recommended, pending further diagnostic confirmation.

INTRODUCTION

The reversed halo sign (RHS), characterized by a central ground-glass opacity (GGO) encircled by a denser rim of air-space consolidation, was initially described in cryptogenic organising pneumonia (COP) cases on high-resolution computed tomography (HRCT) of the chest. Over time, RHS has been observed in various pulmonary conditions, both infectious and non-infectious, thereby presenting a diagnostic challenge. Careful consideration of clinical history and other radiological findings is crucial for clinicians to establish the diagnosis and determine appropriate treatment strategies. In this report, we present a case of a 54-year-old immunocompromised male who had RHS on HRCT chest and was diagnosed with mucormycosis. We also discuss the differential diagnosis, the diagnostic approach and management for this particular case, underscoring the complexity and importance of accurately interpreting the reversed halo sign in pulmonary conditions.

CASE VIGNETTE

A male farmer in his mid-fifties presented with a 10-day history of fever, cough with streaky hemoptysis, and exertional breathlessness. He has a history of smoking, with a smoking index of 250, and consumes alcohol occasionally. He is also a known diabetic and hypertensive patient but has been non-compliant with his treatments. Additionally, he has had a solitary kidney since birth. There was no significant familial or occupational history.

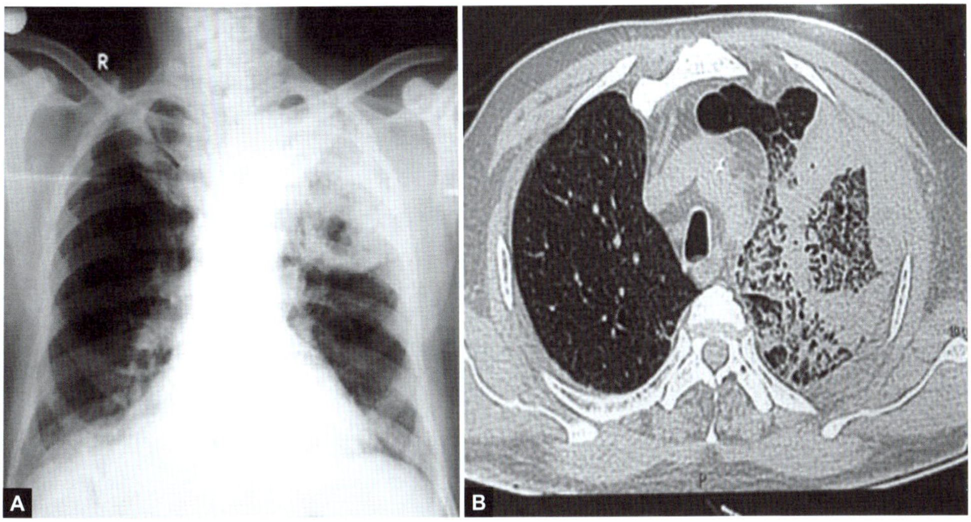

Fig. 31.1: (A) Chest radiograph showing a inhomogenous opacity in the left upper zone; (B) CT thorax showing reversed halo sign in the left upper lobe (central ground glassing with peripheral rim of consolidation).

Upon examination, he was afebrile, with a pulse rate of 98 beats per minute, a respiratory rate of 24 breaths per minute, and a blood pressure of 130/90 mmHg. His oxygen saturation was 97% on ambient air. Chest auscultation revealed fine crepitations in the left infraclavicular and mammary regions. Blood tests showed a low hemoglobin level of 9.5 gm/dl and a total leukocyte count of 12,500 cells/mm^3. His liver function tests were normal, but renal parameters indicated elevated blood urea (102 mg/dl) and creatinine (3.6 mg/dl), with an elevated HbA1C level of 9.2%. A chest radiograph displayed inhomogenous opacity in the left upper zone (Fig. 31.1A). Sputum microbiological analysis did not reveal any infectious agents.

Contrast-enhanced computed tomography (CECT) of the chest showed a central GGO with a peripheral rim of consolidation, indicative of a RHS in the left upper lobe (Fig. 31.1B). A differential diagnosis of RHS, as outlined in Table 31.1, was considered. Given his immunocompromised state (uncontrolled diabetes and chronic kidney disease), and the

Table 31.1: Differential diagnosis of reversed halo sign on computed tomography of the chest

Category	*Disease name*
Infectious diseases	• Pulmonary mucormycosis (most common) • Invasive pulmonary aspergillosis • Histoplasmosis • Cryptococcosis • Paracoccidioidomycosis • *Pneumocystis jirovecii* pneumonia • COVID-19 • H1N1 acute respiratory syndrome • Tuberculosis • *Legionella pneumophila* pneumonia

(*Contd.*)

Table 31.1: Differential diagnosis of reversed halo sign on computed tomography of the chest (*Contd.*)

Category	*Disease name*
Non-infectious benign diseases	• Cryptogenic organising pneumonia (most common) • Secondary organising pneumonia • Vasculitis (Wegener's granulomatosis) • Sarcoidosis • Idiopathic nonspecific interstitial pneumonia • Lipoid pneumonia • Pulmonary thromboembolism • Pulmonary tumour embolus • Pulmonary edema • Hypersensitivity pneumonitis • Lymphocytic interstitial pneumonia
Neoplastic conditions	• Bronchoalveolar carcinoma • Metastatic disease • Lymphomatoid granulomatosis

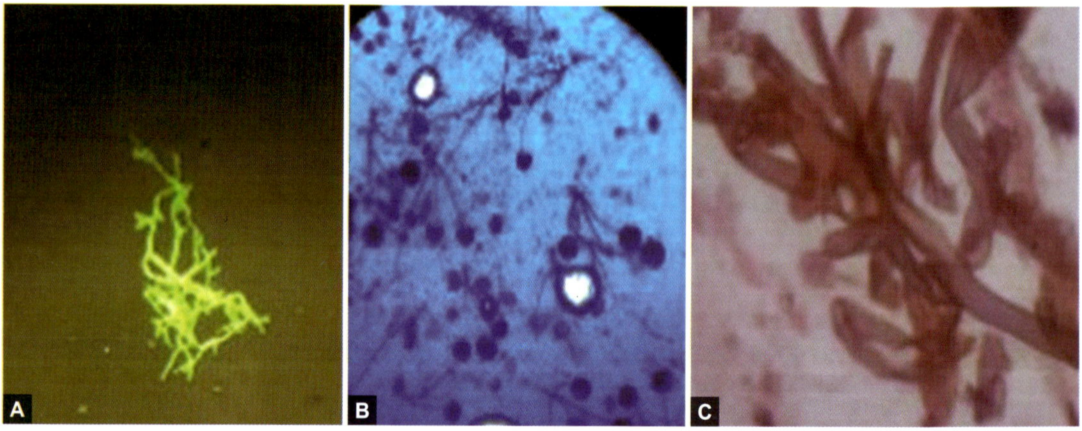

Fig. 31.2: (A) KOH—calcofluor white mount, 100X showing broad aseptate hyphae with right angle branching and ribbon-like folding; (B) Lactophenol cotton blue mount, 100X showing erect branched sporangiophores with spherical sporangia and rhizoids; (C) H&E stain demonstrating broad aseptate hyphae.

presence of RHS on the CT thorax, an invasive fungal disease, likely mucormycosis, was suspected. He was started on empirical antifungal treatment with isavuconazole, pending further investigation.

Patient underwent bronchoscopy and BAL which revealed presence of hyphae resembling zygomycetes, confirming the diagnosis of pulmonary mucormycosis (Fig. 31.2). Due to chronic kidney disease, isavuconazole was preferred over amphotericin B, and a surgical resection of the affected lung was planned.

DISCUSSION

Reversed halo sign (RHS) is a distinct radiographic pattern identified on computed tomography (CT) scans of the lungs. It is characterized by a central area of ground-glass opacities (GGO) encircled by a ring- or crescent-shaped rim of consolidation within the lung parenchyma, RHS was initially described by Voloudaki et al in 1996. They observed crescentic and ring-shaped opacities around areas of ground-glass attenuation in patients with cryptogenic organizing pneumonia. The term "RHS" was later coined by Kim et al in 2002 to describe similar radiographic findings. In 2008, the Fleischner Society defined RHS as a focal, rounded area of GGO surrounded by a more or less complete ring of consolidation.

The RHS is also known by other names, such as the reverse halo sign, atoll sign, or fairy ring sign. The term "atoll," derived from the Maldivian word "*atholhu*," refers to an island with a central lagoon encircled by a coral reef, mirroring the RHS's radiographic appearance. "Fairy ring," a term from Gaelic mythology, is used interchangeably by some authors to describe RHS. However, it is important to note that in the fairy ring sign, the centre of the ring shows normal-appearing lung parenchyma, as opposed to the GGO central to RHS.

RHS is associated with various diseases, both infectious and non-infectious. Its presence in immunocompromised individuals is particularly concerning and often suggests an invasive fungal infection. Presence of RHS warrants a thorough investigation to confirm the diagnoses.

Differential Diagnoses for Reversed Halo Sign

A. Invasive Fungal Diseases

In the context of invasive fungal diseases, RHS is more frequently associated with mucormycosis than invasive pulmonary aspergillosis. This is likely due to the more aggressive nature and greater angioinvasive capacity of *Zygomycetes* species compared to *Aspergillus* species. RHS typically emerges due to infarcted lung tissue at its centre, surrounded by a significant amount of hemorrhage at the lesion's periphery. On histopathology, there is a central infarction, potentially revealing multiple levels of pulmonary arterial or venous thrombi filled with numerous fungal hyphae. Commonly observed in the acute phase of infection, RHS is known to evolve over time into either an air crescent or a cavity.

Clinically, the presence of RHS in conjunction with symptoms like concomitant sinusitis, previous voriconazole prophylaxis, and the presence of multiple nodules ($\geq$10) or pleural effusion in initial CT scans may indicate mucormycosis rather than aspergillosis. Additionally, RHS has been reported in cases of endemic fungal infections such as Paracoccidioidomycosis, Histoplasmosis, and Cryptococcosis, as well as in *Pneumocystis jirovecii* pneumonia, albeit less frequently.

B. Organizing Pneumonia and Other Interstitial Lung Diseases

Organizing pneumonia (OP), particularly ryptogenic OP (COP), is the most common noninfectious condition associated with the RHS. In COP, RHS's central GGO results from alveolar septal inflammation, while the denser rim is due to inflammation or granulation in the air space. RHS appears in about 12–19% of COP cases, often resembling a 'pebble into a pond' pattern where inflammation spreads outward from a central point. While RHS is a notable feature in COP, it does not distinguish between cryptogenic and secondary causes, requiring investigation into possible underlying factors like medication, radiation exposure, or connective tissue diseases.

RHS is also seen in lipoid pneumonia, typically following inhalation or aspiration of lipid substances, and occasionally in other interstitial lung diseases (ILDs) like NSIP and sarcoidosis. In sarcoidosis, RHS might indicate non-caseating granulomatous inflammation or secondary OP. The presence of small nodules or a nodular consolidation rim within RHS in these conditions often points towards a granulomatous rather than an organizing process.

When RHS is present, features like a thicker rim (about 1 cm), reticulation within the rim, and associated pleural effusion can help differentiate fungal pneumonia from OP, as these signs are more indicative of fungal involvement.

C. Bacterial/Mycobacterial Infections

RHS has also been observed in various infections, including community-acquired pneumonias like pneumococcal pneumonia, psittacosis, Legionnaires disease, and mycobacterial infections. It remains uncertain whether RHS in these infections signifies secondary organizing pneumonia as part of the infection's resolution or a direct manifestation of the infectious process. The presence of nodular walls or nodules within the RHS halo is strongly indicative of granulomatous diseases, particularly tuberculosis.

D. COVID-19 Pneumonia

In recent studies focusing on COVID-19 pneumonia, the reverse halo sign (RHS) has demonstrated varying prevalence. A notable variant observed in COVID-19 patients is the bull's-eye sign (BES), also referred to as the 'target sign'. This radiological feature is characterized by a central ground-glass opacity (GGO), encased by a ring of normal lung parenchyma, and subsequently bordered by a ring of ground-glass consolidation.

Contrasting with RHS, which primarily manifests in the peripheral and lower lobes of the lungs in COVID-19 cases, BES is more frequently observed in either central or peripheral lung regions, with a predilection for the upper lobes. There have been documented cases where RHS and BES appear concurrently. The pathogenesis of the bull's-eye sign is likely attributable to centrilobular and perilobular inflammation, sparing the remaining parts of the pulmonary lobule. While the complete clinical implications of BES remain to be fully elucidated, its presence should heighten clinical suspicion for COVID-19.

E. Pulmonary Vascular Disease/Vasculitis

RHS is also seen in some cases of pulmonary vascular diseases such as vasculitis, and particularly in pulmonary infarction secondary to thromboembolism or tumour emboli. These lesions, typically subpleural, can precede cavity development and represent an intermediate stage before cavitation in conditions like granulomatous polyangiitis. In such cases, testing for anti-neutrophil cytoplasmic antibody (ANCA) and obtaining a histopathological diagnosis can aid in identifying vasculitides.

F. Neoplastic Diseases

Malignancies which can have RHS on CT scans are lymphomatoid granulomatosis, lung adenocarcinoma, and pulmonary metastases. The central GGO in these cases typically signifies central necrosis, while the peripheral rim often reflects the angioinvasive nature of the tumour, especially in lymphomatoid granulomatosis. The emergence of new RHS lesions post-chemotherapy may suggest secondary OP. Additionally, a predominant

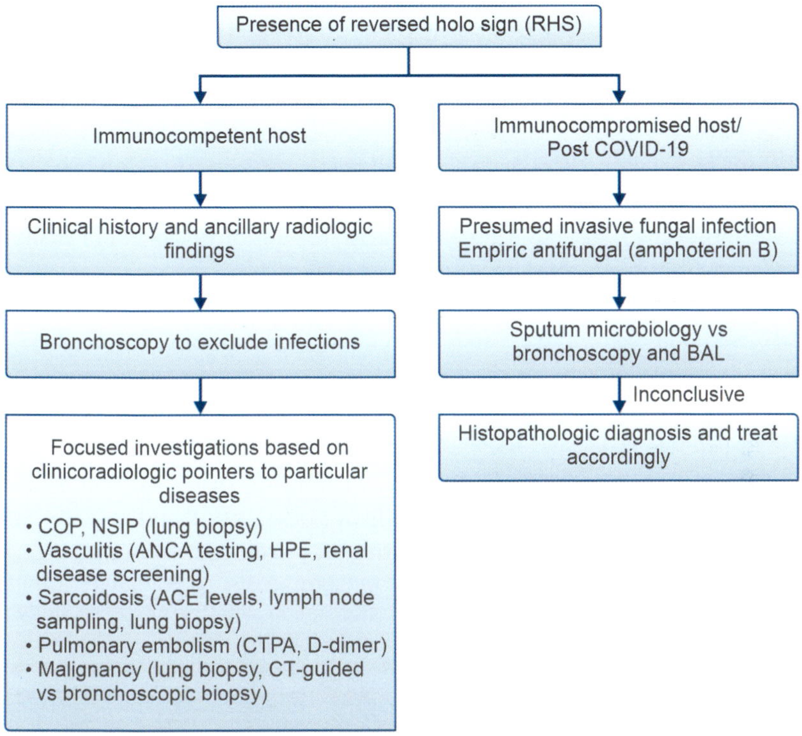

Fig. 31.3: Flowchart showing approach to reversed halo sign (RHS).

COP: Cryptogenic organising pneumonia; *NSIP:* Nonspecific interstitial pneumonia; *ANCA:* Anti-neutrophil cytoplasmic autoantibodies; *HPE:* Histopathologic examination; *CTPA:* CT pulmonary angiogram; *ACE:* Angiotensin converting enzyme.

ground-glass appearance within nodules is usually associated with slower tumour growth and may indicate a lepidic growth pattern in adenocarcinoma. Recognizing RHS and its implications in neoplastic diseases is critical for accurate diagnosis and effective clinical management.

Clinical Approach to a Case with RHS

In managing RHS, a tailored approach is vital, considering the non-specific nature of this sign. We recommend an algorithmic approach as outlined in Fig. 31.3. When RHS is identified in an immunocompromised patient, immediate initiation of liposomal amphotericin B is advised for presumed mucormycosis, while awaiting further investigations. The investigation of choice for an RHS is flexible bronchoscopy-guided bronchoalveolar lavage (BAL) and lung biopsy, with CT-guided or surgical lung biopsy being alternatives. In immunocompetent individuals, a lung biopsy is recommended to establish the diagnosis prior to starting treatment.

Liposomal amphotericin B, at 5 mg/kg per day, alongside early surgical intervention, forms the cornerstone of pulmonary mucormycosis management. Regular assessment of treatment response, typically at 4–6 weeks using clinical and imaging criteria, is crucial. Posaconazole or isavuconazole serves as maintenance therapy post-initial response, although the duration of treatment lacks consensus.

FURTHER READING

1. Maturu VN, Agarwal R. Reversed halo sign: a systematic review. Respir Care. 2014 Sep;59(9):1440–9.

2. Voloudaki AE, Bouros DE, Froudarakis ME, Datseris GE, Apostolaki EG, Gourtsoyiannis NC. Crescentic and ring-shaped opacities. CT features in two cases of bronchiolitis obliterans organizing pneumonia (BOOP). Acta Radiol 1996;37(6):889–892.

3. Godoy MC, Viswanathan C, Marchiori E, Truong MT, Benveniste MF, Rossi S, Marom EM. The reversed halo sign: update and differential diagnosis. *Br J Radiol*. 2012 Sep;85(1017):1226–35.

4. Al-Waely NKN, Fayadh NAH, Shati SG. Analysis of reversed halo and bull's-eye signs in patients with COVID-19 pneumonia on CT scan. *Journal of Emergency Medicine, Trauma and Acute Care*. 2022(3):9

5. Cornely OA, Alastruey-Izquierdo A, Arenz D, Chen SC, Dannaoui E, et al. Global guideline for the diagnosis and management of mucormycosis: an initiative of the European Confederation of Medical Mycology in cooperation with the Mycoses Study Group Education and Research Consortium. The Lancet infectious diseases. 2019 Dec 1;19(12):e405–21.

Index